COMPLEX HERBS-
COMPLETE MEDICINES

COMPLEX HERBS-
COMPLETE MEDICINES

A Merger of
Eclectic & Naturopathic Visions
of Botanical Medicine

Francis Brinker, N.D.

Eclectic Medical Publications
Sandy, Oregon

The information in this book is intended to supplement the education in botanical medicine of doctors, pharmacists, and other health care providers. It is not intended to be used as a basis for self treatment. Individuals with serious medical conditions must be properly evaluated and appropriately treated by a competent practitioner or diagnostic and prescribing team using the best combination of approaches available.

For permission to reproduce selections from this book, write to:
Eclectic Medical Publications
36350 SE Industrial Way
Sandy, Oregon 97055

Printed in the USA
ISBN 1-888483-12-1 paperback
Library of Congress Control Number 2003114579

Production by Nancy Stodart
Book and Cover design, Composition by Richard Stodart

DEDICATION

To the Creator of all, Who Is Love,
beyond our limited means of understanding,
Who generates light/warmth, earth/water,
plant/foods, animal/companions, and spirit/messengers
To manifest power and gentleness, glory and mystery
In the exquisite development of life.

In appreciation for the goodness of the plant mediators
perfectly designed with captivating chlorophyll
Powered by light, to unite carbonized air with water
forming sweet nourishment to energize our activity,
Thereby releasing in their breath the essential oxygen
to sustain our life with this ethereal food.
Nature's green ambassadors diversely transform earthen elements in water
into elaborate nutrient riches that fund our growth.

With compelling generosity, these vital resources provide true medicines
for our health when balance is lost
To buffer the stresses we face, alleviating the disturbances
resulting from deprivation and damage, neglect and abuse.
With flowers and fragrance to lift our spirits
by awakening profound emotions,
The beauty and inspiration from these sublime creature comforts
embellish our experience with a subtle euphoria.

In gratitude for the gift of plants in our life, serving our human nature
which unites the physical with the spiritual,
So that we can at once be at home in both worlds,
to experience the shadow and light of existence,
To the One source of everything good, true, and beautiful
I offer thanks and praise.

Francis Brinker, N.D.

"The angel then showed me the river of life-giving water, clear as crystal, which issued from the throne of God and of the Lamb and flowed down the middle of the streets. On either side of the river grew the trees of life which produce fruit twelve times a year, once for each month; their leaves serve as medicine for the nations."

Revelation, 22:1-2

CONTENTS

PART TWO
Changing Perceptions and Preferences—
Popular Herbs in American Traditions

List of Tables, Terms and Illustrations

PREFACE

What is an herb? In botany the understanding of herb is a plant with a fleshy rather than a woody stem, which, after the plant has bloomed and set seed, dies down to the ground. However, the word "herb" has other meanings that expand the concept. The word is derived from the Old Sanskrit *bharb*, meaning "to eat;" this eventually became the Latin *berba*, used for "fodder." The early English used the word herb as synonymous with vegetables. Later, this was restricted to parts of vegetables that grow above ground. In medicine an herb refers to a plant whose properties allow its use as a medicine. Some are also used as seasonings. In the culinary arts, compared to spices herbs are mild fresh or dried leaves, while spices involve more pungent seeds, roots, fruits, flowers, and bark. Generally, an herb is a plant or plant part valued for its medicinal, savory, or aromatic properties. In all of these cases, an herb is a fresh or dried plant or its useful part. Herb descriptions all involve the intact substance of the plant, including its fiber but sometimes excluding the water. A plant extract is not an herb.

What is a drug? The term drug has different meanings in different times and contexts. Legal definitions and common understandings vary. Most people consider drugs as medicines or substances of abuse, as nonfood items that affect function and sometimes behavior. Herbs and their products are caught in the middle of this web of nomenclature. In the following discussions of herbal medicines, confusion may arise as to the proper designation of these products. A brief explanation is necessary to help guide the reader through this maze. The word 'drug' was derived from the Dutch work *droog*, meaning "dried," and from the Anglo-Saxon *drigan*, indicating "to dry." As recently as a hundred years ago in the pharmaceutical profession, drugs were understood as the dried herbs from which medicinal extracts were produced. This is apparent in the many quotations taken from writings by the president of the American Pharmaceutical Association at that time, the Eclectic pharmacist John Uri Lloyd.

During this same period naturopaths were calling themselves drugless practitioners and using common dried herbs and their water extracts, considering them as foods. By naturopathic reckoning, toxic herbs, alcoholic tinctures, concentrated extracts and isolated compounds from botanical remedies were drugs. This belief was supported by the fact that at that time botanical agents comprised half of medications listed in the *United States Pharmacopoeia* (*USP*), the official American drug compendium. In addition, the *USP* contained many isolated compounds derived from plants. In the naturopathic context most nonaqueous derivatives of herbs used as drugs were undesirable. Synthetic medications, referred to as "coal tar derivatives," were an anathema.

With the passage of time, many alcoholic extracts became accepted by naturopathic doctors as also providing in large part the desirable complex nature of the whole herb. Such preparations as juices, teas and tinctures can be considered native extracts. Native extracts are liquid fractions prepared by simple extraction procedures from the fresh or dried herbs and are consumed without further alteration of these forms. Another term often used to describe these native extracts is "crude extracts." Nontoxic herbs and their native extracts are no longer considered as drugs, and their use remains commonplace among the general public. Ultimately, they became so popular that a law was passed to assure continuing access to these and other nutrients. In 1994 the Dietary Supplement Health and Education Act (DSHEA) included herb products under the official designation as dietary supplements in the United States. Herbs and their derivatives are now being included in the *National Formulary*, a publication of the USP Convention, even though they are not considered as drugs.

The past fifty years has seen an increased medicalization of American culture, along with an increased reliance upon synthesized pharmaceutical medications. Those botanical derivatives that are now officially designated as drugs in the *USP* are almost exclusively concentrated subfractions or isolated components, many of which have been altered at the molecular level for patent purposes. Even the use of concentrated extracts remains rare in American medicine, compared to European nations and Germany in particular. The emphasis on pharmaceutical extracts of botanicals in Europe has led to increasing clinical studies of these concentrates and has allowed for their official approval there as drugs. These phytopharmaceutical drugs are often concentrated subfractions of native extracts, produced by multiple purification steps using toxic chemical solvents. Yet, when these products are imported to the United States, they qualify under the DSHEA regulations as dietary supplements and are referred to as herbs. Such concentrated fractions for all intents and purposes are increasingly like conventional pharmaceutical drugs, the isolated compounds typically preferred in American medical practice.

The reduction of an intact complex herb to a native extract using water and/or ethanol represents the first level of fractionation of botanicals. A diminished complexity results, but these traditional selective liquid extracts are quite appropriate for specific conditions. The reduction of a native extract to a concentrated fraction allows a lower dose in exchange for even more limited activity. The final stage of reduction to a purified chemical compound provides a greater selective strength. Typically, an isolate is more rapidly absorbed and reaches greater tissue concentrations, but the greater bioavailability and potency is often associated with elevated risks as well.

Each person is confronted with important life choices each day. When it comes to health care and medicinal agents, such choices abound. Each individual must decide whether their preference should be for the greatest nutrient and phytochemical complexity as found in the whole herb or a reduced content available with native extracts. Or, are the concentrated fractions or their isolated drug constituents more desirable? It becomes more confusing when the extract is called a herb and the fraction is referred to as an extract. It is exasperating when the fraction is marketed as an herb. Dried herb, extract, fraction or isolate, each form at some time likely called a drug, all with a living plant as their source. How close to the source do you want to be? This book provides information to help understand the differences, so that decisions can be made with a better grasp of the issues involved.

The second part of this book looks at examples of different herbs whose products are popular in America. The uses of the different types of product forms are discussed from a historical perspective. This is intended to show both how our understanding of the herb, its extracts, and its fractions and isolated components has developed and how the uses of the different forms are in some ways similar and in other ways different. The emphasis on the acknowledged activities and uses for each of the forms provides a means for recognizing the unique features of each. While each form has some features that are similar, each also needs to be understood in terms of its own peculiar nature to appreciate its optimal applications in health care. Since the whole is greater than the sum of its parts, the potential found in the living plant remains the basis for each different form.

ACKNOWLEDGEMENTS

For those who in their lives discovered the healing power inherent in nature and its plants, who through their experience and dedication to natural health practices have expanded the applications of these enduring gifts of creation, and who by their instruction have led others to appreciate and apply these lessons of living and healing, recognition for their contributions is only proper. Unfortunately, the names of many of these investigators, care givers, and educators are lost to history. On a personal note I must mention those especially deserving of my gratitude who served as my guides and mentors, inspiring me by their life's work.

Dr. John Bastyr stood as a stalwart advocate and informed practitioner of natural approaches whose successes were always tempered by humility. Dr. William Turska advanced the frontiers of naturopathic practice in the face of fierce resistance, defying the limits of conventional thinking. Dr. William Babnick cultivated strength in his robust lifestyle and demonstrated an unabashed drive to overcome perceived limitations. Dr. Richard Stober proved to be an effective innovator in his daring interventions. Dr. Harold Dick guarded as treasures the curative principles he was taught and proved by his efforts that they are indeed precious.

All of these naturopathic physicians were unique in the ways they each utilized different methods of natural healing, together with ordinary herbs and their extracts, in extraordinary fashion. They devoted themselves to patients and students in sharing the value they found in their profession. These men have now passed on, leaving the future of naturopathic practice in other hands, many of whom they influenced profoundly. As long as naturopathic medicine is maintained and advanced, their memories will be honored along with those who went before them.

The work to advance naturopathic practice continues with efforts by many involved in the field of botanical medicine production and education. This book considers some outcomes of these efforts. There are a number of individuals without whose help the work on this book would not have come to full fruition. A number of discussions with Dr. Ed Alstat and David Lytle on integrating concepts of naturopathic and Eclectic botanical practice served as the impetus for this approach. The encouragement, support, and copy editing of Charo Waite were significant contributions to the completion of the process. Michelle Young also provided timely help with editing, while Dr. David Kiefer provided useful feedback with his textual recommendations. Nancy and Richard Stodart have again proven invaluable in their technical and artistic assistance. Ultimately, any aspect of the text that may be found inadequate is due to the oversight of the author.

INTRODUCTION

Medicine As Food

Among those who utilize natural approaches to health, an oft-quoted dictum attributed to Hippocrates is "Let your food be your medicine and your medicine be your food." This statement appears redundant, unless some actual distinction between foods and medicines is intended. Where plants are concerned, the distinctions can get blurry.

Many naturopaths and other nutrition experts believe that with proper diet, digestion, and assimilation health can be preserved and pharmaceutical medications avoided. This has been shown to be true for a large number of individuals who are dedicated to consuming only those foods that are truly nourishing, in amounts that are neither inadequate nor excessive, and in combinations that optimize their utilization. However, often these people also practice other important and necessary health habits that support digestion, circulation and elimination including relaxation/rest/sleep, exercise/stretching/massage, deep breathing/hydrotherapy/fasting, and other supportive regimens. This total approach to health goes beyond simply eating right. Herbal medicines are also often a part of this natural approach to health.

Another way of understanding the first part of Hippocrates' statement is the utilization of foods therapeutically. This generally involves not only eating foods specific for certain health conditions but also selectively concentrating certain nutrients in the diet. Food is typically thought of as a source of essential nutrients for growth and sustenance. This includes sources of carbohydrates, protein and fats, as well as vitamins and minerals. Whole foods are much richer in other components that support normal function than just these isolated elements. To name a couple of obvious "non-nutritrional" adjuvants found in food plants, fiber and flavonoids have been shown to contribute to overall health benefits. One approach to concentrating certain components like flavonoids (while eliminating another–the fiber) is accomplished through drinking juices of fruits and vegetables. This allows consumption of much larger quantities of both flavonoids and essential nutrients than could be obtained by eating the intact plant part with its fiber.

In some cases people and doctors rely heavily on supplementing food consumption with vitamins, minerals, essential oils, amino acids, and other nutrient components found in food plants. For water-soluble vitamins and amino acids these are safe in relatively large amounts since they are readily eliminated. The minerals, oils, and oil-soluble vitamins have a greater risk of disturbing functions since they are typically xviii Complex Herbs—Complete Medicines

stored in fatty or other tissues of the body. Purists believe that synthesized forms of nutrient supplements and elemental minerals are less efficiently and/or harmoniously incorporated in natural physiological processes than those found as part of a biological matrix. Nutrient intake available when whole complex foods are consumed is quantitatively less than is commonly consumed in manufactured vitamin/mineral supplements. Megadoses of nutrients used medicinally typically involve amounts of compounds unavailable through consumption of foods and may be injected to insure adequate bioavailability. Those knowledgeable in nutrition agree that such medical intervention with nutrients is no replacement for a balanced diet of nutritious foods.

With regard to medicinal herbs, these plants were treated by some as concentrated foods that were used in small quantities to both fortify the diet and also provide non-nutritional support. Before the discovery of vitamins, the 1905 book *Natures Healing Agents* by the late Physiomedicalist, Swinburne Clymer, described herbs as nutritionally beneficial because of their rich mineral content. Now we know that the non-nutrient components in herbs usually provide the greatest functional enhancement.

The distinction between food and medicine is often based on intent. Foods like garlic, parsley, cranberry, cayenne, burdock, celery, oats, shiitake, raspberries, nettles, dandelion, bilberries, ginger, thyme and many others have medicinal properties. Some of these, like celery, began as strong flavored medicinal herbs that were later converted through selection into milder food herbs. The designation of these plants as medicines has to do with the intent of their use, and the regulated dosage, frequency, and duration that describe their utilization. Is this what is meant by the second part of the ancient quotation? Similar to foods being used therapeutically, some medicinal plants can provide a basis for nutritional support. As with foods, the most whole and complex form of a nontoxic plant provides the greatest bioactive content.

The question should be considered: what herb forms constitute medicines as food? This may vary from one plant to another or even between parts of a plant depending upon its inherent potency. In the case of May apple (*Podophyllum peltatum*), the fruit is a food, and its rhizome resin is a toxic drug; neither the sweet fleshy fruit nor the purgative and escharotic root would be considered a medicinal food nor a nutritive herbal medicine. Historically, for many plants the complete medicinal portion of the plant and/or its water extract has been considered both nourishing and medicinal based on the complexity of components or their selective water-solubility. Even native alcoholic extracts have, until the last century, been construed as primarily medicinal in their content and application. Concentrates of medicinal plants have required both professional processing and authoritative monitoring.

The complexity of an intact herb provides combined effects that cannot be achieved by separated fractions of the plant. Even conventional drying significantly impacts the effects of an herb by altering the complex inter-relationships that exist chemically and energetically in the living hydrated matrix. These complexes are expressions of the dynamic vitality of the plants. Plants rarely produce static crystalline compounds. Exceptions involve structural and/or defensive compounds such as needle-like oxalic acid crystals. Concentrations of substances not soluble in water typically occur on the surface of plants as non-living resinous exudates, again to protect the plant or conserve its water to sustain the essential living dynamism. The difference in phytochemical expressions between a living plant and one that is dried is analgous to a living animal and one that has died. The means for functional activity is substantially altered. When natural phytochemical relationships in a live plant are reduced to dessicated, hardened, and/or crystalline forms, they have become essentially devitalized. The structural integrity of natural complexes can be relatively retained by flash-freezing.

Some believe that if medicines are derived from nontoxic herbs, these can be considered as foods. Water extracts do provide the polysaccharides, proteins, minerals, and many vitamins found in the plant. Concentration and isolation of other beneficial though nonessential plant components can further enhance health. On the other hand, applying pharmaceutical chemical solvents to food plants can extract other powerful agents that rank as potent drugs, such as capsaicin from cayenne pepper. So, by concentrating compounds from herbs, maximum tolerable limits can be exceeded.

Modern pharmaceutical development and medical practice should never attempt to lay claim to the title of traditional medicine, a phrase conventional doctors often like to mistakenly apply to their approach to practice. A transition occurs as an herb is processed that diminishes its food quality and accentuates its medicinal utility. Letting "your medicine be your food" implies staying close to the natural whole form, at least the water-associated content as found in juice and teas used traditionally. Native extracts made with dilute alcohol can be expected to increase some effects, especially when utilizing fresh herbs, while losing others, more so when the herbs are dried. The concentrates of dried herbs with exaggerated pharmacological activity and reduced component content produce a stronger impact that may include excessive disruptive effects. The focused influence more readily overwhelms a physiology that has developed through the ages to manage exposure to smaller amounts of compounds available in the context of complex mixtures. At times in severe illness this potency is necessary, but as a standard of care it tends toward overkill in cases of ordinary maintenance or support.

In the process of developing phytopharmaceutical drug fractions, the resulting solid extracts are often identified by the name of the plant from which they are derived as if they were the plant. The fact that these pharmaceutical extracts are sold in the United States under regulations that define them as dietary supplements make the deceptive tendency to describe them as herbs even more appealing. Since dietary supplements don't have to meet the same regulatory requirements as recognized drugs, these hybrid products have become identified in the marketplace as herbs. As a consequence, the standards applied to these products are now expected of those products that truly are herbs or their native extracts and not just chemical fractions or derivatives. There has been a paradigm shift in recognizing and accepting what is a herbal remedy and what is not. Botanicals are now perceived more as drugs than foods, and many believe that they be manufactured and regulated as such. The status of herbal products now is comparable to Frankenstein being established as the standard of what constitutes a legitimate human.

The need to accurately characterize herbal products is necessary and is long overdue, if we are to appreciate the actual herb preparation being discussed. A real herb is a whole living plant. A medicinal herb is the therapeutically active portion. When dead and dehydrated, it should be called a dried herb. If a tea is made, it is a native water extract of the plant, native in the sense of original and natural. Soaking in dilute alcohol results in a native hydroalcoholic extract, often referred to as a tincture, which is a fraction of the herb. With the water, alcohol, or other solvent removed, it becomes a solid extract. A specific portion removed from a native extract is a chemical subfraction of the herb. Isolating a specific component results in a purified compound, typically the form regulated in medicine as drugs. A purified compound, chemical subfraction, concentrated solid extract, or native liquid extract is not an herb; these are all more or less limited derivative fractions of the medicinal herb. [See pp. 52–54.]

This text will consider the differences between forms of plant products. The intent of examining the different forms is to resist the notion that one type is always superior to the others. In fact each type of product has its own value and limitations. The factors that determine which is most appropriate involve both the patient's therapeutic requirements and personal preferences. Compliance is always a necessary consideration, since any medicine will fail to work if it remains in the bottle. In general a hierarchy of preference based on need and intent may influence choices. If someone hopes that the remedy that they are using is both medicinally effective and physiologically nourishing, this suggests a product that is closer to the whole natural state, or at least a traditional native extract. As with food, for prevention, maintenance, or tonic purposes those forms closest to the whole living plant are attractive. For non-threatening subacute conditions or when digestion is compromised, native liquid extracts also appear appropriate. In some acute illnesses or medical crises, more concentrated fractions, or even injectible isolates, are obviously advantageous. Yet no rule of thumb applies to all cases and considerations.

The over-riding issue for all of these different types of products is that the starting material, the foundation of all good herbal medicine, is a healthy living plant whose medicinal portion is appropriately harvested and processed to yield the optimal therapeutic content. Beginning with the correct medicinal herb of good quality is the standard on which the most effective botanical medicine is based. That is why the *United States Pharmacopoeia* and the *National Formulary* have consistently included monographs with quality standards for the whole powdered herb as a prerequisite for inclusion of extracts of this herb. This acknowledges that producing standardized concentrations using low quality herbs as starting material does not translate into a product of superior quality or potency. There should be no controversy about that.

Ultimately, the standard of high quality is the fresh plant part that contains the desirable features. This is the form that rightfully deserves to be described by the plant name. Whatever is made from the fresh part should be described in relation to this form. Dr. Ed Alstat likes to use a common food to illustrate this issue. Grapes (*Vitis vinifera*) are known to be powerful contributors to health as demonstrated by Johanna Brandt and her "grape cure,' in which the whole fresh grape was consumed with its skin, pulp, and seeds. Visit any grocery store and find in the fruit aisle fresh red and green grapes with and without seeds. Another aisle has raisins, dark and golden. Moving through the store you can find white and Concord grape juices. In the condiment aisle will be red wine vinegar. In the freezers are found frozen concentrated grape juices. Many states allow a liquor section where many varieties and vintages of wine will be available, along with distilled brandy. Now, if grapes were like most herbs, these products would all be called "grapes." Does it matter if it's raisins or red wine that you put on your bran for breakfast?

What are some of the differences in these various forms of grapes? In 2000 Karadeniz and others found that compared to fresh Thompson Seedless grapes (*Vitis vinifera* cv. sultanina), loss of the major phenolic acids were on the order of 90% in sun-dried raisins and air-dried dark or golden (treated with sulfur dioxide –SO_2) raisins made from these grapes, with golden raisins retaining the most. Procyanidins and catechins in the raisin samples were completely degraded, while the flavonol content was not greatly influenced. Spanos and Wrolstad in 1990 looked at juice processing of Thompson Seedless grapes. They found that SO_2 addition gave higher levels of phenolic acids and procyanidins but not quercetin glycosides, while enzymatic clarification hydrolyzed the latter two. Heating during bottling and concentration reduced procyanidins, while storing concentrates for nine months at room temperature markedly lowered phenolic acids and completely destroyed procyanidins and quercetin glycosides. Seedless grapes lack certain anti-oxidants to begin with. Of the thirty types of oligomeric procyanidins in grape seeds, Souquet and others found in 1996 that these are limited to the seven in the skins of Merlot grapes (*V. vinifera* var. Merlot). Furthermore, the grape skin and seeds with their procyanidins and the skin's anthocyanins, phenolic acids, and flavonols are removed in the production of white wine. These phenolics make up important taste and health components that vary among Bordeaux red wines such as Merlot, as described in 1984 by Salagoity-Auguste and Bertrand. Sources, parts, and processing matter greatly.[1]

From Traditional Forms To Technological Transformations

The role of plants in the economy of human health has been central from the beginning. Familiar herbs that were readily available would be gathered in season as needed. It could be consumed by chewing or applied fresh as a poultice. Mastication and pulverization were the first forms of processing herbs. Those roots or barks and some stems or leaves that were too dense to adequately chew or pound for consumption needed to be softened or even extracted to derive the benefits, so these were roasted or cooked in water. Cooking was likely the second form processing.

Issues of necessity and convenience demanded that important medicinal plants be available when traveling or living at a distance from their origin and out of season. This required preserving herbs by the only means necessary in early times –drying. The selectively dried part of the plant that was most potent or desirable was conveniently transported and stored for use when needed. This was the third form of processing plants for consumption. Once a plant part was dried it often became very difficult to consume except by inhaling its vapors over coals or smoking. Using it internally was difficult without rehydrating. This often required soaking or boiling the herb for consumption or external application, another means of implementing its use.

In illness when the stomach rebelled from consuming foods or medicines whole and entire, the ease of consuming only fluids led to the preference for water extracts over whole plants. The water extracts of herbs were then utilized, and these could be used as washes or soaks to treat local and topical conditions. The decoction became another means of processing herbs based on preference or necessity. The extracted herbs could be eaten by others or discarded after decocting. As water began to be used extensively for extraction of both fresh and dried herbs, observations were made that cold or hot water could be used for this purpose in place of cooking, or decocting, the

1. F. Karadeniz et al. Polyphenolic compostition of raisins. *J. Agric. Food Chem.*, 48:5343-50, 2000.

M-H Salagoity-Auguste and A.Bertrand. Wine phenolics—Analysis of low molecular weight components by high performance liquid chromatography. *J. Sci. Food Agric.*, 35:1241-7, 1984.

J-M Souquet et al. Polymeric proanthocyanidins from grape skins. *Phytochem.*, 43(2):509-12, 1996.

G.A.Spanos and R.E.Wrolstad. Influence of processing and storage on the phenolic composition of Thompson seedless grape juice. *J. Agric. Food Chem.*, 38:1565-71, 1990.

plant. Infusions were found to be preferable for certain delicate plant parts such as aromatic flowers or leaves.

Since most medicinal plants needed to be stored or transported in their dry form, water extracts became the standard means of using them. Water acts not only as a solvent for extraction but functions as the medium of life on this planet. It should not be surprising to find that many if not most compounds in living plants that are soluble primarily in this medium are very important to the over-all contribution of botanicals to health. Furthermore, the removal of water by drying in the air or ovens results in chemical changes not found in the context of the living liquid cell structure. While water is essential for transporting bioactive compounds, it also provides a medium for their conversion and dissociation as they are processed by drying and extraction. Yet it has long served cross-culturally as the optimal means of utilizing herbs that are not available whole and fresh or convenient to use dried.

By the time history records the developments of early civilizations, other solvents besides water were being used. Wine and fermented grain beverages (ancestors of modern beer) were found to more effectively extract the activity of some herbs, and these solutions could be kept for many days without spoiling. These were in use throughout Mesopotamian and Egyptian medicine and later spread among the Greeks. In the days of the Roman Empire, Galen introduced vinegars to effectively extract and preserve certain medicines, most likely those containing alkaloids that are more effectively removed in with an acidic solvent. Still, these natural fermentation products were used much as water had always been: as solvents to make macerations (cold infusions), hot infusions, and decoctions.

The development of Islamic culture brought with it advances in medical practices, an expanded *material medica*, and extensive alchemical experimentation. Al-Razi (Rhazes) drew upon the Hippocratic emphasis on diet and hygiene, but also was a strong proponent of administering drugs in their most effective forms. He especially preferred pills over liquids. This advancement was enabled with the employment of sugar for coating pills. Ibn Sina (Avicenna) was responsible for introducing a number of spices and extracts and thereby making dosing easier. The discovery of distillation of volatile components provided concentrated flavoring agents that could ameliorate the taste of unpalatable herbs. These distilled oils, together with the use of syrups, provided a pleasant means of administered bitter pills and draughts.

Distillation of alcohol was first brought to Europe under Islamic influence in Spain. Contemporary Spaniards Raymond Lully and Arnold of Villanova brought their studies to the medical school in Montpellier where they distilled wine into *aqua vitae* or "water of life." Those such as Albertus Magnus expounded on alcohol distillation in the context of alchemy studies in the 13th century. While this development was recognized as an important achievement, it was not extensively applied in the practice of Western medicine until the 16th century when Paracelsus advanced the use of tinctures of plant and mineral origin. He believed in the practical application of alchemy for use in medicine. By extracting and preserving the colored principles (tincture) and aromatic oils more effectively than with water or wine, Paracelsus believed he was able to better capture the essence of some plants. So concentrated alcoholic extracts of herbs were a landmark of the beginning of pre-modern mechanistic medicine in the West.

The desire to strengthen the effect of plants by concentrating their extracts reached its extreme in the isolation of alkaloids beginning in the early 19th century. This was met by an attempt to retain some plant complexity while concentrating native extract. One method of both increasing and standardizing the extract strength was the preparation of fluid extracts by percolation and evaporation with heat to provide a 1:1 herb to extract ratio. In the American Eclectic medical reform movement desire for convenient dosing through concentration led to the development by Dr. John King of certain resinoids and solid extracts. The commercial production of these and similar products almost led to the downfall of Eclectic medicine.

The late 19th century in America saw a number of pharmaceutical fads grow and diminish. The replacement of alcohol with glycerin in extracts had a number of notable successes, but failure to adequately extract and preserve as broad a range of compounds as effectively as alcohol led to its use more as an additive than a replacement. Due to its value as a sweetening solvent, it played a role in the popularizing of secretive formulas known as the "elixir craze." Remnants of this movement still exist today in the soda industry. Meanwhile, homeopathic medicine was gaining in popularity while using dilutions of mother tinctures of 1:10 strength made from fresh plants. The Eclectic doctor John Scudder borrowed the notion that fresh plants make the most effective extracts when prescribed specifically in small material doses.

King and Scudder convinced the young pharmacist John Uri Lloyd to apply his skills in refining the specific medications as used and taught at the Eclectic Medical Institute of Cincinatti. In a pharmaceutical manufacturing business with his two brothers, Lloyd developed and refined extracts of mostly fresh plants that proved to be both of high quality and refined potency. Through the use of specific solvent ratios, creative reagents, and a special distilling apparatus he invented that required little heat, Lloyd was able to provide a wide range of liquid botanical extracts that exceeded in practice those agents that were found official in the pharmacopoeias of his day. Unfortunately, with his passing in the late 1930s, the transfer of his business with consequent loss of his formulations, and the growing popularity of synthetic medications, the production of this line of products ceased.

The period of the 1940s to the 1980s led to few innovations in botanical productions. In Germany Walter Schoenenberger produced fresh plant juices of a variety of popular herbs supplied in sealed bottles without the addition of chemical preservatives. However, most natural product development occurred in the realm of pharmacognosy, where plants were considered mainly as sources of drug compounds. After studying activity of extracts and their fractions, isolated compounds with desirable activity were studied. Ultimately, these were converted by molecular manipulation to produce new semi-synthetic compounds that could be patented, thus protecting the investment of research and development in their therapeutic applications.

In Germany the use of plant extracts had remained a part of conventional practice more so than in other Western nations, especially America. The demands of the government that these products be treated like conventional drugs led to the establishment of the German Kommission E that studied traditional use and research to identify those herbs and forms that could be approved and regulated as drugs. Their concensus led to the development of extracts that met the increasing technological demands of medical and pharmaceutical science. Standardization of extracts based on the marker content of representative phytochemicals became the means by which a certain standard of consistency could be achieved. Consequently, the content of these marker compounds tend to become steadily elevated by increasingly concentrating the extracts and/or using chemical solvents to maximize their extraction in contrast to established procedures based on liquid water/alcohol extracts. This attempt to provide more potent herb-derived products through reductionism by quantification and uniformity has led to increasing controversy over issues of quality versus quantity. Use of toxic solvents requires that the liquid extracts be rendered into solid form, requiring the additon of binders, fillers, anticaking agents, and other additives when providing tablet formulations.

While liquid extracts of dried herbs using ethanol, or their solid extracts that are manufactured using toxic chemical solvents, have historically been preferred for their ease of production, storage, use, and concentration, they fail to derive the full potential benefit available in the whole fresh plant. They also introduce chemical changes based on the fluid medium. While water extraction allows enzymes to break down some active components, alcohol precipitates these enzymes along with other proteins and polysaccharides that are also active. Concentrating extracts further alters and/or eliminates components found in the living plant. This is not to say that extracts are not valuable for the scope of conditions for which they have been effectively applied, but they do not represent the full spectrum of important active components.

The preservation of components found in fresh herbs was greatly enhanced when physically freezing plants and suspending their chemical animation became possible on a large scale. The unwieldy bulk of frozen herbs and the need to maintain a frozen storage environment made this advance impractical for widespread application to medicinal botanicals. However, through the technological advance of removing water from the frozen plant material under pressure by another physical process described as sublimation (changing ice directly from a solid to water vapor), freeze-drying, or lyophilization, was discovered. Thus, the preservation of the phytochemicals present in high quality, whole, fresh botanicals became not only possible but convenient. Dispensing these herbs in encapsulated powder form has achieved a level of efficacy and simplicity not possible previously without this innovative technology that relies on the properties of physics rather than chemistry.

The choices of the present include all of those historical developments that are still found appropriate and effective. For each herb, each patient, and each condition the best form is dependent on the specific requirements of that case. This book will help bring to light the main advantages of each form and help delineate the limitations inherent for each as well. In so doing, two contrasting belief systems will be explored: "If an approach is old, it must be good," and "If a method is new, it must be better." Ultimately, the value of complex herbs and their products will be examined with the acknowledgement that there are many ways and means to effectively use these as medicines, depending on the circumstances, but the fact remains that the complete synergistic, additive and auxiliary bioactivity is only available in the whole unadulterated herb.[2]

John Uri Lloyd and Beyond

"There is but one Chemist, an Alchemist, the Creator of all things. ... Listen! The Alchemist I mention, by means of a little dirt, a little water and a little sunshine, brings life into a seed and it becomes something unexplainable. A little dirt, water and sunshine, then comes a living sprout to grow into its own kind—blossom, fruit —and give of its life current vitality to a new crop of seeds that carry the parent stock to generation after generation. Not one life-carrying seed, even microscopic

---

2. For further information on alcohol as a solvent or freeze-drying, see the following:

F. Brinker, The Role of Alcohol in the Development of Pharmacy. *Townsend Letter for Doctors*, 115/116:230–236, 1993. (reprinted in the *Eclectic Dispensatory of Botanical Therapeutics*, vol. 2, 1995; compiled by Ed Alstat, Eclectic Medical Pub., Sandy, OR.).

F. Brinker, Lyophilization of Fresh Medicinal Plants. *Townsend Letter for Doctors*, 73/74:425–428, 1989. (reprinted in the *Eclectic Dispensatory of Botanical Therapeutics*, vol. 1, 1989; compiled by Ed Alstat, Eclectic Medical Pub., Sandy, OR.; reprint available free upon request).

in size, has man, with all his apparatus and presumed scientific knowledge, ever formed." (John Uri Lloyd, *Eclectic Medical Journal*, 1920, p. 592)

From the beginning of naturopathic practice in America at the beginning of the 20th century, herbs were considered by much of this profession as important adjuncts to the health-enhancing practices advocated by these drugless practitioners. When herbs were discussed and advocated, either the whole beneficial portion of the plant was considered, or a tea made from this fresh or dried part. Herbs were considered important sources of concentrated nutrition that provided the body with what was needed to adequately build or rebuild cells and tissues and efficiently eliminate toxic waste products that led to ill health. The action of the herbs was not seen as the cause of restoring health. Rather, herbs were used as a source of biological compounds incorporated by the body to facilitate necessary repair and restoration. These were especially helpful in chronic conditions that required slow subtle changes that resulted in long-term benefits. This was a view shared by physiomedical doctors of the same era who utilized in their medical practice only those herbs that were nontoxic.

Eclectic medical practice during that same time differed in its approach by using other medicinal agents in addition to nontoxic plants. The designation 'Eclectic' came from the Greek *eklego* meaning 'I choose.' The principle of this medical system was that whatever could be of benefit to the patient should be used. The motto *Vires vitals susteinete*, 'sustain the vital forces,' was established by the founder of Eclectic medicine, Dr. Wooster Beach. This concept was further developed as expressed by Dr. W. Wadworth in his article "What is Eclecticism?" in the *California Medical Journal*. He stated (*CMJ*, 1882, pp. 465-6):

> "We have a *rule* for choosing, deduced from a radical and distinctive principle, ... redeeming it from mere empiricism, and making it rational and logical. Disease is impaired vitality, and consequent derangement of function. This is our maxim. We differ from other medical schools in not believing that disease is a personal entity, to be expelled from the body by belligerent forces. ... We protest against the practice of aiding the morbid forces by directing depressive medication *at* the already impaired vitality, and, confiding in the *vis naturae medicatrix* ['healing power of nature'] and the correctness of her reparative *methods* with symptoms—nature's language—for our *data*, we re-enforce the vital forces.... We cannot help nature by hindering her. We cannot heal her wounds by inflicting additional ones.... To make medicine a *healing art*, is the mission of Eclecticism."

As medical doctors, Eclectics utilized many types of botanical products, often preferring those produced by their pre-eminent pharmacy house, Lloyd Brothers Pharmacists. This company was based on optimizing the Eclectic development of native American plants that led to increased popularity of remedies such as echinacea, saw palmetto and black cohosh. John Uri Lloyd had been hand picked in 1871 by the renowned Eclectic doctors of the Eclectic Medical Institute of Cincinatti, John King and John Scudder, to develop a unique line of remedies designated as Specific Medicines. Lloyd pioneered many pharmaceutical methods including processes (mass action in colloidal chemistry), compounds (atropine sulfate), reagents (Alcresta), and apparatus (cold still processor now on display at the Smithsonian Institution). In the 1880s he taught at the Eclectic Medical Institute and served as its president from 1896–1904. John Uri Lloyd, together with stalwarts like Drs. Harvey Wickes Felter and Rollo Thomas, helped the Ecletic Medical College survive the purge of American medical schools in the early 20th century. His death in 1936 ultimately led to the demise of the Cincinatti school.

John Uri Lloyd was also an instructor at the Cincinnati College of Pharmacy during the 19th century. Lloyd was elected as president of the American Pharmaceutical Association in 1887 and served as a member of the *United States Pharmacopoeia* commission in 1890. His book on elixirs served as the basis for what became the official *National Formulary*. Lloyd's mastery of botanical extraction issues was recognized officially by his peers. He was awarded the Ebert Prize for innovative research in pharmacy three times (1882, 1891, and 1916). Lloyd was the second recipient of the Remington Medal, American pharmacy's highest honor, in 1920. Then in 1934 he was presesented with the First Procter International Award. During his career he established the Lloyd Library, endowed for posterity and an important resource to this day. This institution began a publication, *Lloydia*, which evolved into the current *Journal of Natural Products*.

Lloyd's allegiance remained with Eclectic medicine as he strove to improve the quality of their medicines, especially botanicals. He railed against "medical nihilists" who abandoned the use of medicines due to the poor risk/benefit ratio of standard pharmaceuticals. Lloyd advocated the use of fresh plants over the dried herbs ("drugs") in the manufacture of most of his extracts. He believed that some components of the dried herbs and tinctures or other extracts made from these crude drugs could be considered "dirt," or extraneous matter lacking the overt medicinal activity desired from the plant. For example, he included fiber, gums, and chlorophyll as components that he deemed unnecessary, and so Lloyd eliminated these in the process of refining and stabilizing his extracts. He also considered teas more as folk remedies than professional medications.

What Lloyd failed to foresee was the future development of knowledge concerning some of the strictly water-soluble or seemingly minor compounds lost in the chemical extraction process of even the fresh plants. These compounds typically lacked the therapeutic force that was critical in those days to doctors who were used to treating acute critical conditions with powerful botanical remedies. While many of the botanical products known as Specific Medicines that Lloyd developed and Eclectic physicians employed over the years were highly effective, the process used to produce these extracts eliminated more than "dirt." Modern science has shown through research that many important therapeutic contributions come from compounds resident in the whole herb that are only partially extracted or completely lost during extraction. The processes used to extract plants with solvents fail to exhaust the herb of its beneficial components in their entirety. The fact that most commercial extracts are also produced from dried herbs, having already undergone many chemical changes and losing much of the vital activity provided by the fresh living plant, further diminishes their potential.

The long-held esteem that naturopathic doctors gave to natural remedies such as organic foods and whole botanicals over the chemically-treated and highly processed products made from them has been vindicated by studies acknowledging the health benefits of compounds lost during processing. The founder of naturopathy in America circa 1900, Benedict Lust, N.D., M.D., obtained a degree in Eclectic medicine in 1914. Yet he still held to the use of traditional herb preparations from the Old World. In his recommendations Dr. Lust took the lead from his Bavarian mentor, the hydrotherapist Fr. Sebastian Kniepp. Kniepp described his favorite herbal preparations in the book, *My Water Cure*, which included fifty-one herbs that provided the basis for recommending forty-three teas, thirteen dried powders, nine fresh herbs, nine tinctures, five oils, five volatile oils, one wine, and one resin. The tinctures and oils were mostly for topical use. For constructing a home apothecary, he advised obtaining thirty-six herbs for tea, fourteen as powders, seven tinctures, and seven oils.

In the introduction to a compilation of his writings on herbs (*About Herbs*, 1961) that were published after his death following fifty years of practice, Lust stated: "Mgr. Seb. Kneipp ... regained, especially for the most genuine and truest popular remedies —the modest herbs, roots and seeds—their former fame, now greatly enhanced. The fact which makes the herbs, etc., i.e., their teas or plant juices, particularly effective is the lesser or greater wealth of nutritive salts which are always present in them." Lust included one hundred and twenty three herbs. Of these, he specified specific preparations for one hundred and seven herbs that were best suited for particular conditions. Among the different types of preparations of herbs that he included, Benedict Lust specifically recommended: eighty-nine teas (infusions or decoctions), nineteen fresh herbs, eleven dried/powdered herbs, nine juices, nine tinctures, eight extracted in oil, six wine extracts, three beer extracts, and two vinegar extracts. The proportions of forms he used reflected his "old school" beliefs. Powdered herbs were mixed in water and drunk.

Rather than the pharmacological emphasis employed by the Eclectics, Lust was in agreement with the physiological understanding as expressed by the Physiomedicalist Swinburne Clymer, D.O., in describing his herb-based "natura system." In Clymer's 1905 book, *Nature's Healing Agents*, he declares:

"Under the natural plan or—if you wish—the Divine plan, man continues strong, well, and virile by supplying his body with the elements and only such which it requires to maintain a balance—an equilibrium (health being equilibrium). All these elements are obtainable from the organic (organized) kingdoms, principally the vegetables (this term includes all herbs)."

In spite of their respective interests in utilizing botanicals, Lloyd was in professional conflict with naturopathic principles and practice during his lifetime. As a pharmacist, he saw advantages of pharmaceutical extracts of plants, while naturopaths advocated whole foods and a non-drug physiological approach to healing. However, Lloyd recognized the importance of maintaining the effective interactions between natural complex botanical compounds as vital phytochemical relationships that exist in the living plant, even though he accepted the loss through extraction of seemingly insignificant and unappreciated components. Had he the means to preserve botanical constituents that were inevitably lost during extaction due to insolubility, he could have better recognized the value of contributions made through the influences of those compounds that he had considered expendible. The resolution to the professional internecine conflict between naturopathic and Eclectic doctors arrived later with the science of freeze-drying fresh herbs.

The connection between food plant complexities and medicinal plant activity was not lost on Lloyd, as he illustrated in his essay entitled "Plant Pharmacy," published concurrently in pharmacy and Eclectic journals (*AJP*, 1922, pp. 238-44 and *EMJ*, 1922, pp. 53-8):

"Although we relegate the term to ourselves, can the apothecary who makes preparations of plants say, "I am the pharmacist?" Listen. Undeceive yourself. Every housewife is a pharmacist, every loaf of bread is a pharmaceutical preparation. Do not the pulverized seeds of plants enter into the preparation of bread? Touches not the housewife the science of chemistry as well as of botany? ... Is not the use of sour milk, sodium bicarbonate and cream of tartar in the making of bread a beautiful chemical process? ... Fruits and seeds are used in home pharmacy, and likewise sugar in the making of preserves, jellies, in canning, etc. In fact, old-time pharmacy, with its cordials, elixirs, sweetened mixtures, paste confections such as confections of roses, fig and senna, pillular or in mass, wedges very closely into home culinary manipulations.

"And even closer relationships are bred by systematic observers of foods. Do not our mothers tell us that ripe currants should be sweetened after cooking, because the sugar disappears if they be cooked together? ... Good pharmacy is this. They advise that quinces be not peeled, in culinary (home) pharmacy, because quince flavor lies in the rind. Is not this true of other fruits, such as he orange, lemon, the apple? ... In fact, does not the kitchen very closely parallel the laboratory?

"But, one may say, such as this is not pharmacy; these are no pharmaceutical preparations, but foods, nourishers, supportives of life. To this I would reply, where is higher pharmacy than the making of life supportives or of stimulating products to encourage digestion? The pharmacy of death is not my ideal.

"Have we fairly credited vegetation's service in life functions? Have we not seen "through a glass darkly" when we perceive only starches, sugars, fats and nitrogenous flesh as life-giving supportives? ... Do we not depend on plant life as a mixture, not starch and sugar alone, for our existence? ... Have not we the right, is it not our duty to consider this mighty subject as a whole as well as in detail? We live and have our being but by the grace of vegetations service?"

Lloyd's death and the loss of his patronage in 1936 soon led to the passing of the Eclectic Medical College of Cincinatti, the final bastion of Eclectic education. As a consequence of the subsequent decline of Eclectic medicine, the incorporation of many of the American botanical remedies developed by Lloyd and the Eclectics passed into the hands of naturopathic physicians. The influence of Eclectic medical practice on naturopathy eventually led to its transformation from drugless practice into the practice of naturopathic medicine. A signpost of this transformation was the publication in 1953 by the American Naturopathic Physicians and Surgeons Association of *Naturae Medicina & Naturopathic Dispensatory*, edited by A.W. Kuts-Cheraux. It contained 262 separate botanicals whose prescribed forms were described mostly as dried powdered herbs, native extracts (teas and tinctures), specific medicines, and fluid extracts, and a few also as syrups and volatile oil fractions. In addition to these botanicals, the medicial properties of other botanical derivatives were described: fifteen resin fractions, six oil fractions, and nine isolated components (santonin, the alkaloids atropine and quinine, the volatiles menthol, thymol, and camphor, the digestive enzymes diastaste and papain, and chlorophyll). This text was intended to represent the professional scope of prescribing in naturopathic medicine.

Naturopathic medical practice had expanded with American botanicals and concentrated medicinal extracts, but it retained the use of complex traditional remedies as well. When John Lust, nephew of Benedict, published his still-popular text, *The Herb Book*, in 1974 he included 514 plants from around the world whose uses he described mostly for dried powdered herbs, teas, and tinctures. His book was written for the general public. While some naturopathic doctors had embraced pharmaceutical concentrates and derivatives, others still preferred the common whole herbs or their native extracts. As for the best quality herbs, John Lust's opinion was implicit in these statements (*The Herb Book*, 1974, pp. 26, 28):

"Choose only healthy plants that show no damage from pests or disease. ... Whether you collect wild plants or grow your own, you will want to dry some of them for later use. But drying often decreases the effectiveness of the desirable properties."

In the time since John Lust wrote, a new wave of phytotherapeutic research grew in Europe, especially Germany. The focus in many of these studies has been on phytopharmaceutical products that consist largely of concentrated extracts or extract fractions. The medicinal validation of products derived from botanicals has led to a popularization of these phytomedicinal extracts. The passage in the United States of the Dietary Supplement Health and Education Act of 1994 (DSHEA) has led to the popularization of many of these products as dietary supplements, though they are recognized in Germany as drugs.

Several books authored by naturopathic doctors have contributed to the portrayal of these botanical derivatives as herbs. In his 1995 book *The Healing Power of Herbs* 2nd ed,. Michael Murray, ND, covered thirty-seven plants and their medicinal products. Dosage recommendations were given for one or several forms, specifically twenty-eight concentrated/standardized extracts, twenty fresh or dried herbs, fifteen fluid extracts (1:1), twelve teas, eleven tinctures, three juices, three isolates, and two volatile oils. In 1996 Don Brown, ND, presented the scientific validation of eighteen botanical remedies researched mainly in Europe in his text *Herbal Prescriptions for Better Health*. The forms he recommends on this basis include thirteen standardized concentrates, three herbs, two juices, two tinctures, one tea, and one oil. Both Drs. Murray and Brown were botanical medicine instructors in the Bastyr University naturopathic program in the 1990s where research validation of therapeutics has been largely employed. A shift in emphasis from empirical to science-based evidence has narrowed both the breadth and the depth of botanical products as advocated by these naturopathic physicians.

In contrast Jill Stansbury, ND, the chair of the botanical medicine department at the National College of Naturopathic Medicine for a decade, retained a more traditional approach to the subject in her 1997 book, *Herbs for Health & Healing*. In this text a total of fifty-two herbs are individually discussed, of which five are primarily described as topical remedies. The preparations described for self/home use include forty-six tinctures, forty-three teas, twenty-seven powdered and/or encapsulated herbs, ten fresh herbs, six essential oils, three juices, three solid extracts, two glycerites, and one oil. The main differences in this list and Kniepp's are the seventeen American and Asian herbs included and the larger number of tinctures typical of the American herbal tradition. The contrast between Dr. Stansbury and her Bastyr University colleages is due her traditional naturopathic emphasis on herbs and their native extracts functioning as both foods and remedies, since their inherent complexity includes nourishing and therapeutic aspects.

Since John Uri Lloyd was such an outspoken advocate of botanical remedies and innovative developments respectful of their natural integrity, it is appropriate to consider his observations made during the sixty-five years that he spent working in this field. This is not merely an acknowledgement of the oft-quoted adage 'Those who fail to learn from history are doomed to repeat it.' During his lifetime Lloyd thoughtfully considered the many dilemmas faced by those who were trying to maximize the quality of their various botanical medicine preparations. His opinions ranged far, wide, and deep concerning the many questions that challenge those who look for best means of addressing complex botanical issues. His articles were published in the leading pharmacy and Eclectic journals of the day, sometimes in series, and often reprinted in other journals or at later dates with editorial comments added.

Lloyd italicized certain words for emphasis, and this feature has been retained as he is quoted in this text. For clarification of certain terms that Lloyd employed, these are selectively paraphrased in brackets [like this]. For editorial purposes extraneous, redundant, or excessively technical content from Lloyd's writings has been edited out. Where this has been done, even if for only one word, the missing content is indicated by a series of three dots [...]. Those who desire to read the entire contents of any of the Lloyd citations quoted here may obtain these references from the Lloyd Library and Museum of Cincinnati which graciously provided this author with most of these sources.

Some words that he commonly used must be understood in the context of their meaning peculiar to that day and age. For example, his use of the word "drug" to refer to dried plants not only referred back to the original meaning of the word but was also used by him to elevate the status of plant material, then falling out of favor, as comparable in efficacy to the increasing popular synthetic pharmaceuticals of his time. Now, the term "herb" is preferred to identify these botanical agents with safer natural remedies, in contrast to the synthetic medications currently associated with undesirable toxic drug effects. The language employed by Lloyd in regard to botanical pharmacy must be correctly interpreted if the intent behind his expressions is to be fully appreciated. Therefore, the pertinent definitions are indicated below.

Finally, Lloyd was nothing if not a catalyst for creative thinking about profound issues involving medicine and life. Though he was an authority, he did not claim that his was the final word, but it is proper to give him the final word on this issue from the aforementioned essay "Plant Pharmacy" (*EMJ*, 1922, pp. 53-8):

> "No man can to us say, "I am authority," and by that self-sufficient assertion deny others the right to individual thought. No one, in our opinion, has reached infinity of thought. This privilege I hold as a pharmacist. The pharmacist of the future, this speaker believes, will stand above our heads, he will see clearly what we have never seen, grasp things we have never touched. Deplorable would it be to reason otherwise."

Lloyd's Vocabulary

Colloids	affiliations of noncrystalline organic and inorganic compounds in vital associations involving structural attraction and influence
Crude Drug	the fresh or dried medicinal part of a plant
Definite	reliable, as applied to medicines
Dirt	"matter out of place;" plant components, such as gums or chlorophyll, associated with sediment in liquid plant extracts
Drug	dried plant or medicinal part of plant
Educts	separates; extract fractions or components
Energetic	toxic
Fragments	phytochemical fractions dissociated from their colloidal complexes
Herb	the aerial portion of a non-woody plant
Irregular	outside of conventional practice
Officinal	regularly kept for sale in pharmacies
Proximate principles	active constituents of a plant
Recent	withered plant parts, typically succulent when fresh, that have been partially air-dried to reduce water content but retain their living characteristics
Regular	conventional medical practice
Specific medicines	pharmaceutical liquid extracts usually made from fresh medicinal plants by Lloyd Brothers Pharmacists
Structures	complex colloidal relationships of phytochemicals in the living plant
Ultimates	the most active isolated components
Vegetable	plant, botanical

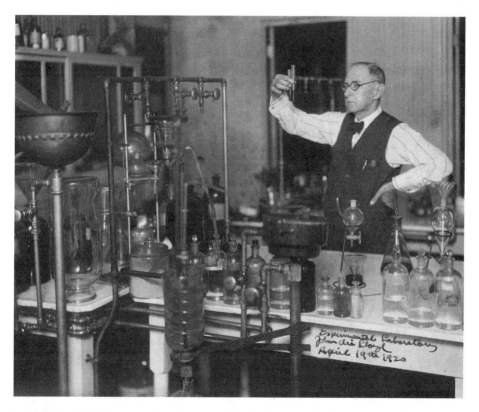

"Rebel in the Laboratory," a photograph of John Uri Lloyd. Courtesy of the Lloyd Library and Musuem. Special Collection 106, Box 1.

References—Naturopathic Botanicals

Brinker, F. The role of botanical medicine in 100 years of American naturopathy. *HerbalGram*, 42:49-59, 1998.

Brinker, F. *Formulas for Healthful Living*, 2nd ed., Eclectic Medical Pub., Sandy, Ore., 1998.

Kuts-Cheraux, AW (ed.). *Naturae Medicina and Naturopathic Dispensatory*, American Naturopathic Physicians and Surgeons Assoc., Des Moines, Iowa, 1953.

Lust, B. *About Herbs –Medicines from the Meadows*, Thorsons Pub. Ltd., Wellingborough, Northamptonshire, Engl., 1961.

Lust, J. *The Herb Book*, Bantam Books, New York, 1974.

Murray, MT. *The Healing Power of Herbs*, Prima Pub., Rocklin, CA, 1995.

Stansbury, J. *Herbs for Health & Healing*, Publications International Ltd., Lincolnwood, Ill., 1997.

References—Life of John Uri Lloyd

Cook, RB. John Uri Lloyd—pharmacist, philosopher, author, man. *J. Am. Pharm. Assoc. (Pract. Pharm. Ed.)*, 10:538-44, 1949.

Ellingwood, F. Biography of Prof. John Uri Lloyd, Ph.M., Ph.D., Ll.D., Sc.D., *Ellingwood's Therapeutist*, 10:1-6, 77-81,159-162,235-238,307-311, 1916.

Flannery, MA. John Uri Lloyd: The Life and Legacy of an Illustrious Heretic. *Queen City Heritage*, 50(3):3-14, 1992.

Flannery, MA. *John Uri Lloyd—The Great American Eclectic*, Southern Illinois University Press, Carbondale & Edwardsville, Ill., 1998.

Flannery, MA. John Uri Lloyd (1849-1936). 2001 Kremers Award address. *Pharm. Hist.*, 43(4):119-123, 2001.

Nellans, BH, ed. John Uri Lloyd—Selected Biographical Sketches. *Eclectic Medical Journal*, 96(5): 179-230, 1936.

Tyler, VE and Tyler, VM. John Uri Lloyd, Phr. M., Ph.D. *Journal of Natural Products*, 50(1):1-8, 1987.

References—Quotes from Lloyd

BOOKS

(AMM) American Materia Medica , Therapeutics and Pharmacognosy (1919 ed.), by F. Ellingwood with J.U. Lloyd, Eclectic Medical Pub., Sandy, OR., 1994.
   Colloids and Colloidal Compounds in Pharmacy, pp. 13-26
   Pharmacy and Pharmacognosy, pp. 49-65

(EFE) Elixirs and Flavoring Extracts, William Wood & Co., New York, 1892.

(EAR) The Eclectic Alkaloids , Resins, Resinoids, Oleo-resins and Concentrated Principles, Bulletin of the Lloyd Library (No. 12), Cincinnati, Ohio, 1910.

ARTICLES

(AJP) American Journal of Pharmacy

Structural plant relationships, 77:385-92, 1905.

Empirical fallacies (and others), 93:627-32, 1921.

Plant pharmacy, 94:238-44, 1922. [reprinted in EMJ 82:53-8, 1922]

Alcohol in pharmacy, 94:519-27, 1922. [reprinted in EMJ 82:367-72, 1922]

Before vitamins!, 106:42-3, 1934.

(CEMJ) The California Eclectic Medical Journal

The debt we owe empiricism, 2:249-53, 1909. [reprinted in EMJ 88:251-4, 1928]

(EMJ) Eclectic Medical Journal

Tinctures made from fresh herbs, 36:260-2, 1876.

Green tinctures, 36:310-14, 1876.

Specific medicines are definite, 36:503-4, 1876.

To what do our medicinal plants owe their value?, 36:551-3, 1876.

Green tinctures, 37:23-4, 1877.

Specific tinctures and fluid extracts, 37:306-9, 1877.

Gelatin, 39:545-6, 1879.

Pure tinctures, 40:159-60, 1880.

What are the conditions necessary to successfully conduct percolation?, 40:258-61, 1880.

Improvement, 41:15-6, 1881.

Office pharmacy, 41:252-3, 1881.

Office pharmacy—tinctures from roots (recent), 41:302-5;356-8 1881.

Precipitates in fluid extracts, 41:441-452, 1881.

Office pharmacy—emulsions, 41:499-502, 1881.

Precipitates in fluid extracts, 42:441-9, 1882.

Infusion and decoction, 45:415-6, 1885.

Polypharmacy, 47:70-2, 1887.

The season begins, 47:259 61, 1887.

Water and medicine, 48:216-8, 1888. [reprinted in 80:207-9, 1920]

A pharmaceutical problem, 48:428-31, 1888.

Influence of heat, 49:27-9, 1889.

Decoctions and infusions vs. alcoholic preparations of plants, 49:372-5, 1889.

"There are tablets and tablets." 57:574, 1897.

Homeopathic pharmacy, 58:525-7, 1898.

Homeopathic mother tinctures, 60:66, 1900.

Organized water as a food, 62:596-600, 1902.

Homeopathic tinctures, 63:49-50, 1903.

Incompatibles, 64:123, 1904.

The art of pharmacy, 64:473-4, 1904.

A little glycerin, 65:617-620, 1905.

Apocynum (old domestic name, dog's bane), 69:454-6, 1909.

Standards of excellence, 69:683-5, 1909.

Quality versus quantity, 74:113-5;169-73;225-9, 1914. [reprinted in 91:45-7;87-92;131-6, 1931]

Animal versus vegetable—organic versus inorganic, 75:613-7, 1915. [reprinted in 80:53-7, 1920]

Strength versus quality, 76:285-8;341-5, 1916. [reprinted in 91: 173-7;215-9, 1931]

Concerning colloids, 76:397-403, 1916.

Chlorophyl complexities, 80:1-3, 1920.

Strength versus quality, 80:363-6, 1920. [reprinted in 91: 257-60, 1931]

Plant constituents, 80:591-5, 1920. [reprinted 81:539-43, 1921]

Variation in color of galenicals, 81:53-6, 1921.

Plant pharmacy, 82:53-8, 1922. [reprinted from AJP]

Plant dirt—no. 1, 82:265-8, 1922.

Infinities in pharmacy, 82:326-36, 1922.

Alcohol in pharmacy, 82:367-72, 1922. [reprinted from AJP]

Plant dirt—no. II, 84:51-4, 1924.

Concerning medicine and medicines, 89:593-6, 1929.

[Quality versus quantity, 91:45-7;87-92;131-6;173-7;215-9;257-60, 1931]

Chlorophyl, 91:341-2, 1931.

Concerning chlorophyll, 92:91-3;183-5, 1932.

Plant drugs—to what do they owe their medicinal value?, 92:229-32, 1932.

Natural products vs. separates, 92:323-6, 1932.

Comparative strength, 93:425-7, 1933.

Plant constituents and structures, 94:443-6, 1934.

(ET) Ellingwood's Therapeutist

Chlorophyll, 3:119-21, 1909

(JAPA) Journal of the American Pharmaceutical Association

Vegetable drugs employed by American physicians, 1:1228-41, 1912.

Solvents in pharmacy, 6:940-9, 1917.

Solvents in pharmacy part II, 7:137-49, 1918

Activities of W.J.M. Gordon, 14:1118-20, 1925

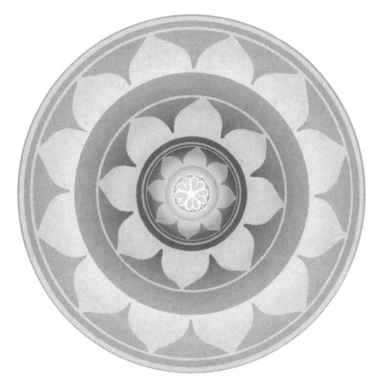

PART ONE

THE CHALLENGE OF COMPLEXITY —
DISTINCTIONS BETWEEN HERB PRODUCTS

1
CHOOSING THE MOST APPROPRIATE
HERB PRODUCT

Why Herb Products Rather Than Single Compounds?

Using plants as agents for health is as old as life on this earth. The art of their application has been refined through the ages, but the affinity of humans for plants has formed beneficial relationships that exist on many levels. Not the least of these involves the vitality and healing. Almost a century ago, John Uri Lloyd expressed it simply (*CEMJ*, 1909, pp. 249-50]:

> "Listen, man of science, listen to the words of wisdom, spoken once but yet lastingly and forever to all mankind. "Remember now thy *Creator* in the days of thy youth."
> ... Among the earliest remedial agents ... are plant products and plant educts. ...
> The most conspicuous of all remedies, as well as foods, have been those formulated under the influence of vegetable life. The "simples" of the aborigines ... the remedies of domestic medicine, ... the agents that science most values and most studies, have been and yet are, plant structures.

> "The one great bank of wealth that conserves life is the green bank of vegetation that encircles the globe. ... The cherished remedies have they been of all nations. No more are they to be displaced by any artificial substitute than are vegetable foods to be replaced by synthetics evolved by the chemist. ...

> "Nor will a person, if he thinks, under-value the inorganics in vegetable medicines, where either alone, or as integral parts of plant structures they do well their part. ... No balanced mind, informed concerning the records of the remedial agents of the past, or their qualities as known at present, will deny the supremacy of vegetable structures as food products or as corrective agents, in the hands of men qualified to use them intelligently."

The preference in natural products pharmacy and medicine for purified compounds allows scientists more control over the manufactured consistency and precise quantification of the content of pharmaceutical products. Given these advantages, why would the use of a complex medicinal herb be preferred over its most active component? Changes in absorption, metabolism, and excretion are manifested in both the effects and toxicity when the complexity is removed from botanical products. The types of changes and potential outcomes are many and depend on the extent of the alterations made in the herb as it is used whole or extracted, fractionated and concentrated. Lloyd described the rationale of whole plant use to his fellow pharmacists (*AJP*, 1905, pp. 385-392).

"Among the earliest remedial agents, as well as the most useful remedies of the present, are plant products and plant agents. ... No balanced mind, informed concerning the record of remedial agents of the past, and their qualities at present, will deny the supremacy of vegetable *structures* as corrective agents in the hands of men qualified to use them intelligently. The life of man and the health of man depend on the conservation of energy held in the life forces that are locked in vegetable structures, be they called food or remedy. ... They produce changes in organs or in structures by their influence on nerve current or on vitalized matter. They are natural plant *structures*, which experience has taught, as a crude whole, can influence or conserve life *structures*. ...

"The proportions and relationships of the intercellular structures of certain parts of the plants used in medicine vary. ... And so empiricism or observation led to the first attempt to make more uniform preparations from the crude parts used in medicine. ... These energetic chemically-constructed ultimates seemed to indicate that behind every natural remedy lay a definite something that could replace in therapy the parent structure. ... That is was a natural line for enthusiasm to take is apparently supported by the aggressive energies of a few educts and products, such as ... the energetic alkaloids, and a few other products which possess in themselves qualities to remind one of the parent structures. ...

"We observe that medical nihilism, too often the result of such medication, is fostered by continued disappointment in directions where *structures*, not *fragments*, dominate a drug [dried herb]. The great mass of organic remedial agents has no one dominating definite structure capable of either isolation or of yielding, by chemical destruction, definite ultimates. ... In the materia medica of intercellular structures, no one chemically-made fragment that can be broken out parallels the drug as a whole, if one knows the whole drug. ... Inter-structural compounds exist, by their well-known *qualities* are they established in pharmacy and therapy, but a blank are they to the chemist's art. ...Unquestionable evidence taught that *fragments* created out of drugs by chemistry do not parallel the natural intermolecular structures that establish drugs as remedies.

"Much of the present discouragement of Regular physicians is surely due to the use of fragments only. Unwisely they have ignored the claims of plant structures which in themselves are valuable in medicine, but are neglected and discarded because the test tube and reagent of the chemist cannot create from them bodies like unto the poisonous alkaloids, atropine, strychnine, morphine. These men seek the hurricane; the still, small voice has no part in such medication.

"Eclectic thought comprehended the situation in the latter part of the last 19th century, and through clinical experimentation came into possession of a great, rich field which the Regular physician had unwittingly relinquished. It turned toward the evolution of a standard form of clean remedies, as nearly devoid of common plant dirt as possible, which should parallel the natural drugs as a whole, not be a fragment only. ... The one school in American medicine that has given its thought, its culture, its aim in the treatment of disease by structural vegetable remedies is acknowledged to be the Eclectic school. ... Textbooks, materia medicas, works on practice, descriptive both of the drugs and their action in disease, were written. ... The evolution of these Eclectic remedies has been clinical, experimental in human disease expressions (not on animals in health), by a rule which necessitated a long and circumspect study of each remedy. ...

"Due credit is given isolated substances in their useful places. Indeed, the credit of discovering those most valued in American plant life is to be credited to Eclecticism. But we value above all the interstructural effect that comes from life-bound *structures* endowed with their full vital qualities, preserved in assimilable form."

Lloyd was no stranger to isolates. He earned his third Ebert Prize for distinguished research in pharmacy by developing Lloyd's Reagent, known under the trade name Alcresta, for the purpose of separating alkaloids from solutions. Licensed to Eli Lilly & Co., Lloyd's development of an atropine sulfate preparation from Datura led to its manufacture by Lilly to supply the U.S. military during World War I for treatment of eye wounds. He was quite cognizant of the differences between this alkaloid and the plants from which it is derived and other similar derivatives (*EMJ*,1932, pp. 324-5):

"*Separates Do Not Represent the Drug*... Consider Belladonna, which *yields* atropine, but yet does not in nature *contain* it. The process of manipulation produces atropine from Belladonna, but the natural alkaloid atropine exists in the drug Hyoscyamus. However, since Hyoscyamus differs greatly in its action from Belladonna, it is a question as to the textural setting of the alkaloidal structure. In addition, there are associated structures that need be considered as influencing partners of every natural drug. This writer ventures to disagree with the view that Atropine parallels Belladonna, or that Hyoscyamine parallels Hyoscyamus, or that either drug parallels the other, as a whole.

"*Evolution of Drugs*... The evolution of drugs presents some very curious paradoxes. For example, a drug may be introduced originally as a remedy to be used in a certain ailment. As time passes, this use may be discontinued, the drug slipping gradually into quite another field of service. This, however, does not necessarily establish its lack of value in its original field. ...

"The act of manipulation destroys, creates, and recreates, to the third and fourth generation. Nor is this due alone to the heat employed in the manipulation.
... Temperature, time influences, have their play of changes, in the face of the manipulator. He begins with a drug that is a mass of structural uncertainties. He ends with a mass of uncertainties that did, or did not, exist originally. ...

"*Macrotys*—The drug Macrotys (Cimicifuga) is an apt example of the failure of heroic chemistry to parallel natural constituents with an ultimate. ... The bulk of the "resin" (so called) of Macrotys is not a resin, nor is it a complexity that exists in the drug. It is a compound of unknowables, by reason of the fact that the complex mixture of its bodies is split into by-products by action of air and drying, some of these being soluble in water, others insoluble. These changes begin when the drug starts to dry. They continue under atmospheric influence and moisture to practical infinity.

"Perhaps no more typical example could be mentioned than this drug Macrotys (Cimicifuga) of the gradual change of its field of action as employed by physicians. Heralded in 1832 as a great remedy for smallpox, it was revived in 1872 as "superior to vaccination." In 1848, Dr. N.S. Davis of Chicago considered Macrotys to be "the most purely sedative agent we possess." "

In his struggles to achieve a practical solution to the quandary of living plants and their medicinal chemistry, Lloyd determined that separating out the so-called active principles did not provide an adequate representation of the action of the fresh plant (*EMJ*, 1922, 336):

"I would not in this place, ... leaving plant crudities, more than refer to those substances that are accepted to be proximate plant constituents, and of which the dead alkaloids seem now to be unfolding into an orderly unity, and to be yielding a system. These several plant principles are evolved from defunct plants by methods of pharmacy and chemistry. They appear from the nether side of phytivorous demolition, and there is a trackless space between the living plant and these sapless, disarranged products."

The established therapeutic uses of plants or empirical understanding of the adverse effects does not satisfy the scientifically-minded until a tentative "active ingredient" and "mechanism of action" has been proposed and explained. However, this level of understanding is insufficient to grasp the therapeutic implications of the combined components and their activities known from clinical applications of complex plant products. Nonetheless, the conventional medical belief remains that identifying isolated effects of specific components, however limited or direct their actual contribution to its total usefulness or risks, is necessary to establish the validity a remedy. Lloyd, a distinguished analyst of plant components himself, was dismayed by the binding limitations of this narrow perspective (*EMJ*, 1909, pp. 454-6):

"Apocynum, ... as is well known, is one of the standard old Eclectic remedies. It is used in confidence by physicians who know how to employ it, and it is considered invaluable by recognized authorities, who have a life-time's experience in the practice of medicine. Probably the most pronounced objection to the use of this drug is the intense bitterness of the preparations. ... The action of the drug in overdoses is distressing, although in Eclectic doses no toxic trouble is experienced. ...

"Mr. Charles W. Moore, under the auspices of Professor Frederick B. Power, of the Wellcome Chemical Research Laboratories, shows that from apocynum can be obtained a *poison*, and that this poisonous substance is capable of killing dogs in a very short time. This fact will be sufficient, we take it, to introduce the drug to those who seek poisonous drug effects, or some toxic preparation made from it, authoritatively as a remedy. ...

"And now as to one of our reasons for believing that this investigation (made in England) will establish apocynum as a remedy in this country, in a direction where a sevety-five years' use of the drug by physicians who have employed it in disease expressions, and know how to apply it in disease, has failed to make an impression.

"*Listen!* When the ethyl acetate and the alcohol extract from Resin A were administered *per os* to dogs, in doses of five and a half grains [357 mg], the dogs were killed. ... One and a half grain [97 mg] apocynamarin, *per os*, violently vomited the dogs. ...

"We make the prediction that after a physiological crusade, in which its toxicity is thoroughly established (but not that this is the reason for its therapeutic value) there will be no addition whatever made in its present Eclectic therapeutical applications. ... Let it not be forgotten that the common name of this drug, *dog's bane*, indicates the fact that even the common people in the century past needed no physiological experimentation on dogs to teach them that apocynum, dog's bane, will kill dogs."

The reluctance to believe that the value of botanical remedies can be reduced to a single active compound that is representative of its medicinal effects was not peculiar to Lloyd but was commonly shared by many in the medical profession of his day. The isolated component stood at one extreme of medicinal choices, while botanicals and their extracts remained as the preferred conventional means of medication. This preference is illustrated by an anonymous editorial, entitled "Gross drugs versus active principles," from the *New York Medical Journal*. It insists that isolated compounds should not become the sole means of administering medications.

The article was reprinted verbatim in the *California Eclectic Medical Journal* in 1910 [v. 3, pp. 285-7]:

"The time is yet far distant when we can depend upon active principles alone for the curative treatment of disease. The complex of constituents represented by the whole drug substance or a tincture or extract of it cannot be dispensed with. ... This latter day tendency to administer attenuated doses of the alkaloids and alkaloidal principles, glucosides, etc., is in a measure to be deplored. It is important, of course, to employ definiteness of dose with the sure knowledge of effect, but, at the risk of being classed among the empiricists, we must confess to a feeling in favor administering the whole drug, either in the form of powder, extract, or tincture."

The traditional preference for the complexity of herbs and their native extracts was based on repeated clinical experiences. Desirable outcomes achieved by using less concentrated products are also less likely to induce an adverse imbalance from their multifaceted influence. It is here that a word may aptly be said about the concept of synergism. The term 'synergistic' is applied to the combined actions of a number of botanical constituents as they affect the same pathological process or condition through different mechanisms. The therapeutic outcome of the combined actions can be greater than would be expected if the effects of each known active component are added together. (The whole is greater than the sum of its parts.)

An article illustrating the advantage of synergism in complex extracts of the Himalayan plant daruharidra compared to fractions and a major isolated constituent was provided by Bhandari and others in 2000, entitled "Antimicrobial activity of crude extracts from *Berberis asiatica* stem bark" [*Pharmaceutical Biology*, 38(4): 254–7]. Powdered bark was decocted in water, typical of it traditional Ayurvedic use. This extract was also separated into two fractions containing either 7 quaternary alkaloids (including berberine) or 5 non-quaternary alkaloids. Another extract of the bark was made by cold infusion in methanol. The activity of the two native extracts and two fractions against 19 species of bacteria plus *Candida* yeast in test tubes were compared to those of the "main" antiseptic alkaloid, berberine, based upon the minimal inhibitory concentrations (MIC). In relation to berberine, the aqueous extract was as potent for 2 of the species and more so for 15 other species. Its quaternary alkaloids were as potent for 11 and more potent for 8 species as well as non-quaternary alkaloids for twelve and five species. The methanol extract was as good or better than berberine against 6 species and 13 species respectively.

Bhandari and others further demonstrated using the MIC that methanol extract was (or tied) the most effective form against 8 species, the aqueous was best against 8, the quaternary and non-quaternary were so against 6 and 1, respectively, while the berberine was best against only one. The two extracts performed better than the two fractions overall. Compared to the more complex extracts and fractions, berberine ranked last both for the number of species it was effective against and the number against which it was the most effective.

Synergy in living organisms can be due to at least two types interactions. Pharmacodynamic synergy implies the therapeutic effects of different constituents are combined, while pharmacokinetic synergy involves increasing the bioavailability of an active component. In 2002 Marcello Spinella described in a review article [*Alt. Med. Rev.*, 7:130-6] how both of these types of synergistic activities are involved in the therapeutic effects of three popular herbs used for their psychoactive influences. As an antidepressant, the hyperforin in St. John's wort (*Hypericum perforatum*) is a re-uptake inhibitor for serotonin, norepinephrine, and dopamine, while its hypericin, flavonols, and/or xanthones inhibit monoamine oxidase (MAO) and catechol-o-methyltransferase. Its procyanidin components increase the water solubility of the hypericins.

Spinella also describes how the kava (*Piper methysticum*) lactones kavain and dihydromethysticin act in an additive manner to inhibit calcium channels, and this in turn potentiates the GABAergic activity of kava. The combination of kava lactones causes a greater concentration of each in the brain than when they are given individually. In the case of valerian (*Valeriana officinalis*), the aqueous extract stimulates sodium-dependent release of gamma aminobutyric acid (GABA), while inhibiting its re-uptake. Other valerian extracts enhance benzodiazepine binding at the GABA site, and its valerianic acid inhibits GABA breakdown. The combined pharmacodynamic and pharmacokinetic effects of these herbs and their extracts magnify the therapeutic influence of individual components.

In a broader sense synergism includes the systemic effects that may not directly affect the condition of primary concern. Additional components in herbs with activities that enhance digestion, metabolism, elimination, anti-oxidant protection, immunity, and other functions contribute to overall systemic health and thereby help to establish a balanced physiological terrain. Many botanicals, especially in their most complex form as whole herbs, supply minor yet important components with nutrient and tonic actions that can indirectly improve the body's ability to respond to many different types of destructive stresses and challenges. Such indirect effects provide a supportive basis for the direct activities for which each herb is specifically selected. In addition, these direct activities may also be an expression of similar or dissimilar compounds with combined complementary effects, the usual understanding of therapeutic synergism.

Speaking to the Ayurvedic medical tradition, Hari Sharma, MD, explains in his article, "Phytochemical synergism: beyond the active ingredient module," that the problem with acceptance of complex approaches to treatment lie with the limitations of standard medical research [*Alt. Ther. Clin. Pract.*, 1997, pp. 91-6]:

"People never ask what the active ingredient was in the dinner they just consumed. ... The active ingredient model does not stem from a strength of the scientific method, as often supposed; rather, it stems from a weakness –from the inability of the reductionist method to deal with complex systems. ... Medical scientists must radically simplify the real world in order to examine it. A screening test for anti-cancer agents, for instance, looks for cell death in populations of malignant cells, whereas other mechanisms may function to rid the body of malignancies. Whole plant preparations have been found ... to cause them [cancer cells] to differentiate and return to normal healthy cells. ... In establishing a new medical paradigm, it will be no surprise if long-held biases are encountered."

As a consequence of the preference for the complete structures provided by the whole herb, those who rely on the traditional complex herb-based approaches now often operate outside of the confines of limited scientific knowledge and, by extension, conventional practice. The limitations or lack of scientific investigations do not deter them from reasonable use of herbal remedies based on empirical observations. On the contrary, empirical knowledge helps refine the therapeutic choices. By incorporating both types of knowledge, clinical applications can be enhanced. Lloyd expresses the advantage of utilizing empirical understanding thus (*AJP*, 1921, p. 631):

"Remedial agents there are, employed in confidence by observing physicians, though the man of science has not as yet fathomed the secret of their action. Helpless is he [the scientist] to account for phenomena known to his microscope, his biological efforts are fruitless, chemistry fails. The empiricist accepts these facts, he continues to employ the agents discredited by all but those who, by repeated experiences, have learned their uses. With the object of curing his patients, the observing physician walks the forbidden path of an ostracized "irregular.""

Eclectics selected from available therapeutic measures those that were most appropriate for individual patient symptomatology, understood as specific indications. It is with bold indifference to convention that, in so doing, the utilization of botanical remedies was not only sustained by the Eclectics, but further advanced according to Lloyd (*EMJ*, 1932, p. 183):

"In thought and action it should actually be our duty to think outside the beaten path concerning drugs and their action. This, because vegetation is the sheet anchor of our remedial agents. ... Our materia medica is not well known to practitioners of the "Regular" school of medicine. ... Should we accept only that which has been recorded by or is known to the majority of writers, it would be to confess that we are devoid both of imagination, the motive power of progress, and the right of thought creation, mental speculation or practical research, outside the printed page. To be Eclectic, we must be cosmopolitan, not restricted."

Whereas 100 years ago the preference was for natural complexity, the modern bias is for product uniformity achieved by isolating components. Attempts at standardizing botanical extract fractions to single component content compromises both of these approaches. Traditional methods of prescribing matched the diversity of herbs and the complexity of their product forms specifically to individual patients and their disease expressions. Modern conventional protocols match standard products and doses to specific diagnoses, so that uniformity is extended into medical practice. Consequently, the complexity and diversity of individual lives and patterns of symptomatology tend to be minimized in standardized therapeutics. Using any single therapeutic approach exclusively risks being counterproductive, when attempting to manage variations in pathological expressions. Apparent pathology and underlying predispositions both need to be effectively assessed and addressed, employing potency and/or subtly when appropriate.

Recognizing Differences

The extent to which benefits are derived from taking a herb, its extracts, or its derivatives usually depends on which form is used. For any herb its different preparations will produce somewhat different effects depending on how the active components and modifiers contained in these products vary. Each type of preparation, from whole herbs and simple extracts to standardized extracts and concentrated fractions, has been shown to be effective for particular herbs in certain specific conditions. While botanicals are available in many forms based on both traditional use and pharmaceutical reductionism, the most effective preparation for any herb depends on the content of its components and their inter-relationships that together affect solubility, assimilation, metabolism, and excretion.

Lloyd deemed the practical application of the art of pharmacy was most challenging when applied to plants. Yet, it was here that he believed the greatest work could be done. The complexity of component chemical and energetic relationships, or "structures" as he put it, was a ponderous matter to him (*EMJ*, 1904, pp. 473-4):

> "The balancing of a pharmaceutical compound presents difficulties which only one concerned in such perplexing problems can appreciate. This is particularly the case in plant pharmacy. The man who argues differently is, in our opinion, either prejudiced, inexperienced, or speaking at random. Not a single natural vegetable structure is susceptible of analysis by any analyst, regardless of his renown or experience. True it is that certain definite substances may be picked out of certain complex plant structures. Thus, citric acid can be chemically derived from lemons. ... Morphine can be obtained by means of heroic chemistry applied to opium, the inspissated juice of the poppy. But a dozen other alkaloids can also be obtained from the same substances. In addition, materials exist in opium that the chemist's art cannot identify. ...

"In many instances a conspicuous structure of a drug is harmful if it be present in excess. ... To make the best of the art of plant pharmacy means to meet perplexing conditions outside the field of molecular formulae; to study with great care the *qualities* of materials that are perhaps in themselves of no intrinsic value, but which by their presence are either harmful or beneficial; to heed everything that is in the plant, regardless of its apparent insignificance or prominence; and above all, to be patient."

Other factors to be taken into account in choosing the form of herbal product to use include the type of condition being treated and its location, as well as the limitations and preferences of the patient. In the case of chronic conditions treated with doses taken two or three times daily, a solid form may be preferable. The fibers and chemical bonds formed in the drying process cause powdered herbs to release their components more gradually. This results in slower absorption, a feature that is desirable for maintaining a steady exposure to the active components.

Liquid extracts tend to be rapidly absorbed, resulting in spiked peaks, rather than plateaus, of specific phytochemical content in the blood. Larger amounts of circulating active components in the short term are advantageous in acute illness. In acute infections with fever and attendant nausea, the use of small frequent doses of liquid extracts may therefore be more effective than larger and less frequent doses of solid dosage forms. Besides being more slowly absorbed, the solid forms can also be difficult to break down when digestion is impeded by acute illness.

In case of local conditions in the mouth and throad, liquid medications that come into immediate contact with the affected tissue can be expected to have a stronger impact resulting from their direct effect. Solids that are taken into the stomach for before absorption and systemic distribution have a less potent effect on local conditions than liquids that are applied directly, whether in the mouth or elsewhere. On the other hand, liquid extracts of some distasteful herbs may exceed a person's tolerance when used orally, requiring a flavored, solid, or encapsulated form of that herb for adequate compliance.

If capsules or tablets are too difficult to swallow, which is often the case in children for example, a liquid extract may be necessary to use. However, sometimes a powdered herb or extract can be emptied from a capsule into appropriate food or drink, such as applesauce or orange juice. The appearance of such a mixture can be disturbing to the patient, so mixing with darker carriers such as apple butter or in grape juice or prune juice may be required to mask the appearance as well as the taste.

Different products from the same plant will vary in their chemical content due to changes introduced through processing and storage. In addition, absorption is impacted by the form of the plant product and by the method of its administration.

For each type of preparation there will be certain advantages in its use for specific conditions that will be counterbalanced by some limitations inherent in that form. It is necessary to consider the particular needs of each individual and their condition to utilize the proper preparations for the intended effect. Part of this assessment involves issues of compliance including cost, convenience, personal preference, and flavor.

The issues that separate more advantageous products from less appropriate choices have to do with component availability, variability, and absorption. Since botanical medicine effects are based on the content and relationships of their natural chemical compounds, the outcomes derived from using plants and their extracts depend largely on the nature and availability of these complexities in the form of the plant product used.

When considering botanical extracts, an important issue is the solubility of an herb's active compounds. Active resins or oils available in the whole herb but insoluble in water won't be found in significant amounts in teas. These types of compounds are available in liquid extracts with high alcohol content or in solid extracts made with other organic solvents that are too toxic to consume as liquids. On the other hand most plant polysaccharides and proteins, such as enzymes, are available in teas but precipitate from extracts containing high alcohol content. The relative solubility of different types of phytochemical compounds in various extracts is addressed in Chapter Two.

The following Table 1 demonstrates the types of herbal products available, from most to least complex, followed by definitions of these forms. An illustration of these different products as they apply to Echinacea can be seen in Chapter Three on page 189.

Table 1 Herb Product Continuum From Most Complex To Least Complex

---

The order in this list follows a steady reduction in content of plant compounds that may serve as adjuvants, agonists, antagonists, buffers, emulsifiers, enzymes, fiber, metabolism inducers and inhibitors, preservatives, stabilizers, synergists, etc. In general, some carriers (solvents, fillers, binders), preservatives, stabilizers, flavors, and/or other additives are present in most forms listed below. These additives usually range in relative content from the lesser amount with herbs (such as capsules) to greater amounts in native extracts (such as ethanol), simplified fractions and isolates.

MOST COMPLEX	

HERB	Common name
	Scientific binomial (*Genus* & *species*)
	Plant part
	Fresh
	Frozen
	Dried (freeze-dried > shade > sun > oven)
	        bulk
	        cut/sifted
	        powdered/capsule

NATIVE EXTRACTS
(Complex Fractions)
	Fresh extracts:
	        fresh juice
	        bottled juice
	        freeze-dried juice
	        preserved juice
	        green tincture
	        homeopathic mother tincture (1:10)
	Liquid extract of dried plant part:
	        decoction
	        infusion
	        cold influsion
	        tincture (hydro-alcoholic) (1:4–1:5)
	        spagyric extract (hydro-alcoholic plus
	            ash of marc)
	        fluid extract (1:1)
	Solid extract:
	        Standardized concentrate (2:1–10:1)

SIMPLIFIED FRACTIONS
(Extract Subfractions)
	Standardized derivatives (concentrated multiple solvent)
	    fraction (10:1–50:1)
	Fixed (nonvolatile) or aromatic (volatile) oils
	    (50:1–100:1)

ISOLATED CONSTITUENTS (Purified Compounds)	Crystalline drug salts
LEAST COMPLEX	

Glossary of Terms from Table 1 As Used in This Text

HERB: intact plant or utilized structures retaining fiber and complete phytochemical content.

Common name(s): describes herb or, sometimes, several similar herbs.

Scientific name: identifies plant species distinct from generically similar plants.

Plant part: medicinally active portion(s); often distinct parts have different activities.

Fresh: recently separated from entire living plant; cells and tissues still alive and growing.

Frozen: plant content preserved by suspending animation with extremely low temperature.

Dried: removal of water to reduce chemical changes, by either:
1. freeze-dried—freezing plant and slowly heating to remove water vapor in vacuum,
2. shade—slowly drying away from intense light,
3. oven—rapidly drying in high heat,
4. sun—rapidly drying in intense light.

bulk—dry herb parts in whole uncut form.

cut/sifted—dry herb parts chopped into slices or small pieces to increase surface area.

powdered—dried herb parts ground into fine powder to greatly increase surface area.

NATIVE EXTRACTS (Complex Fractions): primary soluble portion of phytochemicals removed from the herb by a liquid solvent and/or heat and/or pressure, used to draw multiple types of compounds out of herb tissue matrix and into solution.

Fresh extracts: liquid portions taken from living plant tissues:

fresh juice—recently expressed watery liquid from one or more plant parts,

freeze-dried juice—fresh juice frozen, then water slowly removed under a vacuum,

frozen concentrate—juice with most water removed, then frozen,

stabilized juice—bottled juice sealed under a vacuum, usually pasteurized (heated),

preserved juice—juice with additives (like alcohol) to prevent fermentation/degradation,

green (specific) tincture—fresh plant part extracted at fresh herb weight to solvent volume ratio of 1:1 using a water/alcohol mixture,

homeopathic mother tincture—fresh plant extracted at ratio of 1:10 with a water/alcohol mixture.

Liquid extracts of dried plant part: complex mixture of plant compounds removed with a solvent:

decoction—solution from simmering cut herb in water at low heat for > 15 minutes,

infusion—solution from soaking cut herb in hot (boiled) water for 5–15 minutes,

cold infusion—solution from soaking cut herb in water at room-temperature for hours,

tincture—extract of dried plant part, dry herb weight to solvent volume ratio usually 1:4 or 1:5, soaked in water/alcohol solvent for up to fourteen days,

spagyric extract—water/alcohol plant extract with ash from burnt marc added back,

fluid extract—water/alcohol extract of powdered plant part, weight to volume ratio 1:1, first soaked and then slowly percolated over several days.

Solid extract: powder obtained from liquid extract by removing solvent with heat and drying:

standardized concentrate—contains most dissolved compounds found in a primary solvent extract and a consistent marker compound content, having ratio of original dry herb weight to final extract weight 2:1–10:1, along with excipients.

Continued

Glossary of Terms from Table 1 As Used in This Text *Continued*

SIMPLIFIED FRACTIONS (Extract Subfractions): secondary extracts of complex fractions to concentrate select compounds; specific chemical portions separated from extracts.
Standardized derivatives: multiple solvent extractions concentrate active component(s) to specific content; ratio of dry herb to final extract weight 10:1–50:1.
Fixed or aromatic oils: lipid fraction removed by solvents (both) or cold pressure (fixed), or distilled with heat (aromatics), concentration ratio of dry herb to oil 50:1–100:1.

ISOLATED CONSTITUENTS (Isolates; Purified Compounds): phytochemicals that have been separated from their complex natural matrices; single molecular components removed from complex mixtures, often by fractionation followed by precipitation.
Crystalline drug salts: single constituents altered through chemical processes that result in formation of drugs with ionic bonds that will dissolve in liquids.

Table 2 Product Content Trends When Moving from Whole Herb to Fractions to Isolates

	Most Complex			Least Complex
	Herb	Native Extracts (Complex Fractions)	Simplified Fractions (Extract Subfractions)	Isolated Constituents (Purified Compounds)
Bioactive Constituents	xxxxxx	xxxx	xx	x
Constituents Lost	x	xxx	xxxxx	xxxxxx
Number of Additives	x	xx	xxxx	xxxxxx

Quality Considerations

Due to concerns about quality, there is a growing divergence in opinion about what constitutes preferable herb products. The quality of plant products begins with the correct identification and selection, as well as proper growing, harvesting, processing, and storage conditions of the raw plant material. In other words, the quality of the product reflects the quality of the starting material, the herb itself. The basis of traditional methods of botanical medicine was providing the best quality herb material possible, and then processing this herb in the appropriate manner to maintain the quality and to provide the proper form for specific uses.

Modern attempts to assure good quality medicinal plant extracts has led some manufacturers and medical proponents to advocate standardization to a chemical marker compound in the plant as the primary means to achieve this end. This approach places emphasis on quantity at the end, rather than quality at the beginning. Standardizing to minimum levels of marker components is more valid if the marker is therapeutically active, and if the marker content is only used as a final means of maintaining activity from the growing to the manufacturing processes. Standardization to a marker compound is inadequate if it is simply used as meager evidence of identity, or a quantification of content based on concentrating the limited activity of the chosen compound. In the light of all pertinent considerations, chemical standardization by itself does not provide the necessary assurances to guarantee good quality.

Even the whole herb can be diminished in quality when high yield of a marker is considered the chief desirable criteria. Traditional use of a herb is based on a natural balance of numerous active components. If one compound is identified the a standard for determining quality or strength, plants that are higher in that compound will be selected for cultivation, or hybridization may develop a new variety with significantly greater content than would naturally occur. However, such unnatural selection or breeding ultimately creates a new herb in terms of the altered content and inter-phytochemical dynamics, in which case the herb has become mainly a vehicle for delivering a particular compound in high concentrations. Such a hybrid would best serve as a source for extracting and isolating this compound for use as a drug, if that component is deemed so desirable.

Some plants have been developed for the purpose of maximizing output of particular compounds in this fashion, and others whose natural composition proves too toxic are appropriately utilized as sources of isolates. In most cases the traditional use as a complex medicinal herb would be compromised by phytochemical selection. This approach to treating plants as chemical factories is analogous to cloning for a desired feature, or growing cell tissue cultures for the sake of the chemicals they can produce. In the chemical-standard approach of defining herb quality by quantity, the natural complexity is lost to the concentration demagogue.

Lloyd emphasized a number of points when considering the issue of the quality of medicinal plants (*AMM*, 1919, pp. 51–2):

"The quality of drugs is all important, but no general rule can be established to determine quality. ... The application of chemical tests is useful in a few instances—a very few—chief among which may be cited ... alkaloidal drugs. ... A few resinous drugs may be approximately valued by their resinous constituents. Extend the list to a limited number of glucoside yielding drugs and a few essential oil bearers, and the list capable of chemical determination is about exhausted. Structure, as shown by the microscope, determines authenticity of name, not quality. ... The quality of drugs must be determined through the personality of the pharmacist, the acuteness and perception of his senses, the experience gained in his labors, the drilling he receives from his methods and the self-instruction that comes from a love of art. But in many cases, even these are not enough, for attention must be devoted to a study of climatic conditions, the influences which localities sometimes exert on drug values, the season of the year in which the drug is gathered and the time that elapses before the drug is manipulated after it is gathered. ...

"My experience teaches me that some drugs must be worked green, other partly dry, others are best when thoroughly dried, while others yet even become most useful after being aged to a certain extent. Thus, as examples, only green cactus, in my opinion, is of value. Freshly dried Iris versicolor is superior to the green, and Rhamnus purshiana improves by age."

One issue that Lloyd did not aggressivly address was wild versus cultivated sources of medicinal plants. It may be that in his day, before the advent of chemical agriculture and known problems with toxic environmental residues, there was not a significant advantage in one or the other. In our day the quality of cultivated herbs can vary widely, and this will be addressed shortly. The same can be said concerning herbs gathered in the wild. Wildcrafted herbs are not necessarily superior or inferior. Their quality depends on a number of issues, and their appropriate use entails a number of additional considerations.

One of the fundamental benefits of collecting herbs in their natural habitat is simply the process of searching and discovering these plants in the places where they live. This leads to an appreciation of the type of surrounding that they call home: shade or sun, hill or dale, isolated or in community, and so forth. The type of soil and surrounding plants tell much about their water and nutrient needs. Getting to know plants in their own terms involves an understanding that is much more profound than merely knowing about them. In assessing their growth pattern, it becomes clearer whether they can be harvested in abundance or selectively. Discriminating which plant or plant parts will provide the desired material without threatening the survival of that plant or its community in that ecological niche is necessary in the practice of conscientious harvesting. A grateful attitude will help in moderating one's enthusiasm for assimilating a superfluous stockpile, when less is entirely sufficient.

Collecting herbs for oneself or others implies a certain knowledge of identifying characteristics of the sought after plants. Only those plants that can be positively determined to be the correct species should ever be consumed or shared. Collection of a single specimen for purposes of identification is entirely reasonable, but it should not be taken internally in any quantity that might be toxic. Even handling plants of unknown identity can be a damaging prospect, so appropriate care should always be taken if contact dermatitis or allergic sensitivity might be a problem. The best means of learning to know plants and their habitats is to accompany an expert into the field to obtain practical knowledge about the best means to obtain what is most desirable and to avoid problems.

A singular advantage of collecting fresh herbs is being able to use them in that form. Usually, only a limited supply can be retained for fresh use, though much more can be tinctured in this form. Often, some will need to be dried for future use as teas. For individual use, the amount required is certainly quite limited. The importance of understanding the viability of a species locally and from a larger geographical perspective is a must. Overharvesting threatened, endangered, or rare plants is not only inappropriate and irresponsible, but may be illegal.

Besides respecting the plant's and your own survival, it is necessary to be familiar with the territory that you are exploring and know the legal rights for collecting herbs there. Permission from owners of private property helps address several concerns. In addition to being advised of the limitations of searching and collecting, information on the area's history of chemical exposure can be readily obtained. Wildcrafted herbs from polluted or chemically treated land are of no advantage over those cultivated under the worst of circumstances. Roadside collection comes under this category. Though convenient, the exposure to heavy metal toxins that accumulate in plants, like cadmium in St. John's wort, is certainly counterproductive. A study of roadside soil and medicinal plants in Lithuania in 1993 by Savitskene and others concluded that collection of medicinal plants growing closer than 200–300 meters (around 270 yards) was not recommended.

Knowledge of agricultural practices or pollution upstream is important along rivers and creeks. The proximity of farms that utilized aerial spraying of pesticides is an important issue to consider. In whatever location herbs are gathered, these concerns need to be addressed. Along with the landowner's permission, a land use background check is essential. On public, government owned property these issues remain pertinent but may not be as easy to resolve. At least determine the legal allowances and limitations that are placed on plant removal from whatever area is utilized.

Those who wildcraft commercially obviously need to comply with all of the pertinent issues being raised here. Some of the most popular herbs are being ravaged in their natural habitats. If one is relying on others to wildcraft herbs, or if a customer is using products produced from wildcrafted plants, there should be some reasonable assurance that those doing the collecting are knowledgeable, trustworthy, and responsible. Otherwise, the risks abound. Collectors who utilize and conserve the same plant communities over the years are able to supply a relatively consistent and reliable source of material. Small privately owned companies can and do provide a wide variety of carefully collected botanicals from the wild. Informed individuals can do the same. For some plants that grow in tremendous abundance over enormous and widespread areas (for example, junipers) there is no compelling reason to attempt to cultivate them for commercial medicinal use even when manufacturing products is done on a major scale.

Large companies, for the most part, function most efficiently by contracting for cultivation. Controlling features like irrigation allow for a more dependable harvest. To maintain product consistency it is useful to rely on the same growers and seedstock that represent a chemotype that is naturally balanced. Blending of the plants at harvest for processing helps assure that a typical range of content can be achieved. Achieving a desirable finished product is most attainable when the process is under watchful control even before the select seed enters the prepared soil.

An important consideration is the quality of the soil in which the herbs grow. In his days before chemical agriculture became the norm an unrecognized risk was the pollution of the soil with toxic waste. In cases where toxic mineral content was excessive, this could often be recognized simply by the poor quality appearance of the plants. Mineral nutrient deficiency is more typical now, with the lack of complex replentishment of commercial agricultural soil. The use of organic matter in the past not only enriched the nitrogen, phosphorus and potassium content of the topsoil, but it also provided many other mineral nutrients that were carried by the plant into its own organic matrix. These were then mostly passed on to those who used the complex herb and its water extracts to provide trace amounts of compounds necessary for optimal health. Organic agriculture supplies more than simply pesticide-free produce.

This was shown recently by Virginia Worthington in her review of literature documenting nutrient content of food crops.[1] She found evidence for significantly more vitamin C, iron, magnesium, and phosphorus and significantly less nitrates in organic crops than in those grown conventionally. A number of statistically nonsignificant trends were also identified. Though in less quantity, better quality protein was found in organic crops. Organic food plants had on average a higher content of nutritionally significant minerals (boron +40%, calcium +30%, chromium +80%, copper +10%, iodine +500%, iron +20%, magnesium +30%, manganese +50%, molybdenum

1. "Nutritional quality of organic versus conventional fruits, vegetable, and grains," *The Journal of Alternative and Complementary Medicine*, vol. 7, no. 2, pp. 161-173, 2001.

+150%, potassium +10%, selenium +370%, sodium +20%, vanadium +1=%, and zinc +10%) and lower amounts of some heavy metals in the majority of studies (lead in 7 of 12, cadmium in 6 of 11, mercury in 3 of 5, and aluminum in 4 of 5).

Pesticides are yet another issue that should concern everyone who is conscientious about maintaining or improving their health. Chemical compounds used to destroy or reduce biological life-forms have an impact on common life processes. Though these compounds are studied and their approved use regulated to help reduce the risk of overexposure and untoward effects, these studies are done using the individual chemical toxins. Their effects in combinations over time produce unstudied, unknown, and possibly unimaginable outcomes. Such combinations occur with concurrent applications, unintended exposure through environmental permeation, consuming multiple food sources containing different chemical compounds, and our drinking and irrigation water supplies.

Organic sources of both food and therapeutic herbal products are desirable not only to reduce our own individual exposure to a multiplicity of pesticides and their insidious effects but to help limit environmental contamination. The ever-increasing exposure of our air, water, and soil to widespread use of enormous quantities of agricultural chemicals threaten not only our own health. These concentrated compound impact our communities, the wildlife, and life-sustaining organisms inhabiting the soil (fungus, molds, earthworms, etc.) that make available the required nutrients that sustain plants and all life. The ecology of the interdependent network of organisms demands that we reduce the unnatural chemical load on plants, animals, and ourselves.

In a number of ways chemical agriculture resembles pharmaceutical supplements and medicines. The use of isolated nutrients as dietary supplements to address nutrient deficiencies is a convenient method and effective in the short-term, but long term health demands appropriate dietary intake of whole foods. As used in conventional medicine, drugs antagonize biological deviations, such as antibiotics for infectious disease. However, such drugs don't address complex physiological causes, such as a compromised immune function, to help assure disease resistence and long-term health. While drugs may be tolerable in limited doses when given in isolation, combinations with other drugs can lead to adverse unexpected effects. Likewise, the use of simple fertilizers or pesticides while farming does not result in healthy soil or disease resistant crops, and combinations of herbicides and pesticides can result in adverse health outcomes that are not apparent with these agents when used alone. Once we have become dependent on the exaggerated action of chemical additives to our soil or to our system, it imbalances are created that require additional care and attention.

Though in general many people have their own personal preferences, weighing the advantages and disadvantages of wildcrafting and cultivation involves issues that vary from one individual herb species to another. One major concern, mentioned previously in passing, can determine the necessity of cultivation in certain cases. This involves the danger of eradication of a species or variety in the wild. Commercial and urban development, deforestation, agriculture, over-grazing, and over-harvesting have all contributed to the destruction of plants within limited ecological niches where they have existed for hundreds and thousands of years.

The growing popularity of certain therapeutic herbs has led to increasing stress on their survival within their normal geographical ranges. This has long been a concern for a number of medicinal American species such as American ginseng (*Panax quinquefolius*) and goldenseal (*Hydrastis canadensis*). More recently, the demand for black cohosh (*Actaea racemosa*) has placed it in jeopardy. While local areas of *E. angustifolia* are threatened over its widespread range covering the Great Plains, some threatened or endangered minor species of echinacea with extremely limited distribution (for example, *Echinacea tennessensis*) are unfortuneately taken from the wild in its place.

In such cases and in places where a species disappearance is even remotely possible, the reasonable preference must be for cultivated sources over these wildcrafted herbs until the natural populations have greatly recovered. In some cases the utilization of other medicinal herbs should be preferred when a therapeutic substitution is possible. To assure the recovery of threatened and endangered species, much education, discipline, and vigilance will be necessary. A non-profit corportional called United Plant Savers is working to identify "at risk" plant and develop strategies for their long-term protection.

Comparative Doses

One of the most egregious assumptions in using herbal products is the notion that two products made by different process from the same herb are somehow equivalent representatives of the herb. To try and determine equivalent doses of two different extracts is virtually impossible, since, based on differences in the complete content and proportions of active components in the extracts, the effects produced by these extract will be different. Lloyd describes this issue well, having faced it many times throughout his long career. He uses a simply designed illustration with a few common plant alkaloids to insure a clear understanding, so that the greater implications as applied to complex plants may be even more vividly perceived (*EMJ*, 1933, pp. 425–7, 1933):

> "Among the letters from physicians that come to the writer's desk for reply, no
> inquiry is more frequently made than the request for the comparative dose of
> different preparation of the same drug. At first thought it would seem that a reply

would be simple, as it might be if the different preparations were merely extractions of varying strengths. But if we take into consideration the limits and possibilities of solvents, with knowledge of the diversity of products of the same drug that may be produced by different processes, it becomes apparent that comparative doses with the object of producing identical effects cannot always be given.

"It should be borne in mind, as it is hoped the following ... will demonstrate, that *no two plant extracts, made by means of different solvents and processes can be exactly the same.* To illustrate, let us perform a few simple, test-tube experiments with three common alkaloids, sanguinarine, berberine and quinine. The first two are colored alkaloids that may be easily visualized. The salts of sanguinarine are brilliant red, while the base is white. The common salts of berberine as well as the base are brilliant yellow. Quinine is colorless except for a blue florescence when in acid solution.

"For a solvent we will choose water rather than alcohol, because the latter in different proportions would add greatly to the complexity of the experiment. It must be understood that to extract any constituent from a plant it must be soluble in the menstruum used. To retain a solution unaltered after it reaches the physician, it must not only dissolve but it must stay in solution with the other soluble constituents of the plant. This is a problem of considerable complexity that need not be further considered at this time. ...

"Let us consider a hypothetical pharmaceutical product made from a purely imaginary plant, in which all three alkaloids occur in considerable and equal amounts. We will first extract with ammoniated water. The product will be yellow in color and will contain berberine, but no appreciable amount of the other two alkaloids; for of the three alkaloids present, only berberine is soluble in alkaline water.

"Next we extract with water very weakly acidulated with nitric acid. The product will contain all three alkaloids ... freely soluble in weak acid. Certainly this product will differ in medicinal quality from the previous extraction which contained only berberine. If another extraction is made with water strongly acidulated with nitric acid, it will be found to contain the full amount of quinine and but small quantities of berberine and sanguinarine. ... Plainly this liquid differs greatly from either of the two that preceed.

"The simple example cited will serve to show that the choice of menstruum used in extracting a vegetable drug makes a vast difference in the so-called "strength" of the preparation, but much more. It is a difference in the proportions of the therapeutic constituents. It is even possible that constituents dominating one preparation may be absent from another extract of the same drug. Obviously, a comparison of doses that will produce the same therapeutic effect is impossible.

"It should be understood that no plant is as simple as the imaginary example cited, and that no menstruum will extract all constituents from any plant. Such a menstruum would approach the mythical "alkahest," or universal solvent. It is the art of pharmacy to extract the desirable constituents in balanced proportion and to eliminate the constituents that are antagonistic or for other reasons undesirable."

Concentrates

A mistaken assumption is constantly being promoted that a therapeutic equivalency exists between a certain weight of a whole herb and extracts made from that same weight. Based on the fact that any extract provides only a fraction of the total herb, and only some of any total component content, this clearly is not the case. Even if the whole herb contained only one biologically active component (a situation that is virtually unknown), no commercially employed extraction process will completely exhaust the herb of its content of the active compound. The most common means of making herbal liquid extracts (referred to as tinctures) is with a process known as maceration. When herbs are soaked (macerated) in a solvent made of a mixture of water and alcohol (ethanol), the extraction process stops when the concentration of a compound in the solvent equals the concentration remaining in the extracted herb (equilibrium), known as the marc. Relatively complete extraction of certain components in the herb can only occur under these conditions if the amount of solvent is great and little herb is used, resulting in an extract that is extremely weak. Even this will only occur if the compounds in the herb are completely soluble in the ratio of water to alcohol used. When using a water/alcohol mixture as the extracting solvent, a complete solubility, and therefore extraction, does not occur for any single compound, much less all of the components simultaneously.

The process that most closely approaches complete extraction of certain components of the herb is called percolation. Percolation is typically applied to the manufacture of concentrated fluid extracts. By allowing a slow, steady flow of solvent to pass through the ground herb loosely packed in a column, the fresh solvent added to the top of the column is much more effective in extracting the components than when it reaches the bottom of the column where it is concentrated with extracted components. Even using this method, to completely remove the remaining active components from the herb in the bottom of the column, the final portion of extract is so dilute that it must be concentrated after the extraction is complete. This process employs the application of heat to drive off the excess solvent and reduce the volume. Heating the extract is destructive to many compounds, thereby changing the content and rendering the extract less complex and less potent. As a consequence the extract does not provide all of the original component content and activity present in the whole herb amount that was extracted. Study of the essential oil content in thyme and its extracts has shown in general that the greater the degree of concentrating the extract, the lower the percentage of original content of the whole herb is contained in the final extract.

While this deficit in the retention of content by concentrating extracts is recognized and acknowledged, an associated error in logic is being propagated in the meantime. This faulty reasoning takes as a standard the effective dose of a concentrated herbal extract and then attempts to determine the equivalent dosage of the whole herb calculated on the basis of the degree of concentration by weight that has occurred. In other words, a 5:1 extract whose dosage quantity (for example, 100 mg) represents components extracted from a greater weight of whole herb (in this case, 500 mg) is regarded as five times more potent (a fallacy). As a consequence, it is believed that to get equivalent activity using the whole herb, five time as much of the herb must be used (a further fallacy). It is on this faulty premise that the proposed dosage equivalency of whole herbs compared to extracts is misrepresented to the public and practitioners alike.

Further assumptions are made when considering the traditional dosages of the liquid extracts (Specific Medicines) used by the Eclectic medical doctors in the late 19th and early 20th centuries. These were generally made with fresh plant materials, thus requiring larger amounts of starting material due to water content. The Eclectic emphasis was on phytochemical balance rather than concentration, on quality rather than quantity. Therefore, when the Eclectic botanical authority Dr. Harvey W. Felter is quoted as stating that these extracts are eight times stronger than 1:5 tinctures, it is based more on clinical effect than mathematical reductionism. As the complete statement by Felter in his *Eclectic Materia Medica* (*EMM*) suggests, he was concerned with typical tinctures made with dried herbs (*EMM*,1922, p. 30):

> "The drug strength of Specific Medicines, on an average, is about eight times that
> of the old-time commercial tinctures, although, as already stated, by reason of their
> origins and manipulative processes, comparisons are impossible."

What must be considered for dosage equivalency is not the degree of concentration by total weight that has been achieved through processing, but the quantity of the active components in the original whole herb compared to those in the extract, as well as their diversity, ratios, and interactions within the herb matrix. This is more of an empirical-based clinical judgment than a mathematical assessment. To again quote Felter (*EMM*, 1922, p. 39):

> "The doses given under each individual drug are those found to be within the range
> of the *maximum* and *minimum amounts for most adults*. The determination of
> dosage for gross effects is, to a large degree, a personal matter with the prescriber

and depends very largely upon his individual experience and his skill in determining the needs of the patient."

Drop Size

Another point of confusion regarding equivalent doses is the matter of translating traditional drop doses to their metric equivalent. The old method of using a drop of water as a standard (minim) has at times been misapplied as the standard for all liquid extracts. There are 15 drops of water (minims) in every milliliter (ml). However, the cohesiveness of water is changed when it is combined with other solvents or with solutes (substances dissolved in solution). Pure glycerin is closest to water with 17 drops per ml. Pharmacy grade alcohol (95%–96% ethanol by volume) has 37 drops per ml. When pure ethanol is added to water in equal parts (50:50) to make dilute alcohol, it more than doubles the number of drops per ml (34) that is found for pure water. This was described in Remington's *Practice of Pharmacy* 6th ed. (1916) which documented the number of drops of different types of liquid extracts. The numbers of drops per ml ranged from 11–27 for syrups (avg. 19), 27–37 for essential oils (ave. 32), 28–38 for tinctures (avg. 33), and 30–40 for fluid extracts (avg. 35).

Unfortunately, it has been stated in some popular texts that there are 20 drops of hydroalcoholic extract per ml. The confusion leads to a series of potential mistakes in over-estimating the appropriate dosage size. Using as an example a dose of 60 drops for a hydroalcoholic extract, those who use the minim size of a water drop and apply it to a tincture would believe that this would be equivalent to 4 ml. This is interpreted by others who recognize a small reduction of drop size to be equivalent to 3 ml (60/20 = 3) which is still too large. More accurately, 60 drops of a typical tincture with about 50% alcohol would actually be a dose from 1.6–2.1 ml or 1.8 ml on average (60/33 = 1.8). By miscalculating the size of a drop, some modern writers have misrepresented the size of traditional doses by making them larger than the accurate equivalent amount in milliliters.

Individual Variability

When an *average* dose is determined, this constitutes an effective amount for most people, assuming average weight and "normal" metabolism. The inadequacy of this dose for many people is apparent when we consider the issues influencing an effective dose. The modern "gold standard" for establishing an effective dose is considered by most to be a placebo-controlled, double-blind, randomized clinical study. The tested medicinal product is considered to be effective when therapeutic relief is provided for a significantly greater number of subjects than were helped by placebo (i.e., the product is better than "make believe"). The dosage from such a study is often subsequently reported as the "effective dose." However, this does not infer that it is the "optimal dose" for every individual. In fact, in the active product group of clinical studies there are generally three categories of subjects: those responding well, those not responding well, and those with adverse effects. Based on individual differences in the way each subject absorbs, metabolizes, and excretes the active components of the product, it can be assumed that those who did not respond did not receive and adequate dose, while those with adverse effects received too high of a dose. Unless dosage adjustments are made as part of a follow-up in such a study, the effective dose cannot necessarily be considered the optimal dose. An appropriate follow-up with dosage adjustment can help establish an effective dosage range that will include amounts that are both safe and effective for a larger number of people when the dose is individually adjusted.

One reason why a single standard dose is used in many clinical studies is because of the relatively large dosage of the concentrated form being studied. The difficulty of producing a suitable placebo in liquid form arises from the sensible qualities, especially the taste, of the active product being studies. A solid dosage form in capsule or tablet is much easier to mimic with a similar-appearing placebo, so solid products are typically used in clinical studies. Most of these solid products are extracts, that is, the herb has been extracted with a liquid solvent that is then removed, resulting in a concentrated product. This concentrated product is usually an amount that would be considered a single dose. Therefore, adjusting the dose in a study of this type of product would essentially involve doubling the dose. If the product is sufficiently concentrated so that adverse effects are a concern, doubling the dose is undesirable. Consequently, when the dose studied is found to be significantly more effective than the placebo, the issue of most effective dose and dosage/range is ignored.

The need for individualizing the dosage of any medication should be fairly obvious. Differences in the ability to absorb and assimilate botanical compounds are based on the digestion, intestinal bacterial conversions, and cellular transport mechanisms that vary between individuals. Dosage forms also affect these processes. Yet variations go beyond absorption efficiency. Even with nutrients, consumption requirements are not the same from one person to another. This was aptly described by Dr. Roger Williams, the noted nutritional biochemist, when he stated in his book, *Biochemical Individuality*, "Every individual organism that has a distinctive genetic background has distinctive nutritional needs which must be met for optimal well-being." As applied to medications, genetic polymorphism is the term that describes this variability between individuals. In this regard, certain genes determine each person's ability to metabolize foreign substances, based on the activity of specific isozymes. This is true for each isolated medicinal substance consumed. With the multiplicity of active compounds in a complex herb or its native extracts, the ability and rate at which these many substances are broken down and excreted can differ between people. It should be no surprise then that issues other than age and weight come into play.

The issue of optimal individual dosage can best be addressed by utilizing dosage units that do not represent half of more of the total dosage. For solid forms, this allowance is best achieved by using the whole powdered herb. The lack of concentration allows for moderate increases in the dosage by consuming one more capsule per day. A simple means is by incrementally increasing the dose frequency. For example, when two capsules of herb are as effective as one concentrated extract tablet, if two tablets daily are inadequate, then two capsules could be taken morning and evening with one capsule consumed in the afternoon. On the other hand, when adverse effects are encountered with the concentrate, instead of taking just one concentrated extract tablet daily, one herb capsule could be taken taken three times daily, thus reducing the dose and spreading the effect more evenly over the entire day.

The easiest means by which to individualize doses is to utilize liquid extracts. These can easily have the amount varied by size or frequency. If the extract is a tea, dosage size may be altered by the tablespoon, ounce, or quarter cup and/or varying the number of times consumed daily. Depending on the strength and measuring device being used, tincture doses can be altered by the number of drops, droppersful, or milliliters. It is because of the ease of adjusting doses that liquid extracts are often preferred, especially if mixtures are involved. On the other hand, due to the undesirable taste of some herbs and/or the loss of active components in making liquid extracts, some prefer the use of the whole powdered herb as tablets or in capsules.

If the desired components are not effectively extracted using water, vinegar, glycerin, alcohol, or a combination of these, then a toxic chemical solvent used for extraction must be evaporated to produce a concentrated solid extract. The doses for solid extract are relatively small, and the tablet content includes a number of additives as binders, dispersents, and/or preservatives, or capsules will contain fillers. Such a product resembles a drug more than an herb. The natural complexity is reduced to a selectively configured chemical entity. One problem with solid extract dosing is the relatively large increment necessary when increasing or decreasing the dose by one tablet or capsule, since this is likely equivalent to several capsules of the whole powdered herb, or many drops of its native extract. Individualized dosing is replaced by standardized doses.

Bioavailability

Even when considering only a single component, the issue that ultimately determines comparative doses is bioavailability. In the case of herbal product complexities, consuming more of a compound does not mean that more is being utilized unless in both forms the compounds are absorbed, assimilated, and retained in the same way. It is entirely possible that a form can contain less of an active component and have greater activity from that that constituent, if it is more completely digested, dispersed, and delivered to the intestinal mucosa, more efficiently absorbed from the digestive tract through enhanced mucosal uptake/transport, less rapidly metabolized, deactivated, and excreted, and/or more effectively interfaced with the cells where it is needed. In a complex mixture, congener compounds can reduce bioavailability by binding the primary active component in the gut, increasing its metabolism, enhancing its excretion, or blocking its cellular uptake. Other congeners can counter these effects and thereby enhance its bioactivity. Each compound in a mixture can potentially affect the others in these ways. The actual impact of these influences, when comparing different products of the same herb, may or may not be significant in regard to the therapeutic outcome.

Bioavailability is often described in the literature by the amount of a compound present in the blood over time, but this does not necessarily indicate that the measurable content in the blood will be utilized in the same ways by the target cells if other components happen to influence its kinetics. For example, "inactive" volatile components may improve the assimilation of an active component into cells, or other components may affect the retention of a compound in its active form within the cells. So anytime the co-existing components in a botanical product are altered, the kinetics of the active component(s) can likewise be changed, and the effectiveness of the dose is altered. While relative bioavailability may be measured by serum content, actual bioavailability is best reflected by therapeutic outcome. A complex product form may appear to be inferior by theoretical assessment, but it may work as well, or better than, one that has undergone modifications to concentrate a component or to improve the measurable absorption of that particular component deemed as representative or primary. Knowledge about relative bioavailability of isolated compounds cannot be assumed to apply absolutely to complex mixtures that defy complete pharmacokinetic analysis.

Combinations of Multiple Herbs or Extracts

An herbal combination is ideally formulated to specifically address the health of an individual. The herbs are selected according to the activity of the herb and its constituents as these apply to the underlying causes and presentation of the condition. The herbs that seem most appropriate to resolve the condition and relieve the symptoms of a particular patient are chosen over other similar plants. However, since several plants or their extracts are combined to produce a more complete desirable effect, the multiplicity of components of one can interact with those of another in ways that are sometimes unforeseen, so that the combined action may be either more or less than what is accomplished by a single herb.

Mixing herbs in capsules or for teas is often done commercially for broad influence on a particular condition or system. Encapsulated dried herb powders containing combinations of a half-dozen or more herbs contain so little of each that, for effective therapeutic activity, often many capsules would need to be consumed. While the phytochemical complexity is extreme in these cases, individual phytochemical content per capsule is minimal. Effective amounts of the bioactive components are more easily consumed in tea preparations, assuming the desired components are sufficiently water-soluble. Simple water extraction reduces the phytochemical complexity. With simple extract combinations it is theoretically possible that the reduced phytochemical content of each extract allows for less total complexity and bioactivity in a combination than is found with a single whole herb. However, the speed and degree of absorption is likely improved.

Usually, hydroalcoholic tinctures are the most favored type of herbal combination product for individual prescribing. These can provide a broader range of bioactive components found in the extracted herb, though in less complete quantities. This form is especially convenient for preparing individualized combinations, since a custom formula can be so easily proportioned, prepared, and dispensed simply by adding individual tinctures together in a bottle. Dosage with liquid extracts can also be easily and precisely adjusted. With liquid extracts flavor can be a concern, especially for those who are sensitive to bitter herbs, so additional extracts may be included to improve the taste.

While some traditional formulas in one form have been shown over time to empirically work well together, another form does not necessarily produce the same effects. In addition, modern combinations that appear desirable on paper may be less so in reality. Unless the person developing the formula is expert at recognizing not only patient needs but also undesirable interactions on the basis of components known to be present in the herbs but diminished or concentrated in their various extracts, the outcome can be disappointing or disturbing. Such a prescription can actually lead to less effective therapy than using the single herbs appropriately.

The emphasis on using only products made from single herbs as opposed to compound formulas was one aspect of prescribing that set the Eclectics of the late 19th century apart from Physiomedicalist doctors and others who utilized combinations. Lloyd describes the prior situation of the mid-19th century (*AMM*, 1919, p. 59):

> "About this date all physician were prone to prescribe mixtures –compound syrups, compound powders, compound tinctures, compound extracts, etc., and, indeed, the tendency of Eclecticism was towards medication by means of *complex mixtures*.

"Then came Prof. John M. Scudder, who united with several Eclectic physicians and rebelled against polypharmacy medication. They asserted that physicians should study the action of single drugs, and if mixtures were to be prescribed, should, when possible, make the mixtures when prescribing for the patient. ...

"This innovation, the use of selected remedies for direct medication, was strongly opposed at first. ... But gradually it was seen that the opponents to ... polypharmacy (shotgun medication) aimed to further a pleasant and advanced therapy."

The problem of incompatibles arises when combining herbs with a complex array of components and activities. The major causes of incompatibility are chemical, pharmacological, or pharmaceutical. A good example of chemical incompatibility is precipitation caused by the combination of two components that form a chemical bond rendering the compound insoluble. This is most commonly encountered with tannins that can precipitate alkaloids such as caffeine, ephedrine, yohimbine, berberine, lobeline, etc. When combining several individual tinctures together, precipitation can result if extracts with low alcohol content (< 30%) are mixed with tinctures having high alcohol content (>70%). The resultant combination with around a 50% ethanol concentration may not retain all of the compounds in solution that require the lower or higher amount of alcohol, forming a sediment in the bottom of the bottle over time.

Sedimentation from combining extracts occurs more or less with any variation of initial alcohol content among the liquid extracts used together in a mixture or with combinations of interactive components that result in precipitates. For this reason all liquid herbal formulations should be shaken well before dispensing the dose (either by pouring or using a dropper) to mix any sediment in the bottom of the bottle back into the fluid volume. The solution may then appear cloudy or have small particles floating in the liquid. If a dropper is being used, it is important to fill it for use after the bottle has been shaken; otherwise, the fluid inside the dropper won't have mixed with the rest of the bottle's contents. If sediment in the bottom is not mixed by shaking the bottle before each use, little of these components will be available if doses are taken near the surface of the fluid. As a result, their concentration will become greater, and maybe adversely excessive, as the amount of liquid in the bottle diminishes and reaches the bottom.

Pharmacological incompatibility occurs when two herbs with opposite actions are combined, such as a stimulant (for example, kola nut) and with a sedative (for example, valerian). Normally, this is avoided if one of the actions is desired for therapeutic purposes. Occassionally, this sort of antagonism can be intentional to reduce an effect that may produce adverse results. For example, the spasmolytic effect of fennel on circular muscle fibers in the gut is often used with stimulant laxatives like cascara sagrada that may produce cramping.

A pharmaceutical type of incompatibility is not based primarily on reducing content or activity but rather on rendering a preparation unsightly or otherwise unappealing. This can be due to separation of components by layering and/or uneven turbidity caused by insoluble or gelatinous content, so it may be secondary to chemical incompatibility. Some types of components that are normally pharmaceutical incompatibles can be utilized together when the proper technique is applied. Certain mixtures result in an unappealing conglomeration of ingredients when not properly blended. This is especially true of lipophilic, or fat-loving, products such as oil when mixed with water. To produce an appealing blend of these seemingly incompatible substances, an emulsion must be made. Lloyd describes these (*AMM*, 1919, p. 63):

> "*Emulsions* are mechanical mixtures of oils and water, the admixture being facilitated by the influence of some body capable of affiliating them without chemically altering the oil. ... Powdered acacia or powdered tragacanth are usually employed for this purpose."

Lloyd was very specific in his instructions on how mixing of these combinations was to be done effectively (*EMJ*, 1881, pp. 500–502):

> "In making emulsions, as in all other departments of pharmacy, system is required. ... Proceed according to rule, and not by guess. ... What is an emulsion? Emulsions are simply mixtures of aqueous solutions and a substance, such as oils, balsams, chloroform, etc. ... The milky juice of the asclepias or of the euphorbia is a natural emulsion of the vegetable kingdom. In making emulsions, to an extent, we copy from nature. ...

> "To make the emulsion of an oil or of a liquid balsam: - Pour the entire amount of oil, or mixed oils, into a capacious wedgewood or porcelain mortar. The flat bottomed form is best. Then mix with the oil one-half its weight of powdered gum arabic. ... After mixing these together, add as much water by measure as was used by weight of the gum arabic. ... Rub together and then add another portion of water (the same amount), and rub until a smooth, even emulsion results. To express the proportions plainly: one part of oil; one-half part of powdered acacia; one part of water I portions of one-half part at each addition. After the emulsion is made according to the above process, add the other ingredients that may be directed by the physician. ...

> "Precautions: The mortar and pestle, and the graduate used for measuring the oil, must each be perfectly dry. The water must be measured in a clean graduate; under no circumstances should the oily graduate be used. The oil must be poured directly into the bottom of the mortar, and not upon its sides or upon the pestle as it rests within the mortar. It will be found that much of such oil as may be splashed upon the sides of the mortar or upon the pestle, will not be mixed with the acacia, and

will float in drops upon the surface of the emulsion. Alcoholic liquids should always be added after the other ingredients. If alcohol be added to an emulsion containing but little water, the oil will separate to a greater or less extent.

"Remarks: ... It will afford an interesting line of experiments for pharmacists to investigate this subject and to note the difference in appearance and stability of emulsions prepared from the same materials, excepting simply the operation and proportions of mixing. In some cases it will appear as though the oil separates even with any formula, upon the addition of the first proportion of water. ... When the second proportion of water is added, the two layers disappear, and a beautiful creamy milk results. Emulsions prepared as I suggest will keep without separation for any reasonable length of time, often for months."

Local Remedies

The advantages of particular herb forms with internal consumption are generally greater than with topical application due to the effectiveness of the digestive process. When not taken orally, whole complex herbs or their extracts are not efficiently absorbed. The skin acts as a protective barrier against unintended adverse exposures from external agents. Though the mucous membrane of the alimentary tract also acts as a barrier, the digestive process is designed to facilitate absorption of many molecules. While diffusion of compounds occurs in both tissues, the cells in the intestinal tract also actively take up some compounds with selective transporter proteins. Since herbs consumed orally undergo structural breakdown, liquification, and prolonged exposure to permeable mucous membranes, external applications on relatively impermeable skin must mimic these influences to maximize absorption.

The systemic, or whole body, effect is often not very powerful when herbs are used topically. However, local effects are greater than can be achieved when only using herbs orally. Very often the optimal therapeutic effect of treating a local condition with herbs involves taking the whole herb or its partial form in extracts internally while using the appropriate form locally as well. The superficial surface of the skin is composed of dead cells. Therefore, local product forms must enhance availability of compounds to improve absorption through the skin to be effective topical applications. When treating the skin or other surface tissues, the need for a liquid vehicle to carry active compounds of the herb to the tissue is evident. Therefor, a necessity to promote diffusion of compounds through the skin is to present them at the surface in a liquid interface. In cases of topical applications, fluids are essential components in all preparations, whether water, gels, alcohol, glycerin, or oils. The juice of pulverized fresh plants or soaked and rehydrated dried herbs may likewise be used in local applications.

The perfusion of blood and lymph fluid near the surface of the skin helps to improve the local dissemination of compounds that pass into the surface tissue. This can be done through the simultaneous application of heat or by applying a liquid or semisolid form with a friction rub. Rubefacient herbal compounds such as alcohol-soluble cayenne resin will also increase blood flow and fluid content in the skin. Where the integrity of the skin has been compromised by an irritation, cut, wound, scrape, sore, bruise, or inflammation, the local absorption can be expected to be greater. In cases of open lesions the sensitivity is much greater, and exposure to particulate matter from dried herbs should be avoided by utilizing a barrier of natural fiber such as cotton, linen, or wool.

Local applications are not only used on the skin but also on mucous membrane surfaces in forms such as inhalants, gargles, douches, or enemas. The particular needs and limitations of each case determine what form is most appropriate for a given individual. Some local treatments are used to cause reflex responses elsewhere, affecting nerve conductivity and blood or energy flow. In most cases local treatments are intended for limited surface areas of the body, so less detail will be used to describe them in this text. In conjunction with the discussion of herb product forms for oral use, the descriptions of external or other local applications will be included with similar internal products, going from intact herbs and domestic extracts to more reduced commercial extracts and fractions.

2
TRADITIONAL AND MODERN HERBAL
PREPARATIONS AND DERIVATIVES

Whole Complex Herbs

In regard to its medicinal use the term 'herb' refers to any part of a plant used for its therapeutic properties. In this context the word 'herb' does not distinguish a non-woody plant from a woody-stemmed one, nor does it refer only to plants growing in soil rather than marine or hydroponic forms. The concept of herbs has even been broadened to include non-botanical organisms such as mushrooms (fungi) that lack a plant's ability to photosynthesize, and whose genetic similarities are in some aspects closer to animals than plants. Such distinctions in nomenclature are of more significance to the study of botany than to botanical medicine or herbalism.

In natural medicine herbs are the medicinally active plant structures, distinct from plant extracts, concentrates, or active components that represent only a fraction of the activity present in the herb from which they are derived. So, in this sense, the phrase "whole herb" is used when referring to the medicinal portion of the plant with its fiber and its entire phytochemical composition. Likewise, the phrase "complex herb" is employed here to refer to the complete plant part used medicinally before extraction. Only in the whole complex herb is its chemical matrix intact. The therapeutic and physiological activities are broader, while the impact is modified. Involving the whole herb alters the availability of some constituents. Absorption may be slower for certain components, yet associated compounds may enable them to be more readily assimilated. The metabolic processing and elimination of constituents can likewise be affected, depending on the influence of co-factors in the herb on enzyme systems and membrane transporters.

Even John Uri Lloyd, the innovative botanical pharmacist par excellence, recognized the value of the unsophisticated raw herb (*EMJ*, 1889, p. 372-3):

"From time to time I am confronted with the fact that elaboration in pharmaceutical work is not always improvement, real improvement. I accept without question that the primary object of the pharmacist should be the therapeutical value of his products; elegance of physical appearance being very important considerations, but they are secondary. That I am a zealous advocate of pleasant medicines, presentable forms of remedies, and dislike, even detest, useless dirt in pharmaceutical preparations, even to the point of becoming ethically irregular, is known, and I candidly admit that in some instances a crude drug seems to me superior to any known elaborated product of it. …That I may be criticized by some of my co-laborers in pharmacy for drawing attention to these truths is probable. They are facts, however, and should not be covered under a bushel, and I bow to the necessity that compels an expression of my opinions where humanity may be broadly benefited."

In other words, though he recognized their superior benefits in some cases, inhererently Lloyd was not in favor of using whole herbs because he did not consider these to be professional products of applied pharmaceutical science. Another problem with whole herbs for Lloyd involved the penchant of Eclectic doctors to often rely on botanicals that were potentially quite toxic. The content of extremely potent alkaloids, for instance, could be reduced when making an extract, whereas the proportions of the more toxic and the less active components could not be manipulated in the whole herb by pharmaceutical means, other than by air or oven drying to reduce the potency. Lloyd describes as appropriate the application of techniques to modify the potency of certain components when their activity is too great (*EMP*, 1904, p.474):

"In many instances a conspicuous structure of a drug is harmful if it be present in excess. Here comes the necessity of the pharmacist's art, for by means of the study of neutral solvents, or other kindly touch, the structural life of the complex being may be conserved, and yet its harmful part harmonized in its relationship to its home fellows."

The concept of a complex herb contrasts with the long-held perception of herbs as simple remedies. The use of herb in formulas in Europe following the practice of Graeco-Roman humoral medicine led to single herbs being designated as 'simples'. With the experimental alchemy practiced by notable medieval physicians and apothecaries, intricate extraction processes became the rule of the day. The less processed 'herb simples' employed by the general public in folk medicine were considered disreputable by the arrogant learned even of that time. As modern technologies of pharmaceutical manufacturing developed, these reduced the natural herb complexity to simplified refined derivatives. As a result, the complex herbs were perceived as a source of compounds to be isolated and purified, and reference was made to the whole herb as a 'crude drug'.

Due to the phrase 'crude drug', people involved in the science of pharmacognosy (study of pharmaceuticals derived from natural products) tend to misconstrue complex herbs as mainly an undeveloped source from which science will liberate the true value of purified compounds. Alterations of the natural compounds can then be modified, patented and mass-produced, much as chemists isolated fractions and developed kerosene, gasoline, and synthetic pharmaceuticals from crude oil or codeine, morphine, and ultimately heroin from opium poppy resin.

The "purification" process by which industry removes compounds of unforeseen value from the rich treasure house of plants can best be illustrated by seeing how it has been applied to the food industry. Rather than simply removing the wheat berry from the straw and chaff (the nourishing plant part from the inedible ones), the seeds are processed by separating the starchy, glutinous endosperm as white flour from the nutritious wheat germ and the 'non-nutritive' bran. Elimination of the germ improves storage but removes important oils with anti-oxidant vitamin E, and loss of the bran eliminates the important bowel-stimulating effect. Then, in a simple-minded attempt to improve on nature, a few synthesized nutrients are mixed back in above normal quantities, to not only replenish, but 'enrich' the final product whose iron content in thus elevated to potentially dangerous oxidizing levels. Such refinement and enrichment promotes constipation and accelerated aging, while consumers of whole wheat enjoy the full balance of nature's nourishment.

Lloyd in his attempt to refine his pharmaceutical products believed it was important to remove some confounding compounds that he thought were unnecessary for therapy and likened to dirt. Chlorophyll was one such component that he seemed adamant about eliminating. Yet in regard to this he stated (*EMJ*, 1920, p. 1–3):

"Chlorophyll is tasteless; it seems to be inert. … Other products are with the chlorophyll very intimately associated, this either by adhesion or mechanical combination, all of which in natural setting are colloidal. Chief among these we find certain vegetable waxes, fats and oils, … seemingly inert therapeutically. And yet as concerns their presence and their influence on pharmaceutical preparations, they assume importance to a degree but yet imperfectly understood.

"Be it said that the utmost difficulty is experienced by whoever attempts, with the ordinary pharmaceutical processes, to untangle these chlorophyll-affiliating combinations."

As necessary foods, Lloyd showed appreciation in recognizing the value of such seemingly dispensible plant components as chlorophyll (*AJP*, 1934, p. 42–3):

"Begin with the common "garden stuff," eat freely, especially of such as you crave. They carry little, if any, "scientific" qualities, but they are loaded with *supportives* (a term coined by me to apply to such substances). … Turn to the young onion, which I advise you to eat, top and bulb, chopped fine, on a side dish with vinegar, salt and pepper. The young onion carries incalculable '*supportives*' not found in the onion carried over the winter. ...

"To this may be added that the *young onion* carries a colloidal, slippery serum or juice not present, or at least scarcely present, in the full-grown onion; and that the young onion top carries an abundance of the vitalized green know as *chlorophyll*, which word has long been known, but which substance is no more valued in works on medical science than is sand accepted as other than a cumberer of the earth in which the onion grows. ...

"In books scarcely will you find chlorphyll and its brother associates, the green of vegetation (pure chlorophyll in bulk is black), counted worthy of any consideration. But remember, I tell you they are life supportives and life creators of the entire vegetable as well as animal kingdoms."

We know that chlorophyll is the vegetable equivalent of hemoglobin in its structure, the difference being that magnesium rather than iron is its central activating element. The oils in plants not only provide essential fatty acids, such as the gamma-linolenic acid in purslane, but also carry necessary antioxidant fat-soluble vitamins, flavonoids, and carotenoids. While the colloidal magnesium and oil-associated compounds may not produce dramatic acute therapeutic effects, their long-term consumption has profound health implications in helping prevent heart disease and cancer, respectively, among other conditions. Whole complex herbs provide both food for prevention and medicine for healing.

Among the essential issues to consider is the optimal time to harvest certain medicinal parts of plants. While precise knowledge of individual herbs is necessary, Lloyd provides some general advice for consideration (*EMJ*, 1887, pp. 259–61):

"It ... will harm none to acquaint themselves with crude drugs by a little personal attention. I am speaking now to physicians who use vegetable remedies to a great extent, and shall confine myself to this class of medicine.

"HERBS.—If you propose to use an herb in making a medicine, see that it is gathered when the leaves are mature, not young, watery, green, and succulent; not old, dry, decayed, and insipid; let them be rich in characteristics, mature, perhaps even an off shade. ... I have for years stated that my experience is to the effect that herbs must be collected at certain appropriate times. ... A preparation may be very green in color, and still a poor medicine.

"BARKS.—At certain seasons of the year barks will slip easily. These occur at different times, in accordance with the latitude and the season: in the spring when the buds burst, and (in this section) about the last of June again. At these times most barks are collected for commerce, but I prefer them when the sap is out instead of in the tree. They are harder to collect; they are not so nice looking: fragments of wood adhere to the inner side; but they are better. The valuable part of the bark is the "inner bark," the juicy portion. The dry "ross" is to be shaved off and thrown away.

"ROOTS.—When the plant matures, and the juice disappears, gather these portions of the plant. Do not collect roots in early spring, and it is best with perennials to wait until the growth of the season is suspended, and activity has subsided. In the season of rest, between summer life and vigorous outburst in the spring, I have found roots and rhizomae most valuable. If the plant is an annual, do not allow the top to die or wither before gathering the root. As a rule, annuals yield the most valuable roots and rhizomae when the plant is in the condition of maturity that is shown by the perfect leaf. In some instances, as with hydrastis and sanguinaria, all traces of the plant vanish about the time the rhizome is most valuable.

"BULBS should be collected after the plant has lost its vitality, and even has died to the ground. Then they are rich and plump; they dry firm and smooth, and do not shrink and shrivel to insignificance. Then they are highly characteristic.

SEEDS.—As a rule, seeds are preferred in a ripe condition. However, in some instances they are better immature. … If the seed is used just before ripening, it will be found that while the grease (fixed oil) is absent, the peculiar active agent or agents are highly developed. Taking advantage of these lessons, I have for some time eliminated these fats from certain preparations, in the making of which I am forced to use ripe seeds, and have received more than one letter of compliment regarding their excellence from physicians who value beauty, effectiveness, and elegance."

Fresh Herbs

Whole herbs in this form have most often been traditionally consumed as food or condiments in cooking. Used in this way they can be considered as spices, vegetables, or fruit. The features that distinguish their use as medicinal herbs are the intent, regularity, dosage, and/or duration that they are used. The strong flavor of many of these fresh herbs limits their consumption to small amounts, so they may be considered naturally concentrated. Recently, some of their extracts have been described as nutriceuticals due to the common use of the plants as foods. Because of their high water content they can be readily pulverized and may be used topically as a poultice.

Water is a compound essential for life. Life processes depend on its presence, or rather, they are maintained and proceed in its context. The tendency of thinking of water in a plant or in our bodies as separate from the compounds that it contains and sustains is largely erroneous. Water is not present in living organisms except in biochemical relationships that intimately support the transformations, exchanges, and transportation necessary for the dynamic of vital activity. Comprehending the role of water in necessary for appreciating the complexity of the biochemicals that make up botanicals. The chemical "structures" of biochemicals are not line drawings on paper as we have been led to visualize them in academic courses, but energetic relationships dependent on a suitable medium to form interrelationships and conversions. Lloyd drives this point home when he discusses the importance of water in the context of nutrition (*EMJ*, 1902, pp. 596-600):

"The majority of people accept that the function of water in food substances is that of a solvent only, or as an inactive vehicle provinced only to carry food to tissue and bone. ... Water is not seriously considered in the light of an integral part of food by any one, such solid substances as starch, sugar and nitrogenous and fatty tissues being usually cited as the constructive and heat-producing agents. Our works on digestion and on general physiology state that most foods are three-fourths water, and the human body, bones included, over two-thirds water, but yet consider water irrelevant as a nutrient. ...

"The cabbage, the apple, the fruits of our orchards, the vegetables of our gardens, contain in all cases an enormous amount of water, if we consider the fluid part of the mysterious liquids present in vital juice and organic structure as simply water. Here we are confronted with conditions in which relationships between the large amount of water and the small amount of solid are such as to tolerate the view that this water of combination may be a something very different from pure water, or water obtained by tissue destruction. With such complex examples in mind, we are led consistently to inquire whether such dishes as soup and other aqueous liquids, and water-bearing and water assimilating foods, can, as tissue feeders, be in themselves anything beyond simple solutions of solid matters in water. ...

Should we not look on such water, necessary as it is to life, digestion and tissue replacement, as an integral part of food, instead of simply a carrier of food? It is indeed probable that the student of dietetics must broaden his field and consider foods in their structural entirety, rather than from their analytical created ultimates. The method of the analyst now is to first kill the animal or vegetable, then destroy the tissue, then disrupt the molecules. The final result gives him inorganic elements and a few characteristic chemical structures on which he bases his tables concerning food valuations. ... Is it not more rational to accept that the exceptional value of albumen and other nutrients as typical foods rests on water compounds so nearly in accord with tissues craving just such vitalized water-bearing structures? ... May not water be combined in an untold number of liquid organic structures that are as yet invisible, uncrystallizable, unreachable to our senses as organized bodies?

"But enough for the present. In a time to come it may be clearly seen that students of food and digestion have not given sufficient prominece to the one thing that supports life, nourishes life, that feeds all structures, that constitutes the larger share of all organic tissues, but that, strangely enough, in itself is now viewed as a carrier only of something else.

"We feel justified in anticipating that the immediate future will give a more extended view than the circumscribed atomic theory affords, which, to this date, as a stepping-stone, has served the world well. Shall we then perceive that the vitalized water of organized water-bearing foods, and the combined water of such foods as carbohydrates and fats, are the foundations of the real foods for tissues? ...

"Possibly the makers of food products of the future will give less attention to analytical values concerning dead elements and more to vitalized and vitalizing structures in which available water is conspicuous. Possibly it behooves us even now to ask if a closer inquiry into the water molecule, *the vitalized or easily vitalized water molecule* and its many shadings, may not open up a field for the construction of more rational food products."

Fresh herbs do not contain chemicals that exist as discrete isolated compounds in a lifeless fluid. The nature of life is one of relationships, so that compounds exist as a component of an energetic matrix, constantly transforming itself according to the vital demands of the cells and their functions. The pioneering genius of American botanical pharmacy, John Uri Lloyd, described this matrix as a colloidal complex that alters the physical and chemical nature of substances. These substances exist as crystalline structures outside of this living context, that is, when they are dead, dried, and separated. The relationships that exist within living cells make the components respond differently in terms of the subtle quality of chemical interactions. These differences are expressed physiologically as buffers, catalysts or adjuvants in how they impact accessibility, absorption, and assimilation of the active component chemical compounds.

Lloyd states (*AMM*, 1919, pp. 15–24):

"The fact that condition, not weight of a material, is a first consideration in governing therapeutic activity, parallels the fact that physical condition or state of material governs also much in the line of pharmaceutical possibilities. ... Study a plant in the field, or a tree in the forest. Dissect them as one may, the fresh, undried tissues are ever found to be non-crystalline. In their normal settings, gums, resins, albuminates, tannates, acids, glucosides and coloring matters are, in like manner, non-crystalline. ... In their natural settings, even minerals in vegetation become colloidal. They here possess nourishing qualities quite distinct from the same substances in crystalline form. ... Cast off excretions (such as perspiration) carry crystalline salts, while the urine is a prolific field of crystalline research. But the stepping onward of normal biological processes, the transferring of vitality from colloidal cell to colloidal cell ... seems ever to lean upon the movements and actions of colloidal bodies, which in their formation, and transformation, produce derivatives that, if normal, are colloidal. ... Have we not, for decades, learned by experience ... that many plants cannot even be dried without destruction of their inherent qualities, surely not explainable by mere water evaporation?"

Living plants direct energetic qualities that determine the expression of transforming life. These vital organizing principles not only direct growth and constructive change but maintain control of plant chemistry expression through enzymatic processes. These enzymes can be responsible for destructive changes when chemicals are converted in the process of cell death following harvesting or while drying, or when cell structures are destroyed and/or components mixed for extended periods, as in juices or cold and warm water extracts. Consumption of fresh plants by crushing destroys the cellular compartments that prevent these conversions from occurring in the whole plants. The process of energetic transformations in the mouth while chewing is one aspect of nutrition that has never been adequately studied. It is invigorating to assimilate the nourishing energy transferred when eating fresh plants.

The main drawback of utilizing fresh herbs is their limited availability. Unless one is able to grow their own herb garden it is difficult to obtain quality fresh herbs and adequately preserve them. Freezing breaks down some of the living cells, depending on their water content, and this removes some enzymatic barriers. However, much of the cellular structure remains intact. Another problem with some fresh herbs is there powerful flavor, for example, garlic (*Allium sativum*) or cayenne (*Capsicum frutescens*), that can make it difficult to chew and swallow them. Modifying the flavor or removing the water to reduce the size of the bolus for swallowing is sometimes necessary.

Dried Herbs

The most common process which herbs undergo is air-drying or oven-drying. The word 'drug' originated from the Dutch term 'droog' that referred to dried herbs, and this is the term that Lloyd always used to refer to dried medicinal plants. This form is now typically used by the public for making teas or ground and added to foods as culinary spices. Dried herbs are also the raw material for almost all commercial extracts including tinctures, oils, and concentrates.

After removing the visible dirt and undesirable plant matter, the moisture is removed from harvested herbs to avoid contamination and deterioration by molds and fungi. This eliminates the need for refrigeration and also reduces the bulk and weight for transport, decreasing shipping expenses. For air drying it is best to avoid direct sunlight that can break down the light-sensitive compounds. Providing circulating air around the thin layers of drying herbs is necessary for efficient drying, whether this occurs slowly in room-temperature air or rapidly in ovens. The roots and barks of plants are usually sliced in sections or strips and exposed to oven heat at $40–60^{\circ}$ C $(100–140^{\circ}$ F), until they lose close to one half their weight. The flowers and leaves are dried at lower temperatures, typically from $30–40^{\circ}$ C $(85–100^{\circ}$ F) until they lose about nine tenths of their weight. Most commercial herbs are then cut and sifted for sale. While this makes freight costs cheaper and extraction easier, it also exposes more of the herb to exposure to air, light and moisture, increasing degradation and requiring greater quantities for equivalent activity.

To prevent their chemical breakdown and loss of potency, the dried herbs should be stored away from light, air, moisture, and heat above 15° C (60° F). Storage is best in full, brown glass jars with tight lids; sealed plastic bags with the air removed that are enclosed in spaces protected from light (for example, inside opaque paper bags or boxes or in cupboards or drawers) are okay at cool temperatures. The breakdown of some active compounds (for example, flavonoids, carotenes, or anthocyanins) is evident when the vibrant color found in the fresh plant begins to fade and disappear. A reduction in fragrance or taste further indicates lost quality. To assure that most of the potency in dried herbs remains available, stored leaves and flowers should be replaced after one year, while the roots, barks, and seeds may be kept under proper conditions from three to five years.

Powdered herbs sold in bulk should be avoided. Not only is it difficult to be certain of the identity of the plant(s) or other contents that may be in the powder, but the active compounds degrade much more rapidly than when the herb is kept in its whole, or even cut and sifted, state. Grinding to powder not only exposes the herb to heat, but it vastly increases the surface area exposed to light, heat, and oxygen and moisture in the air. Loss of potency inevitably occurs under these conditions.

There are cases when the diminished potency of older dried herbs is to be preferred over their fresh form. Laxative barks containing irritant compounds such as those found in cascara sagrada (*Rhamnus purshiana*) or alder buckthorn (*Rhamnus frangula*) should not be used fresh. In fact these barks are best aged for at least a year after harvesting to allow for conversion of the irritant compound to less potent chemical forms to reduce the risk of intestinal cramping and attendant colicky pain. Similarly, the Chinese root fo-ti (*Polygonum multiflorum*) is a strong laxative when the raw dried root is used, but the cured root is famous for its tonic properties. Simply drying a plant in some cases is adequate for removing irritant properties found when handling or ingesting the fresh plant. An extreme example of this is the fresh root of bryonia (*Bryonia alba*) whose tincture was used by Eclectic doctors in doses of 5 drops or less to avoid toxicity. Recently, the dried bryonia root with less intestinal irritant compounds has been shown to provide tonic or adaptogenic effects when used in substantially larger doses.[1]

As a manufacturing pharmacist, Lloyd was not an advocate of using whole dried herbs. The expectations of medications were that they represent a degree of pharmaceutical elegance to separate them from the traditional whole herb that had formerly been in common use and was part of 'folk medicine.' His concern rested

1. A. Panossian, et al, Plant adaptogens, II. Bryonia as an adaptogen. *Phyromed.*, 4 (1): 85–99, 1997.

largely with the amount that he believed was necessary to consume due to the content of fiber and what he considered inert material, as well as the overall low potency of conventionally dried herbs. As a pharmacist, Lloyd's practice was to eliminate through the use of chemical extraction much of the content of the raw herb that was not acutely therapeutic (*AMM*, 1919, p. 52):

> "The difficulty of administering crude drugs is too well understood to require comment. Naturally the first step in an attempt to facilitate their employment is that of comminution, or powdering them. At the best, powdered drugs, with their great burden of inert matters, are impractical remedies. This fact necessitated the application of manipulative methods, the object being to ... obtain forms of medicaments capable either of representing in small compass large bulks of crude drugs, or of presenting the active parts in more elegant form."

Herb Tablets

The methods for making tablets from whole herbs can vary, but it generally consists of first grinding to powder the dried herb. The powdered herb is then compressed, often together with binders, diluents, coloring agents, flavoring agents, and/or lubricants, and then sometimes coated with sugar, dyes, fat and/or wax. These additives help assure the tablets remain intact and have a uniform appearance.

There are a number of drawbacks to using whole herb tablets. The size of such tablets is often so large as to make swallowing difficult. Besides adding undesirable compounds to the product, the additives and coating can also reduce or slow the digestive breakdown of the whole herb. The process of making tablets involves exposure to moisture and pressure that can reduce the quality of the product.

Not every herb is able to be prepared in this form. Lloyd comments strongly about inappropriate application of this technique (*EMJ*, 1897, p. 574):

> "A clean tablet that carries in itself what it pretends to convey, is not necessarily inferior to a clean pill. A so-called tablet of a substance that can neither be dried nor powdered is an imposition, and credits neither its maker nor the prescriber. Bottles containing so-called tablets of such evanescent substances as cannot be made into tablets, have done more to discredit the tablets than tablet opposition could have done. Doubtless many physicians have thrown out the entire line of tablets because of the fact that they were unable to differentiate between such as carry their full drug values and others useless.
>
> "For this professional dilemma none are more to blame than tablet makers, who, in the light of experience, will recover from their hasty enthusiasm, and eventually drop from their lists such tablets as discredit the name, and who, in doing so, will place the tablet subject on a more solid foundation. There is a place in medicine for medicinally true tablets, and it is a pity that an entire class should suffer in consequence of the bad company of some of its membership."

Encapsulated Herbs

Herbs are also dispensed as powder in capsules. The drawbacks to powdering herbs have been addressed. Freeze-drying greatly reduces the energy needed to reduce herbs into powder and therefore minimizes the chemical breakdown from small heat generated. Dispensed in bottles as hard gelatin capsules, the opportunities for hydration, oxidation, and adulteration are reduced. Disagreeable tastes are avoided, but, like tablets, large capsules may be difficult to swallow for some. Unlike tablets, no additives other than the capsule are necessary. The herb powder provides a "time release" effect with its components in the gut due to chemical binding to fibers and other compounds in the plant. The powders are extracted only by digestion unless taken with a hot beverage. Another option is to empty the capsule into hot water, and then consume the powdered herb and water together. Consuming herb powder is the best way of delivering certain of components such as astringent tannins or demulcent mucilage to the distal portion of the intestinal tract for their local effect.

Gelatin encapsulation was beginning to become popular toward the end of the nineteenth century, a development of which Lloyd approved largely because of its improving the ease and tolerance of administering poor-tasting remedies to patients, enhancing compliance (*EMJ*, 1879, pp. 545-6):

> "Gelatin is very soluble in hot water, and this, with its property of drying into
> a coating impervious to moisture and the atmosphere, led to its being used as a
> coating for certain preparation, such as pills, capsules, etc.; and when we consider
> that it is soluble in warm water and the fluids of the stomach, is perfectly harmless,
> is tasteless and odorless, we certainly must respect the claims of the coating. ...
> The capsules were glossy, tasteless, odorless. They remained unaltered, and such
> disagreeable drugs as cubebs were entirely covered, odor and taste. ... Thus we find
> gelatin employed to coat pills and make capsules, and certainly we cannot ignore the
> claim of the agent, as a nice coating can be given without the application of a long-
> continued heat, as in sugar-coating. ... These points are worthy of consideration ...
> as gelatin-coated pills are coming quite properly into such extensive use."

For those who wish to avoid the consumption of animal byproducts, powdered herbs are now available in nongelatin capsules, or vegecaps.

Local Use

POULTICES

Poultices can be most simply applied when the pulp from a pulverized fresh plant is applied directly to an area and held in place with cotton or other material. Mashing the plant releases the juice that acts as a carrier. Formerly referred to as cataplasms, poultices can also be made with a little boiling water added to powdered herbs to form a paste. The paste is placed over a local area and covered by cloth. Often, heat is applied over a poultice to help increase local circulation and thereby improve absorption by increasing the fluid content in the tissue being treated.

Native Domestic Water Extracts

Anything other than the whole herb is in reality only a fraction of the herb and should therefore never be described by simply referring to the name of the plant. Rather, the type of herb extract should always be designated to more accurately describe not only the form but, by inference, the content of these products referred to as galenicals (*AMM*, 1919, p. 53):

> "Inasmuch as *Galen* first prominently introduced plants into medicine, or at least, because he has been given great credit in this direction, *plant preparations* are often known as *galenical preparations* or *galenicals*, under which term we may include all of them."

The traditional form of consuming herbs as remedies involves using water as a solvent to effectively extract many of the medicinal compounds. These extracts are commonly referred to as teas because of the popular stimulant herb from Asia that has always been used in this manner. In European folk traditions the same herbs used for generations by commoners as teas would be prescribed as more elaborate and fashionable extractives by professional medics. Native Americans cooked fresh or dried herbs overnight on the coals of their fires to be taken in morning while fasting. The ancient and modern method of preparing classic Chinese formulas involves cooking the herbs in water, sometimes for hours. The variety of plants and their various parts used in these traditional concoctions has often led to their description as soups rather than teas.

Even though Lloyd spent his professional career advancing the practice of pharmaceutical science, he did not believe in the need to replace effective preparations (*EMJ*, 1889, p. 373):

> "Do not discard *all* of your infusions and decoctions because the majority of them may be better replaced with more refined drug representatives. ... Do not argue that you can on general principles discard all that is old in favor of the new."

Lloyd recognized the superiority of particular botanical preparations made by water extraction (*EMJ*, 1885, 415–6):

> "The endeavor of pharmacists to supply physicians with convenient form of remedies, commendable as all will admit, yet may result in occasional mistakes. There are some drugs that are, in my opinion, more reliable in the form of infusion or decoction than as either a tincture or fluid extract. It is a mistake to use fluid

extract of either pomegranate bark, pumpkin seed, or althaea. A decoction of
pomegranate and pumpkin seed should be preferred, and the infusion of althaea.
[*EMJ*, 1876, p. 263: "I ... advise any one desiring to administer a decoction of
pomegranate bark for tapeworm, to boil the bark in the water for a period of at
least two hours."] For some years I refused to make either a tincture or fluid extract
of these drugs. ...

"The infusion of epilobium gave to that plant its reputation; the tincture is passable,
but not equal to the infusion. There is an occasional demand for fluid extract of
slippery elm, sometimes for the tincture, and any person who understands this drug
will know that an alcoholic menstruum cannot extract its mucilaginous constituents;
and it is used for these principles only. Cold water is the menstruum to use; and
strips of the bark should be soaked in it until the liquid is ropy and mucilaginous.

"The list might be considerably lengthened, but I think that a sufficient number
of substances have been named to commend to physicians a little care regarding
the form of drug dispensed. ... I have aimed to make practical chemistry and
pharmacy a specialty in my teaching. ... The next step towards a better education
for the physician, in my opinion, is even a larger amount of pharmacy than I have
heretofore given."

Lloyd noted that many herbs built their solid reputations on being used as water,
not alcoholic, extracts (*EMJ*, 1889, p. 373–5):

"As a sialagogue Jaborandi appeared before the medical world under the
introduction of an unquestionable authority, Dr. Ringer, who used it in *infusion* only.
The record of its field of usefulness seems to be thoroughly demonstrated when it is
taken in hot decoction, the reports being that the sweating was increased and more
quickly induced when the *dregs as well as the decoction were also swallowed by
the patient*. Today this drug is practically discarded (although highly commended in
print) and the medical jury that pronounced the sentence relegating it to obscurity
employed the fluid extract of Jaborandi, a preparation altogether different from that
used by its introducers.

"I rebel against such preparations as fluid extract of Kino and fluid extract of
Catechu [due to their "gelatinization" in alcohol (*EMJ*, 1922, p. 372)], and have
displeased some patrons by refusing to make them. Other cases can be cited in
which such inconsistencies occur, but it is unnecessary, although I might say that in
my opinion a decoction of Apocynum is effective where an alcoholic preparation is
useless, and that the elaborate formula of the United States Pharmacopoeia, 1880,
produces a fluid extract of chestnut far inferior to an infusion of chestnut leaves. ...

"If I wished to administer to a member of my family pennyroyal, peppermint,
sage, boneset, or other of most of the domestic remedies, and many drugs now
only known to the profession in fluid extract form, I would surely make "tea" or

decoction, and not give a fluid extract or tincture. I am a maker of fluid extracts and other similar preparations, and hence cannot be criticized by fair minded persons for advising physicians of this Society who are largely my patrons to benefit themselves and their patients, as I do now, at my own expense."

However, it was apparent to Lloyd that there were definite limitations of water's ability to extract some of the important active components to which medicinal herbs owed their activity. The efficiency, palatability, and convenience of the process is something of a concern to Lloyd as a manufacturing pharmacist. (*AMM*, 1919, p. 52):

"*Infusions* and *decoctions* … were subject to grave objections. In the first place water is capable of abstracting but a limited part of the constituents of many active drugs, such as fixed oils and resins. Second, it dissolves most of the gums, mucilages, inert and objectionable constituents of plants, thus making bulky, disagreeable, often very weak remedies. In the third place, it forms solutions that ferment readily, becoming unreliable in a very few hours. There are other objections … such as the fact that volatile constituents are lost by boiling."

The herb compounds that dissolve in water as extractives, or the water-soluble plant components, include nutritive sugars and other carbohydrates that can be digested. In addition, immune-enhancing polysaccharides made up of branches of sugars, as well as proteins. The combinations of sugars and proteins called glycoproteins or peptidoglycans can also be immune enhancing. Long, unbranched polysaccharide chains appear as viscous mucilage in water, while more complex branched molecular chains that hold water as gels are called gums. A wide variety of chemicals with different properties can be attached to a sugar molecule in the cells of herbs to be more soluble in water. These components are known as glycosides. One example of glycosides is saponins that form bubbles or foam when shaken in water. Saponins from yucca and/or licorice are used for this in root beer. Other compounds extracted in hot water include the astringent and antiseptic tannins. In addition, some alkaloids, potent bitter-tasting compounds, including caffeine, dissolve readily in hot water.

As Lloyd noted, it is also important to know what water as a solvent does not extract or retain well. Some alkaloids such as hydrastine in goldenseal (*Hydrastis canadensis*) are not water-soluble. If there is a sticky, resinous coating on the leaves to protect the plant from water loss or being eaten by herbivores, this will resist extraction by water. Other resins in plants such as the pungent oleoresin in cayenne (*Capsicum frutescens*) do not dissolve well in water, nor do plant oils. Many volatile oils and aromatic balsams are not retained in water, especially in uncovered containers. If alcohol extracts containing compounds such as these are added to water, precipitates can often be seen forming on the surface of within the solution, making it appear milky or cloudy. Resinous precipitates may cling to the sides of the container, and other precipitates will settle to the bottom of the container when allowed to sit for a time.

Many compounds are only partially soluble in water, where the amount retained depends upon the temperature of the solution. The warmer the water, the more it it will dissolve, extract, and retain. Also, components that are insoluble in water as isolated compounds or fractions, such as resins and fixed oils, can become partially soluble when extracted from plants since they are dispersed in a matrix of water-soluble compounds. However, the normally insoluble components tend to eventually conglomerate and/or form precipitates over time.

Cold Infusions

Different methods can be used to extract the medicinal content from plants with water. Cold infusions are made by soaking the herb in water at room temperature or slightly warmer, usually to extract mucilage. This slippery carbohydrate is made up of long strings of sugars without side branches, so the molecules slide easily against each other without a lot of physical/chemical/energetic resistance. The length of time required to make these extracts depends on the size and density of the plant particles. For instance, cold infusions may take up to twelve hours for strips of slippery elm (*Ulmus rubra*) bark that have not been cut or shredded. Certain other barks use particular methods (*AMM*, 1919, p. 53):

> "Special directions are employed as in the official infusion of Cinchona, in which cold water, aromatic sulphuric acid and percolation are used; or infusion of wild cherry, in which cold water and percolation are employed. However, the exceptions are limited."

'Sun tea' describes a cold infusion made by setting a clear jar containing herbs in water in the sunshine for a day. This process reduces the amount of tannins extracted from black tea (*Camellia sinensis*) or raspberry leaf (*Rubus idaeus*) and certain other compounds and is favored by those with sensitive stomachs who prefer a mild flavored tea. This process is generally used to produce weak recreational beverages. Enzymatic conversion by water-soluble proteins of some components dissolved in the water of such extracts as sun tea and cold infusions can substantially alter the content and activity of certain compounds.

Since bacteria grow readily in warm water containing any amount of simple plant sugars, the extended time required to make cold infusion extracts allows for the potential proliferation of these microbes. Mucilage is made of polymers of sugars, so demulcent herbs are the most susceptible to this outcome. One means to reduce this tendency is to briefly rinse the herbs (usually pieces of roots or bark) with boiling water to kill the surface bacteria prior to soaking them for extraction.

Hot Infusions

For making a "tea," this is the approach used by most Americans, that is, pouring boiling water over cut or crushed herbs. Tea bags are often preferred for their convenience, but these typically provide a rounded teaspoon of powdered herb(s) for use as a recreational beverage. For medicinal purposes the amount varies depending on the herb, but stronger extracts are usually employed, using closer to a rounded tablespoon per cup (depending on the herb). Loose herbs are preferable to tea bags, since the greater surface area exposure allows the water to more quickly and effectively saturate and extract the active components.

The plant parts used for hot infusions are the less dense portions, usually the flowers and leaves, either fresh or dried. These should at least be cut to increase the exposed surface area, or may be powdered, preferably just prior to infusing in either a blender or clean coffee grinder or with a mortar and pestle. In general certain procedures are followed, and fresh herbs are preferable (*AMM*, 1919, p. 53):

> "These preparations are made of coarsely ground or bruised roots, barks, herbs and seeds. ... An ordinary infusion, the strength of which is not directed by the physician ... should be prepared by the following formula: — "Take of the substance, coarsely comminuted, ... 50 Gm. Boiling water, ... 1,000 Cc. Water, a sufficient quantity to make ... 1,000 Cc. Put the substance into a suitable vessel provided with a cover, pour upon it the boiling water, cover the vessel tightly, and let it stand for half an hour. Then strain and pass enough water through the strainer to make the infusion measure ... 1,000 cubic centimeters. Caution—The strength of infusions of energetic or powerful substances should be specially prescribed by the physician."—U.S.P.

> "Bear in mind that infusions are prone to ferment, and must be repeatedly replaced by fresh ones. In my opinion, infusions of fresh plants that contain delicate constituents are to be preferred to any preparation made from the dry plant, and in cases where the medicinal constituent is a gum or mucilage, insoluble in alcohol, the infusion of the dried plant is preferable to any alcoholic preparation."

Taken as a hot beverage, more compounds can be absorbed faster because of the local increase in blood flow in the stomach and intestines. However, herb teas may also be allowed to cool and be consumed later. Because the herbal components are usually rapidly absorbed from a liquid extract, it is usually best to slowly sip the tea for a steady prolonged exposure, rather than rapidly consume the entire amount. Appropriate exceptions might be the desire for rapid sedative or stimulant effects from herbs with these properties. The infusion should be used during the day it was prepared if it is kept at room temperature. Otherwise, it should be refrigerated and consumed within two days. Otherwise, fermentation will likely occur, and the taste may be spoiled or sour. Refrigerated tea may be re-warmed in a covered container but should not be boiled.

If a powdered herb is used, it is usually filtered from the extract. However, if it is desirable to consume the whole powder but have it partially extracted by water instead of swallowing it as a capsule, the tea with the powder can be consumed if personal tolerance allows. For example, this can be useful for an herb with resins such as ginger (*Zingiber officinale*) whose aromatic properties for dyspepsia are enhanced by its pungent resins. After drinking the tea the cup and mouth can then be rinsed with a little water to remove the residual powder adhering to the container or the teeth. This powder can then be swallowed.

What of the destructive effects of heat on active components of plants? Let us listen as Lloyd explains (*EMP*, 1889, pp. 27–9):

"Perhaps the only rule that is without exception is the rule of exceptions. ... We find many drugs that are rendered valueless by heat. ... The heat of boiling water directly applied for a brief period, is certainly not uniformly destructive to many delicate plant constituents. ... Peculiar ferments or destructive agencies that work rapidly at moderate temperatures are to be more particularly avoided ... than a quickly applied temperature of 212 degrees F. Indeed it seems not improbable that a study of drugs will yet show that some that are injured by drying might often be sterilized ... by application of a quick boiling heat or current of steam. ...

"It is often the long continued action of a boiling temperature or of atmospheric exposure, that finally disintegrates. ... At first it requires but 212 degrees F. to boil the water – in fact it is simply the boiling of water containing a drug, but as this water becomes charged with extractive matters the temperature rises, the solvent changes from water to a more or less viscid liquid, and as the extract thickens the temperature runs to 218 or 220 degrees F., and hence there is actually a higher temperature with the constant progress of concentration or changes attendant thereto. ... We have less cause to fear a properly applied boiling temperature than is now generally accepted, and ... many of our usually unstable drugs are not destroyed by a quick temperature of 212 degrees F. ...

"A universal rule cannot be and should not be applied to the making of any line of plant preparations of this description. ... Neither drying the bark, storing it for years in a dry situation, boiling it in water for half an hour, nor keeping the decoction for seven years [sealed], destroys the value of pomegranate."

Some exceptions apply to the guidelines for infusing certain plant parts. Some roots and barks may be infused if they are first ground to powder. Also, those plants whose leaves have a heavy waxy coating such as uva ursi (*Arctostaphylos uva-ursi*) may need to be decocted, unless they are first powdered like dense roots or bark. However, this process extracts more tannins, as discussed next.

Decoctions

While not employed by many Americans, this may be the most common form of preparing herbs worldwide. As described previously, the extended simmering or cooking of herbs over heat to most completely extract their components is a typical approach in traditional herbal medicine. One reason for this is the preferred means of storing herbs was in their whole form. Once dried, many herbs, especially roots and barks, are difficult to break up or grind down into easily extractable small pieces or powder. Therefore, extensive cooking provided a way to effectively re-hydrate whole plant parts and extract more of their water-soluble components. In addition, it enhanced the breakdown of structural components of the plant cells that would not normally be available through simple infusion or digestive processes. These include some polysaccharides that are best known for their immune enhancing properties such as those found in medicinal mushroom species.

Even in traditional western medicine, decoctions have been advocated as the best method when using water to extract dense, woody material, particularly roots and barks. This is especially necessary if these parts are dried; fresh roots or rhizomes like ginger may be infused if they are sliced very thin. Cooking the herbs extracts more of the tannins, but it also drives off or breaks down many of the volatile oils and simple proteins including enzymes. Strong tannin extracts can upset the stomach if taken regularly or in large amounts, even when prepared as infusions as is the case with black tea that is too strong. Even with herbaceous plants, flavonoids, another type of polyphenol, are best extracted when decocted for 30–45 minutes and yield 20% more when the herb material is ground rather than course cut.

Some of the hard, inedible mushrooms must be decocted for hours to adequately extract their active cell wall components. In general less time is used for herbs (*AMM*, 1919, p.53–4):

> "As a rule decoctions are made by pouring cold water over a coarsely ground or bruised drug, the mixture being boiled for fifteen minutes, cooled and strained. Very few exceptions are recorded. ...

> "Like the infusion, decoctions ferment quickly and must be often made. It must be remembered that while the usual strength of both decoctions and infusions is one part of drug to twenty of the finished preparation, the proportion of all energetic

(poisonous) drugs must be established by the prescribing physician, who alone has the privilege of increasing or decreasing the proportions. At the best, however, both infusions and decoctions are deficient in drug valuation or reliability. If the aim of the physician be to administer much *hot water* and little drug, or large doses of liquids of uncertain strength, they are well fitted to their purpose. Such are the natures of *teas*, which in reality, as catnip, pennyroyal, etc., etc., are infusions and decoctions in which it is immaterial as to whether or not the drug proportions be uniform."

Not all roots and barks should be decocted to maximize their benefits. Exceptions to the rule include the mucilaginous slippery elm bark. A cold infusion of slippery elm bark provides the soothing demulcent effect for dry, irritated mucous membrane surfaces for which this herb is famous. Decocting the bark would extract the tannins that are present, producing an astringent effect that could aggravate dry mucous membranes. Stone root (*Collinsonia canadensis*) is a herb whose root is widely used for treating hemorrhoids. However, the toning activity is greatly reduced when the root is boiled. Taken for dry coughs, wild cherry bark (*Prunus serotina*) has long been used to reduce the tendency to cough; boiling destroys the compounds that are responsible for this effect.

Local Use

COMPRESSES

A compress is simply a medicated cotton cloth applied locally. A fomentation, also called a stupe or hot compress, is made when a cotton cloth is dipped in a hot water extract. The excess fluid is wrung out, and the cloth is placed over the affected area. Compresses are normally covered and kept hot.

BATHS

Soaking a particular body part in water medicated with an aqueous herbal extract or other compounds is the typical means of employing therapeutic baths, or balneotherapy. The temperature of the water may be hot, tepid (neutral) or cool. However, medicated baths usually employ hot water.

ENEMAS

Enemas involve the injection of water in the rectum. Normally this is done with plain, tepid water to promote bowel evacuation or to help control fevers. When medicated enemas are employed, the water is used in smaller quantities and is held internally to enhance local exposure or increase absorption.

DOUCHES/WASHES

A douche is a flushing of a body cavity such as the external ear canal, nose, sinuses, or vagina, using water that may contain herbal extracts or other medications. A wash refers to the flow of water over an external aspect of the body in relatively large amounts. Both douches and washes are usually done for cleansing and/or antimicrobial effects.

GARGLES

Gargles employ medicated aqueous solutions that are used locally in the throat and temporarily retained. Normally, they are not intended to be swallowed. Typically, gargles provide antiseptic medications locally but may also include local anesthetic compounds for relief of irritation. Such applications are known as mouthwashes when limited to the front portion of the mouth.

Native Commercial Liquid Extracts

The first factor to consider that affects the quality of all botanical extracts is the quality of the whole "crude" herbs from which the extracts are made (*EMJ*, 1887, pp. 259–61):

> "First, you cannot make a good remedy from poor material. Do not understand me to say that there will be any great difference in physical appearance; it may appear fair, but nevertheless will be poor in accordance with the inferiority of the drug it is made from. Of first importance is the drug you use. ...

> "The readers of this JOURNAL know that I am more than persistent, regarding this subject. ... Don't say that you are not interested; if you give medicine you are. Don't think that such studies are unimportant. How can we hope to improve without study? ... This subject is not complete. We must make the tincture."

Herb quality demands knowledge and understanding of the factors that affect the quality of each particular herb, not simply herbs in general. The means required to assess specific herbs are not simply laboratory measurements but organoleptic (sensory) qualities that can only be derived from experience. Unlike the current situation where herbal products can be made and sold as dietary supplements by anyone with enough interest and effort to market their wares, in Lloyd's day the manufacture of botanical products was the work of pharmacists. Though he had never attended pharmacy school himself, Lloyd apprenticed in several pharmacies including that of then-president of the American Pharmaceutical Association W.J.M. Gordon in Cincinnati. He later taught in the Cincinnati College of Pharmacy. Through his experience Lloyd recognized the requirements for an adequate education along this line goes beyond mere books (*AMM*, 1919, pp. 49–50):

> "The greatest care must be used by the pharmacist in the direction of drug selection. A crude drug [fresh or dried plant] is the foundation of a pharmaceutical preparation. Poor crude material is productive of inferior medicine, regardless of the care of the operator. The study of applied pharmacy consequently begins with a

study of drugs, and carelessness or ignorance concerning this oft neglected section in pharmacy is to be held accountable for much poor medicine – more indeed, than is generally known.

"The qualified pharmacist must not only be conversant with manipulative methods, but also experienced in the study of drugs. In this direction it is not alone sufficient to be able to distinguish between different drugs (this is useful to guard against sophistication), but he must be able to judge of the intrinsic qualities of drugs. This last is the most important part of the art of pharmacognosy, for while it is easy to learn to identify different drugs it is difficult to obtain the experience necessary to judge of quality shades. ... There are many different qualities of drugs of every description, and, in my opinion, the knowledge necessary to their successful differentiation is only to be gained by patient study and great experience in practical pharmacy.

"For example: The aroma of a fine ripe peach can only be learned by personal experience with peaches. ... Between the fully ripe and delicious peach and those inferior and worthless, lie a chain of peaches—all peaches, but yet of many qualities.

"True it is that in some instances chemical tests may be employed for drug valuations, but these cases (for example Cinchona and Opium) are so few as to scarcely bear any comparison with the great number of drugs in which we have absolutely no recorded method of detecting values. ... Indeed, in my opinion, this much to be deplored lack of facility to become personally expert ... accounts for much defective medicine in the line of plant preparations. ...

"Those best versed in the art understand best the responsibility resting on the man who audaciously ventures to step into this field without the knowledge that comes from long drilling in practical work under the watchful care of an experienced instructor. ... Neither books nor lectures can teach pharmacy in its broadest sense. The foundation that is gained by the fortunate possessor of a systematic college of pharmacy of university education, is not to be undervalued, but it is only a foundation for the recipient to build upon in the future. In my opinion, no man should at this day be permitted to engage in pharmacy manipulation without a preliminary college course of instruction in pharmacy; neither should he be allowed to practice pharmacy by reason of college instruction alone."

The difficulties in assessing the optimal process for extracting each herb can be daunting. This was the work to which Lloyd devoted his life to patiently engage in experiments and share discoveries (*EMJ*, 1887, 71–2):

"I have long argued that the study of pharmacology as applied to plants, is greater and presents more obstacles than the study of pure chemistry as applied to the chemicals used in medicines. ... During the last two or three months I have ... devoted my spare time to the consideration of ... Thuja occidentalis. ... Thuja I found to contain three entirely distinct proximate principles—an oil, a resin, and a tannate—and these cannot be associated together free from inert matters by making a simple tincture by means of any known menstruum. Several menstruums will only extract one or two of these principles, some menstruums portions only of each. ... We have mixtures in single plants. The time is coming, I think, when the making of a preparation by the adopted methods of the present, one drug being used, the rule of thumb process and one menstruation to extract that drug, will be polypharmacy, or at best crude pharmacy. ...

"When I ignored the fluid extracts of the U.S. Pharmacopoeia and the accepted methods of making fluid extracts and tinctures—when I indicated that those medicines were not the height of pharmaceutical excellence—I was bitterly opposed and in exceptional instances abused. ... The result of this independent study has been accepted by many members of the medical profession that we all honor, and who accept the processes I have one by one evolved after careful investigation, to be superior to the processes of the Pharmacopoeia for making preparations from the same plants. Do not understand me to say that the Pharmacopoeia medicines may not be good medicines. ... I simply believe that continued labor and attention must result in progress. ... In other words, we must recognize that plants contain an association of substances, that necessitates for each plant a separate consideration and an intelligent examination."

Many herb extracts are available in stores that are made by simple techniques that have been employed for hundreds of years. These methods use varying concentrations of alcohol as a solvent to extract much of the fat-soluble compounds from plants. These compounds include many *alkaloids, alkamides, resins, volatiles, fatty acids,* and *sterols* that do not extract well or at all in water alone. Alcohol also acts as a preservative to keep extracts or juices from fermenting and degrading. Depending on its concentration, alcohol works more or less effectively for each type of compound (for example, resins versus alkaloids) or use (extracting or preserving). Similar to their water-soluble compounds, plants contain a variety of components that are more or less soluble in alcohol, so no particular concentration of alcohol will effectively extract all of the active compounds from a herb. In no case is even a single component completely extracted.

Once extracted, compounds from the herb are preserved for some period of time by the alcohol. The time the extract retains activity depends upon the herb and the stability of its components. Alcohol does not of necessity assure that the activity of any extract is permanent. Lloyd points out the fallacy of assuming otherwise (*AJP*, 1922, 527):

"Physicians have much with which to contend from variation of medicinal power of many of the fluids that are made from different qualities of drugs and by different applications of skill in working the same. In some important cases they also have to contend with liquids that are reliable when first made, but become worthless through age, regardless of the skill and care of the operator. In most cases these liquids are dispensed in full faith of their reliability, by reason of the confidence we have in the preservative power of alcohol."

Besides its effect on extracting and keeping certain compounds in solution, alcohol concentration also has an impact on what compounds are kept out of solution. Many of the herb components that dissolve in pure water will be denatured or precipitate, falling out of solution, in pure alcohol. The most appropriate alcohol content of an extract is the one that extracts and keeps in solution the greatest amount of the most desirable components for a particular use. The amounts and content of each different compound changes as the concentration of alcohol is varied in the extracts. Essentially, water and alcohol mixtures compromise the final content in one way or another as their proportions vary. In the end no matter what ratio of these two solvents is used, active components are left unextracted in the plant material that remains.

Diluting extracts with alcohol or water can result in formation of precipitates. In answer to a question about whether precipitates that are formed when alcohol was added to specific tinctures (made from fresh plants) would weaken the tincture, Lloyd made the following comments (*EMJ*, 1877, pp. 306–7):

"Everything in a "specific" belongs there. … Our plant contains oils, resins, gums, mucilage, coloring matter, chlorophyll, alkaloids, glucosides, acids, and other principles. Some are soluble in water, some in alcohol, and some in mixtures of alcohol and water to an extent. When we percolate a powdered plant with a mixture of alcohol and water, we dissolve an amount of certain principles which are insoluble in alcohol, or only soluble to an extent, and if we pour an extract of this kind into alcohol, the matter which alcohol can not hold in solution must be precipitated as an insoluble substance. … If the principles which are precipitated by alcohol give the extract a portion or all of its medicinal value, it is impaired when we throw these principles out. … Alcohol dissolves oils and resins insoluble in water. When we add an extract made with alcohol or diluted, to either water or syrup, such substances as are insoluble in these menstruums will be precipitated, and often they are valuable."

Lloyd makes the point that such incompatibilities are not rare, and care needs to be taken to disperse the contents of an alcoholic extract when it is added to water (*EMJ*, 1904, p. 123):

"Staphisagria mixed with water turns milky, an oily substance rises to the surface. Is this as it should be? Yes, for Staphisagria is greasy, very. The separated oil is as natural as if an alcoholic solution of castor oil were mixed with water. … Concerning Podophyllum, … a precipitate forms when it is mixed with water. This, too, is as it should be, for the resin of podophyllum is not soluble in water. The same rule applies to macrotys, jalap, and other resinous drugs. In a similar way, the oleo-resins separate: for example, Iris versicolor, silphium, Rhus aromatica, etc. All such as these should do this very thing, and when such remedies are added to aqueous liquids, the prescription should be shaken before each dose is taken."

Juices

Referred to in pharmacy as the 'succus', this is the liquid extract that is produced in our mouths when we chew fresh plants. The water-soluble components are available in this form, but much of the fat-soluble compounds remain bound to the fibrous matter left behind. The liquid expressed from living plant cells needs to be consumed quickly or enzymatic breakdown ensues. To guard against this, several methods are employed. After mechanical expression of the juice, which is now frequently done at home with modern juice extractors, the fresh fluid can be refrigerated for a short while. However, enzymatic breakdown of components begins immediately, and the flavor and effects can sometimes change dramatically in a short period.

For commercially juiced herbs, flash heating or pasteurizing can be employed to control microbial growth and destroy the enzymes that catalyze chemical conversions of active components. The juice is then poured into vacuum-sealed, sterilized bottles. This method is most often employed for fruit and vegetable juices that are consumed in large quantities. After opening the bottles the juice needs to be refrigerated. Otherwise, sugars in the juice will be fermented by microbes, and the flavor and/or activity will be altered.

As an alternative to heating, alcohol can be added to at least a 22% content to prevent fermentation and denature the enzymatic proteins to prevent breakdown of components. Either heating or alcohol must be used if the juice is to be stored as a liquid. While heating is the method preferred for mass production of fruit and vegetable juices, addition of alcohol is the most common method of preserving herb juices.

A word of caution is necessary regarding the over-consumption of juices. With the removal of plant fiber it becomes easy to consume much larger amounts of plant components that would normally not be possible if the entire plant were eaten. For most fruit juice this allows consumption of large amounts of sugars that are not appropriate quantities for regular use. For some vegetable juices other types of compounds may be taken in excess. For example, chemically-fertilized celery (*Apium graveolens*) contains high concentrations of nitrates that are converted in the body to nitrites. If exposed to large quantities, these provide the basis for carcinogenic nitrosamines. In using herb juices similar caution should be applied. Only those herbs that are regarded as nontoxic should be consumed in the form of juice extracts in large amounts on a daily basis.

Medicated Wines and Vinegars

Wine was used as a solvent in medicine at the time of Christ, as we hear in the Gospel of Mark (15:32): "they tried to give him wine drugged with myrrh, but he would not take it." Wine, as an alternative to water as a solvent, was typically used more by those in medical practice. Wine had the advantage over water as serving both as a solvent and preservative. Its use continued past the time when tinctures were popularized by Paracelsus in the16th century. However, as tinctures became the standard extracts employed in medicine, medicated wines eventually fell out of favor. They were described briefly by Lloyd (*AMM*, 1919, p. 62):

> "Among the earliest pharmaceutical preparations were to be found solutions of drugs in wine. The alcohol therein tended both to help exhaust plants and to preserve the product from putrefaction. ... Among the wines are to be found the common beverages, white wine made by fermenting the juice of fresh grapes freed from seeds, stems and skins; and red wine made of colored grapes, including their skins. These are used in preparing the medicated wines. Eclectic physicians use medicated wines very sparingly, with the exception of the old Eclectic *wine bitters*, which is still a favorite with many."

Vinegars were popularized first by Galen in the 2nd century as a means of enhancing the extraction of certain herbs. It was later learned that alkaloids are more readily dissolved in this mild acidic solution. Since the acid is produced from fermented sugars, further microbial contamination is prevented. The acid also helps prevent their growth. Acetic acid is present in a 4% concentration in this aqueous solution, and these extracts are sometimes referred to as 'acetracta.' Vinegar is still preferred by some, since it is non-alcoholic. Lloyd refers to their limited use (*AMM*, 1919, p. 58 and 63):

> "These not very uniform preparations are similar to tinctures, excepting that in making them either diluted acetic acid or vinegar is used as a menstruum instead of alcohol. The early Eclectic physicians considered several medicinal vinegars with some degree of favor, for example, *Vingear of Lobelia, Vinegar of Sanguinaria,* etc."

> "They were once used freely, but have fallen largely into disuse. The vinegars (aceta) are peculiarly adapted to alkaloidal drugs. ... In the regular school of medicine vinegar of opium or *black drop* was once a favorite. ... In this class may also be placed the *acetous emetic* compound of early Eclecticism."

Tinctures

With the discovery of distillation, Arab pharmacists found a means of concentrating volatile liquids such as alcohol. First described for use in making extracts in Europe in the 13th century, it was not popularized until the 16th century when Paracelsus found it to be a useful means of concentrating certain active principles from plants. After that time it became the standard method for manufacturing medicines through the late 19th century. Tincture remains the official medical term used for extracted drugs. Therefore, many liquid herbal extracts made with a mixture of water and alcohol and sold as dietary supplements are often described simply as liquid extracts.

Tinctures are liquid extracts that are usually made by soaking (macerating) a cut or ground dried herb in a solvent mixture (menstruum) of water and alcohol for one to two weeks. It is agitated daily by shaking to mix the extracted compounds (solutes). Otherwise, these tend to layer out in solution, causing the concentration to be greater in the bottom of the container where the herb is also settled. After extraction has reached equilibrium, the extract is strained, and the marc (soaked herb) is pressed out. The extract and the expressed liquid are then combined and filtered. Another method of preparing tinctures is by percolation. This process is discussed under the heading of fluid extracts.

Tinctures are hydro-alcoholic extracts, that is, the solvent is a combination of water and alcohol in a proportion designated by the ethanol percentage. The percent of alcohol used to make tinctures of different plants or different parts of the same plant depends on which preferred constituents are being selectively extracted. An alcohol concentration of about 25% is used to keep many of the most water-soluble constituents in solution. A 45% alcohol content is an effective solvent for many alkaloids and most saponins. Alcohol in the range of 60–70% is typically used for volatile aromatic components (essential oils) in whole herb extracts. Balsams are extracted with a 75–85% alcohol solution. At concentrations greater than 90% alcohol is most effective for keeping resins in solution. Therefore, the percent of alcohol in an extract does not specify the strength of the extract but suggests the type of compounds that are considered more or less important or desirable, based on their relative solubility at that concentration.

Tinctures are manufactured at different strengths. This is described as a ratio of the weight of the dried herb compared to the volume of the solvent in the extract. Weight and fluid volume units formerly used in America to describe the strength ratio were ounces to fluid ounces. Now, here and in the rest of the world the standard units used to describe the strength of a tincture as a ratio of herb weight to liquid extract volume is grams to milliliters. The standard tincture strength is 1:5, that is, one gram of dried herb is used to make each five milliliters of extract. This is common for most herbs, but a reduced strength ratio of 1:10 is typical for very potent herbs in cases where even very small doses, as low as one drop, could be excessive if the extract was more concentrated.

Tinctures have varied in popularity and have been made by different processes and strengths over the years (*AMM*, 1919, p. 55):

"This class of preparations derived its name from the fact that they were usually of a dark color, or, at least, possessed of a characteristic color. They are ... of deficient strength as compared with extracts and fluid extracts. Formerly tinctures derived from single drugs, if unofficial, were by common consent made to practically represent two ounces of drug to the pint. At present the custom seems to warrant the proportion of one part of drug to ten parts of finished tincture. ...

"Tinctures carry all the substances, both inert and active, soluble in the menstruum used to exhaust the drug, and are consequently prone to precipitate. Excepting with energetic drugs, a large amount of alcohol must be administered in order to get the full therapeutical drug effect of a tincture. Tinctures (with few exceptions) are rapidly falling into disue and are practically discarded in Eclecticism, where very concentrated, exact preparations of plants are now generally employed."

Commercial tinctures are almost all made from dried herbs. Yet this fact, suggestive of convenience, brings with it no assurance that the dried form of a plant provides a superior basis to begin extraction. Let us hear Lloyd's opinion on the matter (*EMJ*, 1876, pp. 311, 313–4):

"Water is intimately connected with the creation of all the component parts of our plants, and experience will teach us that the dissolution of many of these bodies takes place when the water upon which they are indebted for existence, is removed. ... Dried plants are exposed to the influences of moisture and the atmosphere; from the time they are gathered until used a constant change is going on, and although a plant may weigh as much twelve months after, as it did when first dried, this imperceptible decomposition may have resulted in the total destruction of the principles that originally give it its therapeutical activity. ...

"The business of the pharmacist is a study of the handiwork of the Almighty. He is constantly brought face to face with facts he cannot understand. ... Pharmacists cannot calculate. They are operating with intricate combinations of elements, and investigation alone will teach them the properties of the bodies formed by these different combinations. ... Certainly it is true, that it has become a custom to use dry plants for making tinctures; but this fact does not prove they are best adapted to the purpose. ... The U.S. Pharmacopoeia does not recognize a single green tincture. ... We must have light upon this subject, and the way to get light and see the facts of the green tincture business, is to put our own shoulder to the wheel and exert ourselves."

Some highly processed products sold as tinctures actually are made from solid extracts produced from dried herbs and then redissolved in a mixture of water and alcohol. In these cases the percentage of alcohol does not suggest what compounds were originally extracted but only what might be retained in solution. These extremely processed products are a number of steps away from the "crude" and complex but basic commercial extract and function more as limited fractions. According to Lloyd, such fractions may be considered more as products of chemistry, rather than biological material obtained from fresh plants (*EMJ*, 1915, pp. 616–7):

"As men consider structures and not artificial ultimates, it will, we believe, be demonstrated that a study of the dead products broken out of vitalized plant textures is not a study of materials that exist in the plant, but results of the chemistry applied to the plant."

Green Tinctures

Many tinctures can best be made from fresh plants. These are referred to variously, depending on the process used in their preparation, as green tinctures, recent herb tinctures, or specific tinctures. The latter name is taken from the prescribing principles of John M. Scudder and other American Eclectics in the late 19th century who preferred fresh plant extracts. Lloyd elaborates on the difference between these fresh plant extracts and official liquid extracts in the U.S.P. (*EMJ*, 1877, p. 308):

"The officinal tinctures and fluid extracts are made from dry materials. Maceration and percolation are employed. There are no fresh plants used, and in my opinion it is not right to call a medicine officinal, in the form of a tincture or fluid extract, unless it is made in accordance with the pharmacopoeia, from dry plants, and of the officinal strength. And I can not see that Prof. Scudder could have done better than to give the entire line of remedies he desired to have used in connection with his treatise on the specific action of medicines, a name which would place them apart from fluid extracts and tinctures, as he was not in favor of these preparations as found upon the market, and the medicines he used were entirely different. ...

"Great care is required to work fresh plants, and almost every article behaves differently. I am not of the opinion that any one believes "specific medicines" possess any properties not found in the original crude drug. They are only represented by me as superior preparations of very choice materials. First get prime crude drugs, then work with care and use the best processes, and do not believe than any amount of care will make good medicines from worthless drugs."

For Lloyd the essential aspect for making effective extracts was the quality of the plant material, whether fresh or dry. The exceptional factor that distinguished fresh (living) from dried (dead) plant material that he found so appealing was the colloidal, noncrystalline nature of the chemical content. His description of colloids was necessarily vague due to the limited research applied to their nature (*EMJ*, 1916, pp. 400–3):

"WHAT ARE COLLOIDS? — ... The incoming life-structures, the established life-structures, and those passing out of existence, are totally colloidal in their nature. (Cast-off excretions, such as perspiration, carry salts of crystalline opportunities. Urine is a prolific field of crystalloid research.) The stepping onward and the transferring of vitality from cell to cell, and from organism to organism in the support of life, seems to depend wholly upon the movements and actions of colloidal bodies. ... This includes what may be known as the juices of plants and animals, whether formed by secretions in cells, or appearing as a complexity of liquids in the veins or arteries. ... Colloidal are the nourishing structures of the most valued foods. ... To the homely motto, "Nature abhors a vacuum," I would add the parallel, "Life structures abhor a crystal." ...

"Colloids may be classed as I now view the subject in its relationship to life, as formless, vitalized structures, capable of creating, nourishing, and next destroying creatures composed of cell aggregations. ... A colloid (as afore illustrated) is a substance that has no definite form, and under ordinary conditions at least, is destitute of crystalline structure. A colloid may be liquid, it may be jelly, it may be a solid. It may be colorless and transparent, whether liquid or solid, or it may be colored and either liquid or solid, but in it all, if it be a true colloid, there is no definite formation, such as governs bodies bounded by systematic crystalline plates, edges and angles. ...

"Pass now to foods. ... These may be defined under the blanket term "colloids," even though the form as of starches is characteristic. Cast your glance over such as these, and note that all are destitute of crystalline structure; they are amorphous, colloidal. ... The majority of life structures, created by life processes, are colloidal, as well as are the nourishing principles that carry life energies to their upbuilding and upkeeping. ...

"This article is designed only to describe and define a colloid ... *as a class.* An effort has been made to exclude all technical divisions and subdivisions. ... May I not, in summing up the problem as a whole, assume that the consideration of organic colloids is the study of life structures, that a study of the action of colloids concerns the very foundation of life, known as vitality?"

Factors influencing the quality of the fresh material used were also points of keen interest to Lloyd as he discussed the gathering and processing of fresh plant parts for tincturing (*EMJ*, 1881, p. 253):

"We can refer to the list of products of our gardens and fields, and as a rule, will find that all must be collected at the proper season. This is true likewise with such portions of vegetation as are used in medicine, but the fact is not generally recognized. ... As a rule, the reader may argue that specimens of plants should be gathered after the growing season is about over, and before decay begins. This is true of herbs, and leaves. Barks are least likely to be affected by season, but even these should not be gathered when filled with sap."

In his pursuit of preserving the therapeutic properties of good quality fresh plants, Lloyd utilized the best available method prior to the development of processing fresh herbs and juices by freeze-drying. His approach required adaptation to the different types of herbs. He continues with instructions on using "recent" roots, describing the appropriate means of reducing water content of a succulent root (*EMJ*, 1881, pp. 302–5):

"As a rule, roots, tubers and rhizomae should be procured in the latter part of the summer, and during the autumn. It will be found that all succulent roots are filled with sap during the spring months, and from some the water may be squeezed by simple pressing with the hand. Such are worthless, or almost so, as remedies, and should not be procured for making pharmaceuticals. In this article we shall consider under the general name root, such parts of plants as grow under the ground, although strict accuracy forbids the application of that term to tubers and rhizomae.

"Such as Cimicifuga racemosa, Hydrastis canadensis, Collinsonia, and those that are of ordinary size, should be procured entire. This is a point that writers do not mention, and that experimenters doubtless have neglected. However, my experience teaches me that a mistake is made when roots intended for recent material are broken, even for the purpose of drying. They should never be broken if we desire to represent them accurately by pharmaceutical preparations, until they are to be bruised, sliced, or ground for extraction with our menstruum. ...The explanation of my directions that the root be gathered entire, therefore, resides in the simple fact that air alters the properties of the root if it be broken, in a much greater degree than when it is permitted to dry through the skin. Gather, then, the *entire* root if practicable. ...

"Some of our pharmacists use only certain parts of the root. Thus some remove the fibrous roots or rootlets, and use only the main root. ... As a rule, it is not supported by my experience, excepting with hard woody roots, where the bark is to be taken, and I advise the reader to use the succulent roots as they are found, fibers and all. ... I have known men to scrape the bark from roots before tincturing them. The persons who are so nice as this, overstep themselves, for often the brown bark is the most valuable part. Especially is this true of dry roots. ... Let it be remembered, then, if the desire is to represent the fresh root with our pharmaceutical, use the root as nearly in its natural state as possible.

"The article I am writing now is regarding the preparation of tinctures from "*recent material.*" ... Many of our roots, even late in the season, are filled with sap, much of which is free water. This water is not only objectionable on account of dilution of our preparation, but often it prevents the solution in alcohol of the real active principles of the plant. Sometimes it aids in the decomposition of the tincture after it is prepared. Therefore, I find it necessary to separate the roots as much as possible of this superfluous water before preparing from them my pharmaceuticals. ...

"When the green root is gathered wash it carefully and in such a manner as if possible not to bruise or break it. Then place it in a cool situation where there is a constant circulation of fresh air. Observe that the roots are well spread out, and are not in bunches, and in all cases keep them from the direct sunshine.

"In most cases it will be found that with this simple plan, a very large part of the water of the root, after a moderate time, will escape by evaporation through the epidermis. It will be found, also, that to a certain point the loss is not followed by a change in the properties of the root. However, at last the water of combination of the root begins to escape, and now the change in constitution sets in. After this point the further exposure of the root is objectionable, as it is undergoing changes that alter its properties. It must now be tinctured.

"Let the reader then follow the rule, that the root in its entire condition, can be exposed to a cool current of air until it commences to change in color, or give other evidences of decay, as shown by breaking a piece from one of the young roots. When this point is reached it should be known as "recent material," or in other words, material in a condition that can be tinctured to satisfaction.

"Most of our pharmacists have scarcely thought of a line of remedies outside of those directed by our United States Pharmacopoeia. Some have thought of the matter, and considered it impractical because the books were silent on the subject, and, as we well know, some manufacturers have even derided the idea, refused the physicians the desired remedies, worked against the problem of an improvement in this direction, and argued from the "water" and other standpoints, that the medicines could not be made. ...

"In conclusion I desire to impress upon the reader, that there is great room for improvement. I have worked upon the subject of preparations from recent material for many years, and have overcome many difficulties, but others are before us that this generation will likely not have settled."

Having described the best approach of his day for gathering and preserving fresh roots, Lloyd proceeds to elucidate the optimal means of preparing an extract of optimum quality. He makes a point of emphasizing that not only the quality of the botanical material determines the value of the final remedy, but the care and expertise with which it is processed (*EMJ*, 1881, p. 356–8):

"I have particularly requested care in the preparation of material for tincturing. The fact is, good pharmaceuticals cannot be made from worthless drugs. ... Do not infer that the reverse is not also true, for a bad workman may spoil his material; the fact that prime material is used is not a sign that the tincture *must* be reliable. ... When we note the destruction of prime material in any department of the arts without a creditable return, a feeling of shame comes over us, even though we are not personally interested. How much more is this the case when we feel individually responsible.

"If the root be succulent, like that of the common poke, slice it very thin by cutting it across the grain. Use a very sharp knife, and as the slices are made permit them to fall into official alcohol. ... When the slices are within half an inch of the top of the alcohol the proportion of root to alcohol is best, as a rule. Let me particularly refer to the slices of root. They should not be *chunks*, but nice thin sections, about the thickness of ordinary blotting paper.

"The alcohol should be in a salt-mouth bottle (wide-mouth glass-stoppered), and as soon as the proportion of root to alcohol is obtained, the bottle should be stoppered, placed in a moderately warm location, and permitted to remain until the following day. Then reverse its position (turn it upside down) and permit it again to stand for twenty-four hours. In a day return it to its former position. This change in position I find to be the most reliable of any method that I have investigated to thoroughly extract the soluble principles from sliced roots. ...It tends to establish an equilibrium between the soluble solid matter in the root and the solid dissolved matter outside of the root quicker than when the bottle is shaken. ... *Let the operation of daily reversing the bottle be continued for fourteen days*; then pour the liquid from the root, and if it be not clear filter it quickly. Or what is better, pour the liquid from the root into a tall bottle, cork it tightly, and after twenty-four hours decant the clear solution, and then into the decanted liquid filter that which remains and which contains the precipitate.

"Such roots as Cimicifuga racemosa, Collinsonia canadensis, and others of a hard, woody texture, cannot well be sliced. In these cases the root must be placed in an iron mortar, and crushed until it is in shreds, or the state of a pulp. This is then to be slowly dropped into the bottle of alcohol, in small amounts, care being taken that after each addition of the root the vessel be thoroughly agitated. When the root has been added until it remains firm and in a mass just below the surface of the alcohol, the proportion is correct. Some of our readers may ask my reason for adding the root to the alcohol, and not mixing the alcohol with the crushed root. It might seem that little difference, if any, could result from reversing the operation, and stirring the alcohol slowly into the mass of moist pulpy root. I cannot consume time with the argument now, but I can say that it often makes a *very great* difference as regards the permanence and elegance of the tincture.

"After the mixture of crushed root and alcohol is made, stir the contents of the bottle well with a flat stick. Let the motion be such as to cause the mass of liquid and pulp to revolve, and at the same time, by an upward motion of the paddle at the termination of each revolution, bring the material from the bottom to the top. I recommend this process because often the mass of crushed root adheres together, and simply shaking of the bottle moves it about in a lump, and does not thoroughly mix it. Let the process of stirring be repeated daily for fourteen days, then drain the liquid from the pulp. Transfer the pulp to a strong strainer, and squeeze from it all the solution practicable. Pour this last solution slowly into the decanted solution, stirring it well, and after twenty-four hours decant or filter it as we have directed for the former preparation.

"In closing this article I beg the reader to remember that I am compelled to briefly state certain facts that are the result of my experience in this matter. I believe that whatever is worth doing is worthy of attention and care, and I am certainly of the opinion that physicians will find it to their interest to encourage study and attention in every direction which is connected with the preparation of medicines.

"Recently one of the old and successful graduates of the Eclectic Medical Institute said to me, "I have better success than my competitors of other schools from one reason, I use better medicines." Let physicians remember, *medicines are your tools.* If they are poor ... what use is there in prescribing them? What reason have you for talking about doses? Let me impress upon my friends of the medical profession the necessity for all to take high ground in this direction, and insist upon care and attention in the preparation of remedies."

Whereas Specific Medicines were made at a 1:1 strength similar to fluid extracts, many modern green tinctures are of a strength ratio of 1:2 (fresh plant weight to final extract volume). These higher ratios for fresh herbs are used since the volume of water in the plant itself adds to the final fluid content of the extract. The difference in outcome is not so much a matter of relative weight to volume that ultimately is similar to tinctures made from dried plants. The major difference is qualitative due to the matrix of interconnected chemical components that remain together in a way similar to what is found in their natural living state.

Some herbs necessitate being tinctured fresh due to the nature of their active components. Lloyd indicates that concentrated extracts of certain dried plants cannot approach the potency of their standard green tinctures (*EMJ*, 1876, pp. 260–2):

"Some people imagine that the tincture from a pound of green herb only represents the strength of a few ounces of the same herb when dried; that the medicinal strength of our pharmaceutical is in proportion to the solid material of the drug from which it is prepared. ... I will take issue when they say that the medicinal principles of our herbs are relatively in proportion to the solid and unvolatile materials. ... I have also learned that in many cases sufficient exposure to evaporate the water will destroy the medicinal principles of the plant. ... The principles that impart the therapeutical properties to our plants are true chemical compounds. ... Some are easily volatilized, some are so unstable as to render it impossible for man to separate them from their natural relations to the plant without decomposing them, and others cannot possibly be retained even for a few hours by any means yet discovered. ... We must make our tinctures as necessity may require from that which is the most suitable; there can be no invariable rule. If a plant is found to lose its medicinal virtues by drying, that plant must be tinctured fresh."

The value of the type of tincture designated as "green" is not dependent on a green color, as the liquid extract may or may not be green initially or later. An exception to the importance of preparations maintaining the color of the fresh plant is the perpetuation of the green pigment chlorophyll. According to Lloyd (*ET*, 1909, p. 120):

> "It will, on reflection be apparent to many physicians who read the article, that chlorophyll in the preparations on their shelves, often fades. A tincture may change from green to even brown, and still, seemingly, have lost no therapeutic qualities. Ointments, green when first made, become yellow or even brown, but yet remain energetic."

This comment on the color change in literally green tinctures was necessitated by numerous concerns and complaints expressed by physicians who thought the quality of their medicines was thereby diminished or a substitution had taken place. Lloyd's observations (*EMJ*, 1921, pp. 55–6):

> "A plant preparation of a deep green color when purchased stands on the shelf as it is utilized in office practice. As used the air overlying the liquid abstracts alcohol if any be in the liquid, or otherwise changes the solvent. ... It may result in change of color owing to the influence of air on the chlorophyll compounds present. When the bottle is nearly empty – perhaps months have passed – a newly purchased supply is placed by the side of the old, and the contrast in color, most marked, leads the physician to question as to whether there be not a mistake in labeling. ... These questions are not now, however, often asked by physicians of the Eclectic school, most of them being fully informed concerning the fact that the green color of the leaves of plants has no connection with therapeutic qualities."

The tinctures prepared from fresh plants are often light in color. This can be perceived by the uninformed mind as an indication that the extract lacks potency, as if the strength of a preparation is determined by its opacity. The concept that darkness indicates strength was offensive to Lloyd (*EMJ*, 1877, pp.23–4):

> "The true medicinal agents in our plants are generally colorless, or nearly so. ... Tea and coffee contain caffeine, or theine, as it is sometimes called, which imparts the invigorating properties to these two common articles of domestic use. Yet this substance is white. ... Hydrastia [sic], one of the proximate principles of hydrastis c. is white, berberin [sic], the other, is lemon yellow. The dark red color of fluid extract of Hydrastis canadensis is the consequence of an impurity. A true fluid extract of hydrastis, or tincture, should be yellow, not red, not black. Oil of valerian is colorless. The best authorities tell us valerian root depends mainly upon this oil for its value in medicine. Fluid extract of valerian is very dark. It will make a mark upon paper, but that it does so, is because it contains impurities. The active principles of most of our plants are white. Why should fluid extracts and tinctures be dark?"

While Lloyd was concerned with optimally balancing what he described as the plant's "energetic" principles to be used in medicine (compounds such as alkaloids that have the greatest pharmacological potency), he did not have scientific evidence to document that many colored compounds have important physiological activities and influence. Believed by Lloyd to be unwarranted in potent medicinal extracts, chlorophyll and other components unnamed at that time but found in the fresh green plants were recognized by him to be of intrinsic nutritive value as supporters of health and life (*EMJ*, 1931, pp. 341–2):

> "Consider remedies used in treating an ailment (or ailments) then titled "scrofula." These remedies were bunched as "antiscorbutics," ... *things* having antiscorbutic qualities. ... Among these, lemons and oranges may be named as prominent. ... Any vegetable food that came in the springtime was included—yes, suggested—as dominating even these citrus fruit. ... "Eat freely of the early vegetables, prescribe them to your 'run-down' patients. Begin with the common 'garden stuff,' eat freely, especially of such as you crave. They carry little, if any, 'scientific' qualities, but they are loaded with *supportives* (a term coined by me to apply to such substances). ...

> "Turn to the young onion, which I advise you to eat, top and bulb. Chop them fine, or slice them on a side dish with vinegar, salt and pepper. The young onion carries invaluable "*supportives*" not found in the onion carried over the winter. ... The *young onion* carries a colloidal, slippery serum or juice not present, or at least scarcely present, in the full-grown onion; and that the young onion top carries an abundance of the vitalized green know as *chlorophyll*, ... but which substance in no more valued in works of science than is sand. ... In no books will you find chlorophyll and its brother associates, the green of vegetation, worthy of any consideration. But remember, I tell you they are *life supportives* and life creators of the entire animal kingdom."

Research since the time that Lloyd wrote has shown that colored compounds including yellow and orange flavonols and flavones, red, blue and purple anthocyanidins, and red and yellow carotenes are extremely important for health due to their anti-oxidant activity, including anticancer effects, and vasoactive influence. Lloyd frequently noted a yellow color that appeared in alkaline extracts from many plants and finally did isolate the flavonoid component he called eldrin, now known as the quercetin glycoside rutin, from white elder blossoms. He hoped that this would prove to be an agent of significant nutritive value. However, the physiological science of his day failed to recognize any obvious effects (*EMJ*, 1920, p. 594):

> "I sent some of this material to Prof. R. Adams Dutcher, University of Minnesota, requesting that he make a physiological examination of it. His preliminary report was to the effect that, according to a preliminary investigation, it had no physiological action. May I not ask, should a peculiarity of action be expected of a substance pervading plant tissues everywhere? I had vitamins in mind, there was reason to hope that a general life supporter of plant life, serviceable to animals, could be found and isolated. Not a poison of energetic action. This, I accept,

Dr. Dutcher demonstrated as a fallacy in the direction of this substance."

Unfortunately, science was not as far advanced as Lloyd's intuition into these matters.

Homeopathic Mother Tinctures

Mother tinctures are homeopathic extracts of plants and other medicinal substances that utilize a water and alcohol solvent mixture. The homeopathic plant extracts are typically made with fresh herbs in a 1:10 strength (ratio of 1 part plant weight in oz or ml to 10 parts extract volume in oz or gm, respectively) based on the calculated dry weight of the fresh plant. These mild liquid extracts are the beginning solutions for preparing succussed serial dilutions used as the individual remedies in homeopathic prescribing. This approach was developed in the early 19th century as an effective way to capture the vital energy of the living plants.

Lloyd believed the quality of these extracts was good because of the use of fresh plants and the care that was employed in preparing these extracts (*AMM*, 1919, p. 60):

> "These alcoholic preparations are admirable remedies in many respects, but lack the concentration to which Eclectic physicians employing specific medicines are accustomed. ... As a rule the mother tinctures represent much less than the drug used in making them (dry drug taken as a standard), still, aside from their deficient strength, they are excellent preparations. ... Owing to the care in collecting the drug, the fact that in many cases the plant is not dried, and the explicit details of pharmaceutical manipulation, the resultant preparations are very clean and useful remedies. As a rule, they are light in color."

Lloyd did not advocate replacing the use of Homeopathic mother tinctures with his own Eclectic specific medicines made from fresh plants when the former was recommended in a journal article. His comments on this situation were as follows (*EMJ*, 1900, p. 66):

> "Use the preparation named if you wish to credit yourselves and do justice to the author of the paper whose method of treatment you propose to follow. ... Specific medicines are a standard in themselves and so are the Homeopathic mother tinctures. So far as we know, no authoritative comparison has been made between them."

Likewise, he believed in maintaining a professional loyalty to those establishments whose long support and development of quality medicinal products enabled the survival of that form of medical practice (*EMJ*, 1903, p. 50):

> "Physicians of the homeopathic school should bear in mind the fact that their school has been made a possibility by the good work given them by their homeopathic pharmacies. Had it not been for this care, in our opinion there would today have been no homeopathic school of medicine. To have depended on the remedies evolved

by their antagonists or rivals would have been suicidal. To attempt to practice —much less build up an aggressive school in medicine—by depending on remedies found in commerce, would have been fatal. Bear these things in view, you ... who feel like deserting the men who put their shoulders to the wheel in behalf of the school whose diploma you hold. ...

"Let credit be given to those to whom it is due. Let the practitioner ... remember that his pharmacies must needs charge fairly for the care and labor necessary to the proper manufacture of their productions. ... It is vitally necessary for the credit and for the very existence of the homeopathic school, that the old standard homeopathic pharmacies be supported loyally by the homeopathic profession, and that the utmost encouragement be given them to make the very best remedies possible."

Long before the time of Samuel Hahneman, the founder of homeopathy, established precedent has been confronted by innovation. Strict conformity to established methods is considered by farsighted pioneers to be a hinderance to progress. This applies to all types of business including medical practice. Attempts at changing the traditional production methods to improve the quality of extracts used to manufacture homeopathic remedies proved controversial, a point that was not lost on Lloyd (*EMJ*, 1898, pp. 525–7):

"In the upward movement of any society there must be differences of opinion, both professional and business rivalry, and occasional heated discussions concerning methods and means to attain the object. ... Too much stress is often given the detail methods of authorities who originate a movement and make it successful as a whole, and yet who are likely to err ... preliminary to improvements that experience and systematic study may afterward make. ... Science in all directions gives evidence of the fact that improvements are necessary to human progress. ... It is evident that unless Dr. Hahnemann was more than human—infallible—... his methods and his products should from time to time be improved upon by men who make homeopathic galenical preparations a life study. ...

"A century of investigation in pharmacy, and of provings and experimentation in therapy by cultivated and observing men, must add much positive knowledge. ... If the suggestion of a friendly critic is in good form, he would say ... do not become acrimonious, and do not let personalities interfere with your good work. Remember that you are all striving for the same end, viz., to improve your medicines, to assist the medical profession, and ultimately to benefit humanity."

A distinct feature of homeopathic dilutions is the fact that they are regulated as over-the-counter medications, and as such they are allowed to carry therapeutic label claims for treating disease. This is in contrast to other nonprescription botanical products that are regulated as dietary supplements and may only carry claims addressing their effects on normal structures and functions.

Spagyric Extracts

The development of more complex extraction procedures than simple soaking (maceration) of herbs in solvents of water and/or alcohol began in the 16th century with the man often referred to as the father of modern medicine. Theophrastus Bombastus von Hohenheim, more commonly known as Paracelsus, attempted to extract the vital elements of the total plant as completely as possible by using several extraction processes. The methods employed were typical of the chemical manipulations involved in the practice of alchemy at that time. These processes are altered from plant to plant and use water, alcohol, and combinations of both in different orders depending on the plant in an attempt to maximize the active components in the extract. The plant material left over after extraction (the marc) then undergoes a 'calcination' process, usually by incineration, to release the minerals bound in the matrix of plant fiber and associated components. The mineral ash is liquefied and added to the other blended fractions. The entire concentration process takes weeks and is sometimes done in conjunction with moon phases.

The high degree of processing renders additional mineral components of the herb soluble in liquid but is limited by incomplete extraction and the disruption of the biochemical relationships found in the living plant. As with any extraction process, the results are incomplete compared to the content and vital complexity of the fresh plant.

Local Use

INFUSED OILS

To prepare infused oils herbs are soaked in fixed oils at warm temperatures for a prolonged period, usually one to two weeks. For more rapid extraction the herbs are briefly heated in vegetable oils. In some cultures animal fats such as lard or tallow that remain semisolid at room temperatures are used.

Concentrated Commercial Extracts

The desire in medicine has long been to maximize the potency of remedies and thereby reduce the necessary dosage. This increases the pharmacological impact on the patient and allows for more convenient administration. Concentration is achieved by removing more and more of the herbal content to reduce it chemically to a simpler form. Concentration progressively reduces the complexity of the chemical profile and broad-ranging activity found in the whole herb. The resulting product may be described best as a phytopharmaceutical drug. However, under current regulations in America, it is legally sold as a dietary supplement. As a result, its content and use, and therefore its identity, is often confused with the whole complex herb from which it was derived or with traditional liquid extracts (teas and tinctures) of the same herb.

Concentration begins by removing water from the fresh plant; it then proceeds by discarding the fibrous content along with a greater or lesser percentage of the active phytochemicals in making a particular liquid extract. Even this complex extract is but a fraction of the content and activity of the whole herb. Then, by reducing the total volume of a liquid extract, or removing the entire liquid portion of an extract solution, concentration proceeds further to produce what are termed a fluid extract (1:1) or solid extract, respectively. At this point a complex extract exists, but numerous chemical conversions have occurred through the processes of drying, extracting and concentrating that often involve heat. Using other solvents on concentrated solid or liquid extracts further reduces the resulting solution to a less complex form that separates particular types of chemicals into fractions that share a similar solubility. An example of a solvent used to remove a particular chemical class of compounds could be ether for extracting fixed oils. This multiple solvent extraction process results in a more simplified extract fraction by taking part of a part of a part. While concentrating one chemical class or compound, it ultimately dilutes or eliminates the other active components.

Ultimately, the process can be taken to its inevitable extreme of isolating a single compound believed to be responsible for, or at least representative of, part of the herb's therapeutic effects. This reductionistic extreme typifies modern conventional medical practice. By producing extract fractions, natural products manufacturers are mimicking the medical module while avoiding product classification as drugs, eliminating the required research on safety and efficacy for these new phytopharmaceuticals. These products are mistakenly marketed under the names of their herbs of origin, when they are actually more similar to conventional medications. Ultimately, each step away from the living botanical source further upsets the natural balance of compounds found in the whole plant by altering the proportions and relationships of its chemical components.

Lloyd noted the problem of creating a concentrated pharmaceutical extract of an active complex botanical (*EMJ*, 1888, pp. 428, 430):

"One of the problems in pharmacy has been the representation of a crude drug as nearly as possible in one liquid, or in a single powder. ... By means of various chemical reagents and manipulations we can produce alkaloids that are characterized by energetic physiological actions, and which predominate the properties of the crude drug, but, as a rule, in doing this we so demoralize the residue as to leave little if anything of the original plant substance, and hence we conclude that only the evolved products are of value, and we pass in silence the unknown."

The ideal of producing a uniformly potent form of a remedial product from plants has led to historical developments and different attempts at pharmaceutical manipulation of plant extracts. Some of these have been more successful for some plants but less so for others.

Specific Medicines began being produced by Lloyd Brothers Pharmacists in the late 19ᵗʰ century. John Uri Lloyd distinguished these from other medicines at that time (*EMJ*, 1876, p. 503):

> "In his practice, Dr. J.M. Scudder insists upon getting medicines that are prepared from prime crude drugs. The "Specific Medicines" he recommends so highly, if prepared as he demands, are in the majority of cases made from fresh herbs, roots, or barks, carefully gathered in their proper season, preserved in alcohol and used in definite quantities, consequently, the "Specific Medicines" are in every sense *definite medicines*. ... Honestly made U.S.P. fluid extracts are *definite*. Honestly made U.S.P. tinctures are *definite*. Homeopathic diluted tinctures are *definite*, but are none of the above J.M. Scudder's "Specific Medicines." "

Specific Medicines were not just simple tinctures made with fresh herbs (*AMM*, 1919, p. 59–60):

> "Rational or specific methods should use simple representatives of plants that had been gathered in their prime and when in their best condition worked by careful methods. ... the Eclectic medicines known as *Specific Medicines* were thus introduced as a line of remedies, each being labeled true to drug name, each depending for its position on legitimate pharmaceutical skill and care, and, as now prepared, all of them have been developed by years of study and the expenditure of much money in scientific experimentation.

> "Unquestionably the high standing they now occupy results from ... the knowledge gained by the study of crude materials, the proper season for collecting drugs, and the conditions best fitted for their manipulation. ... Each drug is worked in accordance with the process that experience has demonstrated is applicable to the abstraction, purification and retention of the medicinal constituents of that particular drug. The aim has been to exclude coloring matters as much as possible and inert extractive substances also from these preparations. ...They differ from class fluids, such as tinctures and fluid extracts, in that they are not prepared by rule of thumb methods as concerns menstruum and process. With them, the word *quality* is preferred to *strength*. The energetic (strength) part of a drug may dominate a preparation to the destruction of *quality*."

Attempts by manufacturers to provide the same type of product (for example, fluid extracts) for all plant remedies have ultimately failed to deliver superior results in many cases. The so-called 'resinoid' concentrates of mid-19ᵗʰ century American pharmacy typify the mistaken enthusiasm for uniform pharmaceutical products of plant medicines. Fluid extracts are a remnant from this phase of attempting uniform product development. Again, it is useful to quote Lloyd (*AMM*, 1919, p. 20):

"An error common to a superficial, as well as to a one-sided or fragmentary, conception of pharmacy, is that of considering *strength* and *quality* as synonymous terms. As we have said, it is a common error, but it is one established by very high authority. The truth is that, although more or less related, the constituent that gives the factor *strength*, is often less important than are the attributes that go to make up *quality*, which, perhaps more than does strength, tends to high excellence. ... *quantity* is but one factor in many directions that involve both chemical and therapeutical action. The *condition* of a substance is a mighty factor as concerns its action as a *thing*, and necessarily in this case, becomes a dominating agent in its therapeutic application. ... The quality of a drug depends not alone on the weight of the materials; its *physical condition* is all-important. ... To ignore natural structures is to neglect an opportunity in pharmacy. That whilst the ultimates broken out of structures are of value in therapy, the structures yielding the ultimates are possessed of qualities that in many directions make them superior to the artificial products."

In his own business Lloyd also manipulated and/or concentrated selective content of the native, or crude, extracts in manufacturing his Specific Medicines as pharmaceutical products. However, it was common knowledge in pharmacy that the use of heat in reducing the solvent content disrupted and destroyed much of the activity he hoped to preserve from the whole complex herb. To address this concern Lloyd experimented with an extraction apparatus that could reduce the exposure of the native extract to destructive heat and thus improve the quality of the concentrate. He was able to develop a device that allowed not only the avoidance of excessive heat in adjusting the concentration of liquid extracts through removal of solvent, but also to readily recover the alcohol or other solvent for re-use. In 1904 he patented his invention, described as Lloyd's "Cold Still." One of the original prototypes is now on display at Washington, D.C.'s Smithsonian Institution. Thus, Lloyd was able to deliver greater quality and potency with his Specific Medicine liquid extracts than could fluid extracts of the same quantitative strength (1:1) made by conventional methods.

While Lloyd points out the foibles of always looking to extract and concentrate the most active components as the best means of producing medicines, he also emphasized the importance of utilizing these types of products when appropriate. For he stated (*EMJ*, 1929, p. 595):

"The Eclectic who would assert that because his material medica has been evolved from crude drugs in which are structural compounds of great value, and, arguing therefrom, should assert that there is no place in therapy for broken-out products, such as have been mentioned, would make a mistake. This mistake he does not make, for he ostracizes nothing, notwithstanding that he selects what he considers the best."

The practice of concentrating or isolating components of a plant whose effects in its whole state are sufficiently potent raises the issue of increasing the adverse effects from excessive exposure to the active principles. The preference in conventional medical practice for the most potent, and potentially toxic, botanical substances have made the need for exact dosing an essential aspect of pharmacy. It is to avoid the potential toxicity that precise quantification is necessary to provide an established average therapeutic dosage of the active compound being administered. This practice is applied even though this average dose is inadequate for some, resulting in a lack of efficacy, and excessive for others, leading to adverse side effects.

The requirement for exact dosing seems to necessitate the use of single isolated compounds as medicines, even though they may manifest greater toxicity in this form. Interactions between complex phytochemical mixtures in powerful drug plants reduce the predictability of individual alkaloids that can be dangerous when given in strong pharmacological doses. Examples of this difficulty were described in 1987 by Izaddoost and Robinson. Their article "Synergism and antagonism is the pharmacology of alkaloidal plants" [*Herbs, Spices, and Medicinal Plants,* 2:137-58], discusses the problems that can arise with potent or poisonous herbs like belladonna (*Atropa belladonna*), ipecac (*Cephaelis ipecacuanha*), cinchona (*Cinchona* spp.), ephedra (*Ephedra sinica*), opium poppy (*Papaver somniferum*), and green hellebore (*Veratrum viride*).

The extraction and isolation of a plant component were sometimes not as cost effective as synthesis, and the natural form was unable to be patented. Due to lact of patent protection, the exorbitant costs of requisite research on safety and efficacy could not be ventured. Manipulating the dosage form of a single isolated active compound eventually led to the development of its chemical modification and synthesis to replace the natural compound. After becoming accustomed to using precise small quantities of toxic medicines, prescribers came to expect exact dosage information as an assurance of safety and efficacy. This assumpmtion of reliability is not without risk, however, due to the inherently variable individual responses to uniform doses.

The Eclectic medical doctors prescribed many powerfrul plants as non-standardized complex extracts. They managed this quandary by prescribing extracts diluted in water to be given in small (subpharmacological), frequent doses. After an adequate pharmacological effect was achieved, they would then adjust the dose and frequency for short-term maintenance. Aside from cardiotonic botanicals, they seldom used toxic plants for long-term therapy. Their approach addressed individual variability in requirements and in responses to the complexity of the botanical extract being utilized.

When is use of a fraction or isolated constituent necessary? The purifying process becomes essential rather than a matter of preference when the whole complex herb, extract, and/or fraction contain an unnecessary and extremely toxic component. The simplest example of this would be the castor oil seed that contains ricin, one of the most potent toxins known. Since the therapeutic use of its laxative activity resides in the oil fraction and ricin is not lipid soluble, it is obviously necessary to use only the oil to avoid inevitable poisoning from the whole seed. The recent research establishing that podophyllotoxin, in spite of its name, is much safer for topical application to venereal warts than podophyllin (the complete resin fraction of Podophyllum with alpha- and beta-peltatin that was originally isolated by the Eclectic doctor John King) indicates the need to choose the isolated compound over the active fraction in this case.

In other cases the content of an effective compound may be so low in a plant that its action cannot be utilized as such without some degree of extraction, concentration, and/or purification. The methyl xanthine alkaloid theophylline from tea leaves comes to mind as a useful component whose natural yield in the whole leaf or water extract is inadequate to produce the desired therapeutic results. Lloyd concurred with selectively extracting beneficial compounds for a particular limited condition when associated components in the plant caused other unwanted effects (*EMJ*, 1876, p. 552–3):

> "We find substances producing beneficial effects as remedies, associated in the same plant with others equally as valuable for medicines, yet existing in such small amounts that their action can not be obtained until the former has been administered in quantities larger than the system can withstand. ... Then let man display his power and apply for his own benefit those substances experience proves of value to himself, thrusting away those which, although indispensable to the plant, are valueless or deleterious to himself; and where substances existing in the plant, exhibit opposite properties when administered as found in the plant, let man apply his science and if possible improve upon nature, so that when a diagnosis demonstrates an organ to be ailing, we will be enabled to apply a remedy that will act directly upon the diseased part, without being compelled to doctor the entire system for another disease."

Fluid Extracts

Lloyd described the evolution of this term as applied to concentrated liquid extracts (*AMM*, 1919, pp. 53 and 55):

> "Percolation was introduced into pharmacy and with this process of extraction came efforts to concentrate liquid representatives of drugs without evaporation, and to these products the terms *concentrated tinctures, saturated tinctures* and *fluid extracts* were severally affixed. These preparations were all made with alcoholic menstruums,. ... With their advent arose the class known as manufacturing

pharmacists. ... Gradually the terms *concentrated tinctures* and *essential tinctures* gave way to the term *fluid extract*, which becoming the official title in the Pharmacopoeia, has now practically displaced the others.

"These, as has been shown are in reality *concentrated* tinctures, and had the Pharmacopoeia selected that term it would have been as appropriate to the class as the term fluid extract. In some directions it would have been preferable. They are made by percolation, and carry all the constituents, good and bad, found in tinctures. ...

"Fluid extracts are with few exceptions made by percolation according to one general formula, the distinction being the menstruum selected. ... The art of percolation, the nature of drugs, the valuation of product, the study of changes, is, each of them, capable of consuming a devoted life. And yet while the fluid extract at the best is imperfect, it is a useful remedy when fresh and conscientiously made, although thoughtful, experienced pharmacists perceive fully the imperfections, to which I will now briefly allude.

"They are prone to precipitate; they are usually thick with inert matters, both colored and colorless. They are of variable strength, owing both to variation in the quality of crude drugs and the care of the manufacturer."

Developed as a mid-19th century innovation to provide both concentrated and consistent strength medicines, fluid extracts are standardized according to the process of manufacture and the one to one ration of dried herb to liquid extract. The need for consistency was joined to the concept of prescribing simplicity, so that each measured drop (minim) of extract was equivalent to one grain (65 mg) of dried herb. Minims and grains were standard units of measure in those days. In a medical practice that at the time found doctors often supplying medicine to their patients, this consistent strength according to equivalent weight made the prescribing process easier by providing a rapid means to accurately calculate doses. Fluid extracts became so popular due to their concentrated, "standardized" strength that they formed the predominant type of botanical extract in the *United States Pharmacopoeia* and *National Formulary* in the early 20th century. It was this class of extracts that was the most harshly criticized by Lloyd for its use of dried herbs and an inadequate standard procedure applied to all different plants that failed to produce as stable extract. His critique of the process and the product reveal much about the issues that determine quality in botanical products.

Percolation is the standard process by which fluid extracts are made. This procedure involves carefully packing moistened, ground herb in a funnel, covering the upper surface with filter paper, and then soaking this (maceration), usually for a day, in the appropriate water and alcohol solvent mixture. This same solvent is allowed to percolate slowly and steadily through the funnel column and is collected underneath, as more solvent is added to the upper surface at the same rate. The first volume that was macerated is set aside, while collection of the percolate continues until the medicinal content of herb is exhausted. The volume of the final percolate is then reduced by evaporation through heating. It is thereby concentrated to the point that, when it is added to the first macerated percolate collected, the final fluid volume of the total extract in milliliters represents the original dry weight of the herb in grams, as a one ml to one gm (1:1) strength. Advantages to this process over tincturing by maceration are a more complete extraction of active components from the herb, a relatively concentrated product allowing smaller doses, and an easily calculated dose based on the original weight of the dried herb.

Lloyd described the essential features that make the percolation process effective (*EMJ*, 1880, pp. 259–61):

"To arrive at a proper understanding of the laws which govern the solution of substances—that is, the transfer of a solid into a liquid state through the aid of solvents—we should consider first the greatest agent in percolation—the attraction of gravitation. ... Gravity ... is ever tending to draw the liquid most heavily charged with soluble matters, downward through lighter, and thus there seems to be no rest, but, on the contrary, continued change. ...

"Let us turn our attention to *solution*. ... We must accept the fact that below the melting temperature certain solids will, to a fixed extent, assume the form of liquids, if in contact with particular fluids. The conditions necessary to effect and promote this change are: surface exposed to the dissolving medium, circulation of the liquid, temperature, and time of contact between the surfaces of the solid and the liquid. In regard to the first of these conditions, it is invariably found that the rapidity of solution increases with the area of surface exposed. ... The desired increase of surface is most readily effected by pulverizing the solid, thus obtaining irregular surfaces.

"In considering the rest of the conditions upon which solution depends we next observe the action of *currents*. ... In observing closely the process we notice streams of liquid circulating ... in response to the law that fluids of different densities seek their own level. ... Thus continuous currents flow over and down ... and fresher menstruum is constantly taking the place of that more saturated. ... A surface of liquid revolving against a solid ... wears away the solid and decreases the wearing force of the liquid. ... The circulation of the medium becomes gradually less and less distinct, and finally ... disappears. ... The increased amount of surface contact before considered hastens the operation. Thus we find that nature's laws constantly produce circulation while solution is progressing.

"Temperature is most important. With a few exceptions substances dissolve to a greater extent in warm than in cold liquids. ... Heat also decreases the cohesive attraction of solids, their molecules being more easily detached from the mass, and therefore more readily unite with those of the liquid. ... Time is a consideration of importance. An appreciable amount of contact must be allowed between solvent and solid. That solutions require time for action is a principle well recognized and scarcely necessary to mention."

Though more complete extraction takes place by percolation, it remains largely dependent on the relative solubility of herb constituents in this concentration. Disadvantages of this method include loss of volatiles in the concentration process and breakdown of glycosides and labile compounds. However, one of the greatest disadvantages and concerns of Lloyd had to do with loss of components, and therefore activity, due to precipitates that form in the percolate. This occurs largely from the sequential extraction of components of varying solubility that occurs during percolation which is related to the varying solvent potential of the menstruum as it passes through the column. This critical issue led to Lloyd's observations and paper that resulted in his being awarded his first Ebert Prize for innovation in pharmacy in 1882. He begins by alluding to causes of precipitation applicable to all liquid extracts but proceeds on effects that are peculiar to the process of percolation (*EMJ*, 1881, pp. 441–52):

"I considered the principle of percolation ... as though the various menstrua entered the powders intact, and in their passage through the powders dissolved certain materials. ... In continuing the subject, I must bring forward another phase of the act of percolation. This influences the percolate materially, ... a vital point when we connect percolation with the class of preparations known as fluid extracts. In as much as percolation is mainly applied by pharmacists to the making of fluid extracts I shall refer to this class of preparations hereafter. ...

"We find the following from the pen of the late Prof. Wm. Proctor. "The question to be resolved is, can we make fluid extracts that contain all the valuable ingredients of the drugs, that are capable at the same time of resisting the mutual reaction of their proximate principles, and such external agencies of deterioration as heat, light and oxygen, and thus be entitled to the character of permanent preparations." ... Who will argue that however carefully a fluid extract be made by percolation it is a "permanent" preparation? ... The original idea of percolation with two or even three menstruums for one powder and subsequent evaporation and mixing of the percolates is improved upon by the use of, as a rule, *one* menstruum, and little if any evaporation. ...

"Still prone to change upon standing, one of the results is the production of precipitates, and to a very great extent these precipitates result from the reaction between menstruum and powder during the act of percolation. ... Pharmacists feel annoyed and discouraged when they find their bottles partly filled with sediment;

and this trouble (sediments) is the rule and not the exception. ... I shall refer briefly to the theories that have to my knowledge been offered in explanation of their formation. ...

"*Oxidation.*—Certain organic bodies are prone to unite with oxygen and form new compounds, often of an insoluble nature. ... I can not in a large number of experiments find that the precipitation of percolates proceeds any faster in an atmosphere of oxygen or of ordinary air than it does in an atmosphere of hydrogen gas or carbon dioxide. ...

"*Change of Solvent Power of Menstruum by Evaporation.* —If a menstruum be altered in composition by the evaporation of some ingredient which is more volatile that another, a change follows in the solvent power of the menstruum which remains. This may necessitate the subsequent precipitation of organic matter to a greater of less extent, in consequence of its insolubility in the new menstruum, although it was perfectly soluble in the original. ... The subject has been clearly expressed in an article written by Mr. Henry Thayer ... as follows: "These precipitates ... are medicinal principles deposited because the menstruum loses its power of solution in consequence of the evaporation of alcohol."

"*Change of Temperature.* —During low temperatures precipitation results from inability of the cold liquid to hold in solution matter which was perfectly soluble while warm. This fact must be familiar to all pharmacists. ... It is not uncommon to find, with certain preparations, the sides of large fluid extract containers studded with masses of crystals during very cold weather.

"*Chemical change* outside of oxidation undoubtedly often results. ... Sometimes these changes take place gradually until the entire soluble solid material seems to have changed into insoluble; then again the alteration is of such a nature as to lead to the belief that there is no change, until suddenly the entire contents of the bottle solidify. As examples I can name the gelatinous magmas which form more or less frequently in such preparations as fluid extracts of Galium aparine and Chionanthus virginica, and the brown magmas of the fluid extract of that class of astringent plants which, like Geranium maculatum, Stillingia sylvatica, etc., contain an abundance of red tannates. ... These precipitates or magmas, as a rule, refuse to dissolve in a menstruum of the alcoholic strength employed to make the original extract, or in any mixture of alcohol and water.

"*Light.* —The action of light is said to alter certain bodies in solution. ... It is certain, however, that light will affect vegetable powders, and it may affect fluid extracts so as to produce precipitation.

"I have now finished the brief review of the accepted causes for precipitation in percolates. ... The result of my observations and study of precipitates has convinced me that the larger part of the permanent sediments which form in most of our fluid extracts arises from a cause heretofore unconsidered. They are neither the result of decrease of temperature, of oxidation, nor of chemical change. ...

"Heretofore, as far as I can learn, we have accepted the idea that a percolate from a powdered plant is a solution of substances in one solvent, if the act of percolation has been conducted with one menstruum. ... It is also often accepted that the dissolved material of various portions of a percolate is the same, excepting in amount. These conclusions are doubtless erroneous. If we use dilute alcohol (or any other mixture of alcohol and water) throughout the entire process, the menstruum which holds the solid matters in solution is not simply dilute alcohol; and the dissolved matters of a percolate differ in composition and in general properties at various stages of the operation of percolation. ...

"As an example of this fact I will cite Experiment No. 5, which shows the percolate of a fifty pound experiment with Cannabis indica. It will be noticed that the first part of the percolate has a reddish brown color, while the latter part is deep green. The menstruum used was strong alcohol. ... It is not unusual to find a sudden change in the properties of a percolate, and it will be found that after this change the two portions of percolate will precipitate if mixed together. Arguing from such a stand, the term we use regarding the percolate is hardly proper, even though the same be collected in one vessel, for it is a number of different solutions instead of a single solution. The term percolate does not convey the idea of plurality. ...

"As a first consideration, I shall call attention to the fact that commercial powdered plants contain more or less water. ... Some plants are very hygroscopic, and will absorb and hold from five to fifteen pounds of water to the hundred. ... When these commercial powders are submitted to percolation, the first part of the percolate carries the water, and consequently differs from the latter portion in actual alcoholic composition, even though one menstruum is used throughout. As a result, the first portions often contain, of gums and bodies more soluble in water than in alcohol, larger amounts than the last portions can dissolve; and the last portions may contain a larger proportion of resins, oils, and other bodies less soluble in dilute alcoholic menstruum. Thus we find ... the dissolved materials in the first part of the percolate ... may be so great as to be partially insoluble in the entire mixed percolate. ...

"As a consequence, after the full percolate is mixed a gradual separation of each of these classes of substances follows. Naturally, therefore, such an entire percolate is not a single body (as it is obtained), but a mixture of percolates, each of different alcoholic strength. ... In practice the first part of a percolate and the last part, if kept separate, will each for a time hold its dissolved matters more perfectly than if the entire percolate be mixed. ... The foregoing very natural cause for certain sediments in our fluid extracts should be sufficient to induce careful pharmacists to prepare fluid extracts from dry powders where dried plants are used, and while our

Pharmacopoeia is silent upon the subject, we all know that the intent is to recognize perfectly dry powders.

"Let us cast aside now the foregoing cause of precipitates, for together with those I have previously named we may do so and have a class of precipitates that remain to be accounted for. ... I shall now introduce the explanation, in my opinion, for the larger part of ordinary precipitates. Especially do I include such as commence to form as soon or even before the operation of percolation is suspended, and continue to deposit for weeks, months, or even years.

"First, let me call attention to what has been conclusively proven to my mind, viz., the *solvent power of the menstruum actually varies at different stages of the operation of percolation exclusive of variation which could be attributed to the presence of more or less water*. ... That such a menstruum can differ in solvent action is not generally recognized, if at all.

"Dried plants contain several widely differing and closely connected principles. Thus we have gums, and extractive matters related to gums, and which are very soluble in water, and almost insoluble in alcohol, and are variably soluble in different mixtures of alcohol and water. Upon the other hand even the same plant may contain fixed and volatile oils, resins, oleo-resins and resinoid bodies, which are soluble in alcohol and insoluble in water. These bodies, together with other substances which are variably soluble in alcohol and in water such as glucosides, tannates, glucose, sugar, chlorophyll, alkaloids and their salts, and the salts of minerals, furnish us a medley of different materials. Every plant contains more or less of these substances, and when percolation is carefully performed there is scarcely the part of any carefully made percolate which is not saturated with some organic body or mixture, and the slightest alteration of solvent power of menstruum after percolation tends to throw down this body in part or wholly as a precipitate. ...

"From the moment our menstruum enters the powder, it commences to dissolve matters that are soluble in that menstruum. This forms at once a *new menstruum*, and which has the power to dissolve substances that are only partially soluble in the original menstruum. As this liquid percolates through the powder, it takes up more and more of the matters which are very soluble in it and becomes an increased (or occasionally decreased) solvent for substances which the original menstruum could scarcely dissolve. These various bodies in solution alter the solvent power of the menstruum to such a degree as to enable it to dissolve substances which may be perfectly insoluble in the original menstruum. In this manner resins and oils may be dissolved to a more or less extent in a water menstruum, although the purified resin or oil may be practically insoluble in water. ... Thus it is that during the operation of percolation a constantly changing menstruum is passing through the powder even though the original menstruum be unchanged. The percolate in accordance is variable in composition and in solvent powers even if it be spoken of as though it be one menstruum. ...

"*Why the Percolate Precipitates.* —.... By agitation we mix these solutions and a new menstruum results. An equilibrium is established as far as the proportion of liquid and solid matter is concerned, but *not* an equilibrium as regards the solvent action of the new liquid. ... It may be that some of these substances are at once precipitated, or that more or less time is required before they separate. ...

"*Why the Precipitate Continues to Form.* —... It may be asked why an equilibrium is not established in a short time, and the precipitation cease. ... Even with some solutions of definite chemicals, a precipitate, as is well known, refuses to form until the vessel is permitted to stand a certain length of time. ... They may continue to separate during a greater or less period of time and from these bodies alone a series of preciptitates result. Now we come to another point. Let us continually bear in mind the fact that all of the substances which are held in solution are a part of the solution, and any precipitation of dissolved matter alters the solution and the solvent power of the liquid. Thus as these bodies separate, the menstruum actually changes, and as it changes in composition, substances which were readily dissolved by the original liquid become insoluble. ... Thus apparently by a series of steps the percolate changes in composition and in solvent powers, each change being followed by the precipitation of certain substances. In reality the process is almost continuous and often without a line of demarcation. ... In consequence of the foregoing we find that a percolate may be filtered or decanted from time to time, and in each case a sediment will be obtained.

"*Experiment No. 1*, April 19, 1881.—Eighty pounds of Hydrastis canadensis were percolated with a mixture of three parts of alcohol and two parts of water. Of this first percolate and of the fiftieth pint of percolate six fluid ounces were reserved. Two fluid ounces of each were mixed, the remaining four fluid ounces of each being kept separate.

"*Remarks.*—After twenty-four hours the first and second percolates were clear. The mixture had deposited a *brownish* yellow sediment. After four days the second percolate was clear. The first percolate had thrown down a slight *yellow* sediment. The mixture had increased its precipitate. After eight days a *greenish* precipitate appeared in the second percolate; after two weeks the *heaviest* precipitate was in the first percolate. The precipitates at this date, July 7, range as follows: 1st percolate heaviest, color deep yellow; 2nd percolate lightest, color greenish; mixture between, color greenish yellow.

"*Experiment No. 4*, May 9, 1881.—Eighty pounds of Valerian were percolated with a mixture of alcohol four parts, water one part. The percolate was reserved as in experiment No. 1. In twenty-four hours a slight precipitate appeared in mixture. In five days there was a precipitate observed in first percolate. July 7, we find a slight precipitate in the second percolate. The precipitates of the first percolate and in the mixture are about equal in amount.

"*Experiment No. 11*, May 21, 1881—Eighty pounds of Taraxacum were percolated with a mixture of alcohol three parts, water two parts. The percolate was reserved, as in experiment No. 1. In twenty-four hours there was a yellowish-white precipitate in the mixture and the first percolate. July 7 there was a precipitate in the first percolate of one-fourth of an inch in depth, composed of a light-colored lower stratum and an orange colored upper stratum. The mixture contains a thin precipitate, divided like that of the first percolate into a light colored lower stratum and an orange colored upper stratum. The second percolate contains a crystalline aggregation over the bottom of the bottle, and this is perfectly white.

"In commenting upon the afore-mentioned experiments I will say that the powders were thoroughly dried. The result supports my theoretical explanation of the formation of a line of precipitates by simply mixing a percolate, and without calling upon chemical action, oxidation, etc. I can say that many other experiments instituted in like manner gave similar results. ... I must say that it does not seem probable that we shall ever, by percolation alone, succeed in making a line of permanent fluid extracts from dry plants."

Continuing his discussion of the problem of precipitates in fluid extracts as products of percolation, Lloyd noted that due to layering, or strata, of the liquid percolate the process of precipitation was never-ending. This results in a continuously changing soluble content (*EMJ*, 1882, pp. 441–2, 445–9):

"After a certain time under such conditions, a pure menstruum would remain, and all of the dissolved matter would have settled to the bottom of the vessel. Now we know that this point is never reached. Fluid extracts and tinctures ... never reach a point where all of the dissolved matters become insoluble. Upon the other hand, under ordinary conditions changes usually follow ... and the result of these changes is a continuous precipitation. ... Continuous precipitation may be taking place without depleting the liquid of dissolved matters. ...

"If a tincture or a fluid extract be made by percolation, ... there will be a decrease in gravity from the bottom of the container upward. This is in consequence of the well known fact that the denser part of the percolate passes first, and that the percolate grows less dense with more or less regularity as percolation progresses. When such a percolate is permitted to stand, it will resolve itself into strata. ... The collection of strata of precipitates at one or more points throughout such liquids, indicates where the lines of division are to be found. ...

"After a precipitate has formed in a tincture or a fluid extract it is generally accepted as permanent. All will admit that precipitates often continue to deposit for months and even years. ... It has never been stated, that I can find, in connection with this point, that at intervals the precipitate to a greater or less extent will dissolve, yet such is the case. Were it otherwise, a point would be reached when all of the dissolved matter would be thrown from solution, and consequently no further deposition could occur.

"A change in solvent power of the solution must take place before further precipitation can follow, and a change in temperature will be followed by either decreased or increased solvent power, and consequently by more or less precipitation, or re-solution of the precipitate. ... This precipitate during the low temperature settles to the bottom of the bottle, and upon an increase of temperature re-dissolves, giving us a dense layer of solution upon the bottom of the bottle ... until the composition of liquid within the container is again uniform, and the strata have disappeared. Such a state of the affairs can only be reached under an unchanged temperature, and we know that under ordinary circumstances an even temperature for any length of time is impracticable. As a consequence we may expect to have more or less of strata in our containers, and repeated precipitation and resolution. ...

"I shall now introduce the notes of an experiment which illustrates the formation of a precipitate by the gradual admixture of different portion of a transparent percolate, and which will show us the workings of the strata currents under ordinary conditions. May 5, 1881. Eight troy ounces of powdered capsicum were properly moistened with dilute alcohol and packed in a cylindrical percolator. The receiving vessel was an ordinary two gallon salt mouth bottle. Into the mouth of this the percolator was inserted, and to the exit of the percolator a rubber tube was attached. This tube extended to the bottom of the bottle, and the lower end of it was fixed to a cork, so that as percolation progressed, the floating cork would hold the exit of the tube at the surface of the liquid. By this arrangement the percolate was collected in the order obtained and without mixing, the lightest liquid being on top.

"*Description of Percolate.* —The percolate passed transparent from the beginning until the end of the act of percolation. The lower portion of the liquid was dark red in thin section, black as viewed in bulk. From the upper part of this dark layer, the color became gradually less and less in shade, until it passed to a light straw color. This point was reached at a height of four inches above the dark layer; the remainder of the container (6 inches) was of a uniform light straw color. ... This percolate consisted then of three parts, ... the proportion being as 3, 4 and 6. ... The entire percolate had two points of distinct division, one where the color rapidly decreased from dark red to light red, and the other where the change was rapid from light red to yellow.

"*Changes.* — ... In two hours from the time of the cessation of percolation a muddy layer of liquid appeared between the dark red (lower) and light red (overlying) solutions. In four hours the entire light red percolate was muddy, in six hours it had resolved itself into three sections, each with distinct lines of demarcation. After twenty-four hours particles of yellow precipitate appeared abundantly in the upper of these sections and gradually settled to the surface of the second section. ... Finally it collected in large particles and fell through the second dividing plane. As the precipitate passed through this second section it decreased and finally entered the heavy dark lower liquid *where it entirely dissolved*. After seven days the three central strata had resolved into two sections and had become transparent, throughout which were clots of precipitates. The upper portion of the liquid in the bottle was very muddy and gave rise to a constant rain of precipitates that gradually settled through the lower strata dissolving as the passed, until only a very small amount reached the bottom of the bottle. These appearances were maintained for ninety days at which time the liquid in the bottle had become transparent, and of one color and composition; the strata and lines of demarcation had disappeared, a uniform yellow precipitate covered the bottom of the bottle, and a layer of oil globules overspread the surface of the liquid. ...

"*Cause of Precipitation.* —... The precipitate under present consideration followed from the usual cause, a mixing of percolates. The concentrated solution at the bottom of the bottle was gradually transferred to the dilute solution above, and *vice versa*. This caused a precipitation of substance insoluble in the new solvents, and as the greatest change or strain results from the rapid dilution of the heavy solution, precipitation was most rapid at intermediate parts, or the upper portion of the liquid.

"*Resolution of the Precipitate.* —It will be noticed that after the precipitate was formed in the upper part of the liquid, it disappeared as it progressed towards the bottom of the bottle. This resolution resulted from the fact that the lower strata were solvents for bodies that the upper could not hold in solution. ... It must be remembered that the lower solution gradually became more dilute, and that finally its solvent action was so decreased as to permit more or less of the precipitate to reach the bottom of the container.

"The points I desire to present ... may be summed up as follows: —We cannot hope to produce by percolation a line of permanent fluid extracts or tinctures, for most percolates will precipitate more or less owing to aforementioned causes, even without a change in temperature. ... However, an unchangeable temperature is not practicle under ordinary circumstances. ... Thus we find that from natural causes precipitation in fluid extracts made by percolation may continue indefinitely. ... It follows also that even though we may prepare a fluid extract with great care and shake the same until it is a uniform mixture, after a period it may be very different at the top and bottom of a container."

The dark color of most fluid extracts is another issue indicating inferior quality due to caramelizing of sugars from heating the extract that darkens the final product. Lloyd found this objectionable, as he frequently commented on the impurities encountered in this type of medicine (*EMJ*, 1880, p. 159):

"It is not, in my opinion, necessary for all liquid preparations of plants to be black as we must admit so many of our fluid extracts are when made exactly according to the pharmacopoeia. I am convinced that in a large number of cases these dark colors depend upon impurities, and are objectionable. Our pharmacopoeias do not recognize colorless fluid extracts, therefore, if we, by any means, decolorize the fluid extracts, it will be a misnomer to call them by the name fluid extracts. ... And now I advance again the idea that this trouble regarding the dirt in fluid extract may be overcome by using drugs that *do not contain dirt.*

"If yourself or any other reader of this article will take the trouble to examine the fresh roots of such plants as grow convenient, it will be found that almost invariably they are nearly white internally (a few exceptions, hydrastis, sanguinaria, etc.). They do not contain black extractive matters and therefore will not produce black pharmaceutical preparations. Dry these same roots and they turn dark brown and yield dark colored or black liquids. This black coloring matter results, I am led to believe, in the majority of cases, from decomposition of natural constituents of the root and formation of new (worthless) substances.

"This rule to an extent applies to barks, few *inner barks* being dark brown when fresh. ... Herbs also form black extractive matter when dried, and thus yield fluid extracts that are black when the fresh leaf is green, and produces when fresh a green tincture. ... A few years ago the cry was "give us black fluid extracts, they are strong." Now physicians realize that color and value are usually independent. That even distilled water may be blackened by the additon of a little burnt sugar. That the easiest extract to make is the black extract. I shall do all in my power, wherever I am placed, to advance the science of pharmacy, whether among druggists or physicians."

Lloyd was hopeful in finding that the production of fluid extracts improved in some respects over the years (*EMJ*, 1881, pp.15–6):

"We find as a rule the gums of our plants are inert and burdensome to a liquid preparation, and that by a tendency to change they make deposits within the bottle. They make an extract thick, but only in a few cases are they desirable as therapeutic agents. ...We find that in the majority of cases the sediments in fluid extracts are worthless, and where they are not worthless they result from an endeavor of the maker to hold inert gums and extractive matters in solution. ... The very fact of a deposit of dirt two or three inches in depth seemed then to be a credit, for such an extract could not hold the principles in solution. ...

"Pharmacists have been working since that; *they* also must move. One by one changes have taken place. One by one the old and erroneous ideas regarding pharmaceuticals have passed away. Now we seldom find a physician that prefers a liquid representative of a plant on account of the *dirt* it contains."

Overall, Lloyd was dismayed that the pharmaceutical development of fluid extracts in general had proven inadequate in comparison to traditional preparations of herbs (*EMJ*, 1889, p. 373–5):

"I view fluid extracts as one of the stepping stones to a more perfect pharmacy. ... They have ... given us portable preparations, but have in many instances crowded our shelves with preparations very much inferior to the decoctions and infusions, or even the crude drugs, that have been displaced."

Lloyd believed that a botanical extract designed for specific therapeutic application should have removed from it not only those compounds that he considered unnecessary but also those thought to interfere with the particular desired effect. His reduction of the extract content was based on intentionally obtaining a specific activity that excluded other influences (*EMP*, 1904, p. 474):

"The pharmacist may, yes, *must*, consider such bodies as these in the building of his pharmaceutical structures. Too often the presence of certain plant disturbing agents that possess to the chemist no interest whatever demoralizes a plant preparation. Again, on the excluding of certain passive substances that are not mentioned in any work whatever, that are unknown alike to microscopist, chemist or biologist, depends the art of making certain pharmaceutically perfect preparations."

Lloyd advocated for pharmaceutically elegant extracts that improve upon standard procedures applied to make fluid extracts that contain many unattractive residues, or "dirt." He makes a case for eliminating coloring matter and what he considered inert components present in many official pharmacopeial extracts (*EMJ*, 1922, pp. 265–8):

"Dirt has been neatly defined as "Matter out of place." ... The integuments of plants bear burdens that have no place in the pharmacy of medicines, and although present in official fluid extracts, should be properly classed as "dirt.' ... Destructive chemico-pharmacy, that establishes values by destroying natural plant compounds and by picking out a few isolated products attempts to standardize drug values thereby, and claims that these substances dominate the therapeutical energies of the plant, must yet surely demand a cleaner, higher pharmacy than now prevails. ... Believers in active plant constituents should abhor plant dirt in their pharmaceutical preparations; for if their views are correct, the coloring matter in plant liquids and extracts is but "dirt." Take now the official pharmaceutical preparations ... and we find them black, green, or brown, by reason of the presence of much useless coloring matter (matter out of place). ...

"Many colorless plant constituents, useful in the economy of the living plant, must also be classed by us with plant dirt. ... The writer believes that the larger part of officinal plant dirt is not a mysterious unknown, but a reachable reality. It is composed mainly of gum, chorophyll, wax, sugar, glucose, neutral fats, inactive resins and oils, coloring matter and other substances that, colored or colorless, ... seemingly bear no direct connection with the natural, medicinal plant constituents. They have, as a rule, no recognized value in therapy. ... They are but burdens to our official galenical liquids, and unless eliminated, tend to discredit our art."

Lloyd believed that official medicinal preparations of plants should meet strict qualifications for purity that separate them from conventional means used in times past (*EMJ*, 1924, pp. 51–4):

"In the chemical section of that excellent work, the Pharmacopeia of the United States, we find the utmost pains taken to guard against the presence of dirt (foreign substance). Explicit care is taken to give test for impurities in chemical compounds. ... How different the section of that publication devoted to galenical pharmacy. ...

"The chief change in the process of "regular" galenical plant pharmacy, from decade to decade since 1850, has been simply the changing of the alcoholic proportions of the menstrua employed. Here and there glycerin has been added. ... The officinal preparations of plants, such as fluid extracts and tinctures, on which regular medicine depends, may, by means of neutral solvents and excluders, nearly all of them, be made as mobile as alcohol, and in many cases scarcely colored than whiskey, often nearly colorless. They are now, as a rule, nearly black, while there is little, if anything, in most plants in their fresh condition, to produce colored compounds. ... The result is that fluid extracts are unstable and unsightly; they are prone to precipitate and disintegrate, and are far from creditable remedies. ... Regular physicians dominate the Pharmacopeia. They should encourage investigation in pharmacy outside the routine processes laid down in former times. ...

"Unless there be a revival, the practice of plant pharmacy will fall exclusively into the hands of trade manufacturers and chemists (it is fast drifting there now). ... Do not break up by heroic chemistry the natural compounds in which active agents exist in the plants. Take the opposite course, apply pharmacal skill, but retain these active principles intact, as formulated by nature.

"If the bulky plant dirt is thrown out of the preparations of officinal galenical pharmacy, such remedies will replace fluid extracts, and yet be as active as fluid extracts are now. Their therapeutical constituents will remain intact, associated as nature has combined them, and ... they will not produce unsightly liquids. Fluid extracts ... will not precipitate, but will remain transparent, carrying their physiological energies more unchanged than is the case with the present incongruous liquids.

"Some persons will reject this view of the problem as merely a Utopian dream. ... It is well known to our members that so-called active principles are not representatives of plants; it is also known that dirty pharmaceutical preparations may be improved if the plant dirt is excluded; and lastly, that the drug energy of the remedy will remain unimpaired, a discriminatively prepared liquid representative carrying the therapeutical force of the drug."

Solid Extracts

The development of solid extracts was simply a matter of trying to concentrate the liquid extracts of plants to make them more potent, as a means of reducing the dosage to make administration easier. Unfortunately, this approach of representing the activity of the whole herb in concentrated form often backfired in its clinical outcome (AMM, 1919, p. 52–3 and 56–7):

"For more concentrated preparations ... the evaporation of tinctures, decoctions and infusions resulted. The residues were usually reduced to the consistence of a stiff magma capable of being rolled into pills with or without the addition of an excipient, and to these substances the term *extract* was applied. ... When these extracts were fully dried and powdered, they produced the class known as *powdered solid extracts*. But it became apparent to thoughtful persons that extracts often did not, as might naturally be supposed, represent the tincture employed, and then it was discovered that the heat applied and accompanying atmospheric influence affected the remedial part of the remedy deleteriously, indeed even in some cases to its utter destruction.

"When a fluid extract is evaporated until the residue reaches a masslike consistence, a prime solid extract results. ... Solid extracts, therefore, do not contain any therapeutic qualities in addition to those possessed by the tincture. ... For some purposes, however, as in making pills, ... where liquids cannot be employed, these preparations answer a good purpose, although the physician should administer liquid plant remedies if he desires to obtain the full effect of the drug. ... At the best, commercial solid extracts are less reliable than either tinctures or fluid extracts, although when care and skill are employed in their preparation active drugs may yield very energetic remedies. ... Much harm to pharmacy and to medicine has been done, in my opinion, by thoughtlessly believing that the drug values of tinctures and fluid preparations of many drugs can be carried into a dry condition."

Manufacture of solid extract concentrates begins with dried herbs processed into liquid extracts, usually described as crude extracts. From these partial extracts the solvents are then evaporated. If dried completely, like the whole herb these solid extracts can be reduced to a granulated powder and encased in a gelatin capsule. They can also be made into tablets that are typically mixed with binders, fillers, etc., before being pressed into tablet form. Some solid extracts form an amorphous mass, and these can also be coated with sugar or gelatin (*AMM*, 1919, p. 64):

> "*Sugar Coated Pills* ... are excellent forms in which to administer many organic drugs, and also solid extracts, resins, etc. ... Sugar coated pills are made by the simple process of first cutting out the pill mass, rolling it and then coating the pills with a sugar in a candy machine. ... The risk that users of sugar coated pills have to guard against is the effect of the heat that is applied to the pill if it be reduced to perfect dryness after being cut and before it is coated.

> "*Gelatine Coated Pills*—These, in my opinion, are superior to any and all forms of candy or similar medicines. They have the advantage of being easily made our of very moist pill masses, and of being easily coated when still soft and moist, a feat that is impossible to accomplish with some drugs in the heated sugar coating machine. The gelatine excludes the air, preserves the contents of the pill, and is tasteless and harmless.

> "*Tablets* are cheap machine stamped out discs, and became popular very rapidly because of their neat appearance and convenient form. ... Many tablets are fine remedies; others are unworthy of confidence. The fact is though, ... makers of tablets have been very injudicious, and have injured their interest in selecting tablet compounds that on their face are shown to be at once destroyed or much injured in the drying process. ... It therefore behooves physicians to closely scrutinize the natures of the substances that appear under the tablet label. In my opinion certain physicians have been very thoughtless when they have displaced gelatine coated pills by means of tablets. ... No tablet can be made to represent evanescent plant preparations or those in which alcohol is necessary as a preservative."

The strength of these extracts is often described as a ratio of original dry weight of the herb to final solid extract weight, as five grams of crude dried herb reduced to one gram of solid extract would be a 5:1 extract. However, it must be understood the solid extract does not provide the total activity available in the original complex whole herb, but only an extracted portion, the fraction of components depending on the solvent(s) used. So 1 gm of a 5:1 solid extract may only contain as much activity as 3 or 4 gms of the original herb, not all of the major and minor active components from the 5 gms extracted. The more concentrated the extract, the less of the total original activity it usually contains.

One method of preserving fresh juices or water extracts is to freeze the extract before dehydrating them in a vacuum to a solid form. This method of freeze-drying the liquid effectively preserves the components in the original juice or extract. The freeze-dried extract produces a solid powdered form that can be most readily rehydrated in water or other liquids or taken in capsular form. Once the original juice or complex extract is made, the only component removed to form these concentrates is the water.

Solid complex extracts can be assayed to identify the relative content of a particular marker substance to which it can be quantitatively standardized. This process allows for adjustment of extract content in a capsule or tablet to be altered according to the relative concentration of the marker substance by adding more or less filler per batch to the final product dispensed. Thus, the supposed "strength" of the extract is then described as a function of the standardized marker content, that is, so many mg of a particular compound per unit (tablet or capsule).

In standardized solid extracts, the strength may not be described in terms of concentration strength, that is, the ratio of dried herb to solid extract by weight. If it is, the proportion is then usually a range of weight of the original dry herb to the final solid extract, for example, 8–12 : 1. This usually indicates the actual strength based on the ratio of marker in the extract is on average 10:1, but this still does not mean that the extract has ten times the potency as the dried herb. Due to loss of other active components in the process of extraction and concentration, the relative strength of the solid extract to the herb in this example may be on average 6:1. Therefore, relative potency estimated by either extract concentration or marker concentration is unreliable, unless the marker is the major active component. Since the marker is selectively concentrated, if it is not the main active constituent, the extract may have much less strength than indicated by the concentration of marker content.

There are two main differences between a liquid and solid extracts from the same herb. When a complex solid extract is made from a native liquid extract, the solvent is removed through the application of heat. Outside of freeze-drying either juices or native water extracts, this process is typically destructive of some bioactive components. A major difference between many solid extracts and traditional liquid forms involves the solvents used. While liquid extracts must be made with solvents that can be safely ingested in normal quantities (water, vinegar, alcohol, glycerin, and/or vegetable oil), industrial chemical solvents (for example, hexane, acetone, methanol, and isopropyl alcohol) are frequently used in making solid extracts. Since these are inherently toxic, such extracts have never been consumed in their liquid form. Even after the solvent is removed, residual traces inevitably remain. A notable exception is supercritical carbon dioxide, a liquid form of the common innocuous gas utilized under high pressure and sometimes with high temperatures. For all of these solvents there is no precedent for their use, since traditional liquid extracts used ingestible solvents that remove a different complex of components from the whole herb. Therefore, solid extracts made with non-ingestible solvents can only be considered effective for those conditions that have been shown through modern studies to be successfully treated with these specific extracts.

Local Use

PLASTERS

These are prepared by spreading a stiff paste of extracts mixed in a base thinly on or between supportive material such as cloth or paper, sometimes moistened, and applied locally. A few counterirritant commercial plasters made from capsicum and mustard are still available in some pharmacies. Formerly, lead oxide was used as a base, but this has long been abandoned. According to Lloyd (*AMM*, 1919, p. 61):

> "These preparations are so stiff, that at the temperature of the body they are elastic and adhesive, but not soft. Hence when heated and spread on sheepskin or on muslin, and then applied to the skin, they adhere, maintaining their position. By this means remedies incorporated into the plaster may be held firmly in contact with the skin."

Commercial Fractions

Extract Subfractions

The desire to provide concentrated extracts that can be easily administered in small doses without having to taste the intense flavor of some herbal compounds provided the incentive to developing pharmaceutical alternatives to liquid extracts. In the 19th century this led to the earliest attempts at isolating alkaloids in chemistry and producing semi-solid concentrates in pharmacy. An early version of concentrates that were partial fractions of the more complex liquid extracts were developed and popularized by Eclectic doctors, beginning with Dr. John King. These fractions were designated as 'resinoids' because they were developed by adding saturated alcoholic botanical extracts to cold water and collecting the water-insoluble precipitating mass that formed. However, the failure of these products to achieve consistent therapeutic effects compared to the complex crude extracts from which they were derived rapidly led to their being discredited as unreliable products.

Through the process of concentrating fractions of the complex extracts, many important compounds and co-factors that enhanced the effects of the original extracts were lost. The reputation of Eclectic medicine in the mid-19th century suffered from this attempt to equate quality with concentration by reducing the complexity of extracts (*AMM*, 1919, pp. 58–9):

> "It was impossible to carry the full, or even the partial, therapeutic values of most plants into a dry condition. ... The "resinoids" became typical of the results of deplorable pharmaceutical processes. They were products that had no rational home. Neither alkaloids, extracts, nor ultimates, they found themselves discredited pharmaceutical incongruities."

Concentrating active fractions in an attempt to represent the whole complex herb was intended primarily as a means to lower the dose and thereby ease the burden of administering the medicine to the patient. The lesson learned, however, was that concentrates produced a burden of their own due to their chemical force, resulting in physiologically disruptive effects not encountered with milder and more complex botanical products. Aggravations produced by concentrates were exaggerated in patients whose resilience was already compromised. Lloyd describes in retrospect his assessment of the experience (*EAR*, 1910, p. 41):

> "Comes now the lesson taught by the half century of turmoil in and among the alkaloids, resins, resinoids, and oleoresins. Shattered ambitions, blasted hopes, disappointments generally, ... dispelling of the illusion that a fragment can parallel the whole, if the whole be intelligently comprehended. Eclectic physicians learned from an experience not easily forgotten the lesson that dried fragments of drugs are not representative of drugs.

> "The administration of violent ultimates and large doses to shock the system ... gave way to kindlier methods. The doctrine of humanity to the disease-weakened sufferer, not brutality to the helpless, once more revived and became not merely ideals in theory, but logical facts in a successful practice. The original Eclectic motto, "Vires Vitales Sustinete" (Sustain the vital forces), so often lost to view by some people involved in the fallacy of the nineteenth century alkaloidal-resinoidal ultimates, became, as in the days of the fathers, a legitimate Eclectic watchword. By a final, natural *evolution* the school, after facing disaster, passed safely through the crisis."

Concentrating extracts by isolating fractions, usually for purposes of standardization to high levels of active markers, is derived from the concept that quantity = strength = quality. This belief has long been a determinant of manufacturing pharmaceutical products from botanicals. It was one of the major fallacies that John Uri Lloyd contended with all during his professional career. The issue was so important that he twice issued a series of articles in the *Eclectic Medical Journal* on the subject. It began with an article in 1909 that he incorporated in 1914 into the first of three articles entitled "Quality versus quantity." He continued this series in 1916 with two articles in the *EMJ*, parts 4 and 5, entitled "Strength versus quality", and he completed the series in 1920 with article number 6 of the same name. The need to stress the issues discussed therein was such that the entire series of these six articles from 1914-1920 were reprinted in 1931 (*EMJ*, 1931, pp. 45-7(I), 87-92(II), 131–6(III), 173–7(IV), 215–9(V), 257–60(VI)):

> "I. October, 1909, I wrote an editorial titled "Strength versus Quality." ... I reproduce the same as follows:

> "Strength versus Quality. —An error common to a superficial, as well as to a one-sided or fragmentary conception of pharmacy, is that of considering *strength* and

quality as synonymous terms. ... The truth is that, although more or less related, the constituent that gives the factor *strength* is often less important than are the attributes that go to make up *quality*, which, perhaps more than does strength, leads to high excellence.

"Let us define *strength* as a dominating something that stands out boldly, and which, in toxic drugs, produces a violent or energetic action, as does the poisonous something that produces death when an overdose of a toxic drug is administered. Let us define quality as a balanced combination of other something, with just enough of the toxic agent to make a complex product that, as a whole, has wider functions than are possible if the single death-dealing substance dominates. But we need not confine ourselves to toxic drugs, for, from all time, in many familiar directions, such as tea, coffee, spices, tobacco, etc., standards of strength have been differentiated from those of quality.

"For example, the *strength* of wine lies in its alcoholic proportion, but the *quality* of wine depends on the attributes imparted by accompanying congeners, such as water, potassium salts, ethers, acids, tannates and such. These, if balanced, the one in proportion to the other, produce wine of varying qualities. ...

"Nor is a standard of strength difficult to attain, whereas that of excellence, based on quality, is too often vainly sought, or reprehensibly neglected. It is easy, and not, as a rule, expensive, to double or treble the amount of the strength principle of a compound in which the congeneric substances that make for quality are elusive. ... An apprentice in pharmacy can, from *dried root* of gelsemium, make a preparation very poisonous by excess of the alkaloids, but yet very deficient in quality as contrasted with a preparation of the recent root of less alkaloidal strength.

"In our opinion, the attempt to standardize a preparation by a single dominating constituent is but a struggle towards a pharmaceutical standard of excellence, in which *therapeutic quality* should be the ideal. This fact Eclectic physicians have recognized for more than half a century. —Lloyd, *EMJ*, October, 1909.

"Colloidal chemistry is based upon the fact that quantity is but one factor in many directions that involve both chemical and therapeutic action. The condition of a substance is a might factor as concerns its action as a thing, and necessarily, in this case, becomes a dominating agent in its therapeutic application. ... The *quality* of a drug depends not alone on the weight of the materials; its *physical condition* is all-important. ... And yet we have not as yet reached colloidal structures that stand in liquids without settling, that pass through the filter paper, that are so finely dispersed as to even receive the name, "*colloidal solutions.*"

"II. ... The kernel of it all has, however, been to the effect that plant pharmacy is not a superficial problem, but a mighty study, based on the art of natural structural aggregations that exist in plant complexities, the art of the chemist being largely restricted to the destruction of these natural structures, together with the study and description of the factors evolved there from. I have continually urged the utilization of neutral solvents designed to liberate and to separate structural entities that are so easily affected by heroic chemistry, be it of any form or description. I have been irresistibly forced, with increasing evidences before me, to conclude that the art of pharmacy in the direction of plant complexities is the reverse of the art of the applied chemical processes of the past.

"The pharmacist's province in plant structures seems thus to me, primarily, the investigation and preservation of the qualities of natural associates that need be preserved as such, and differentiated from each other, with the aim of utilizing those that are useful. The art of the chemist seems to be that of applying destructive processes to plant structures, by means of such reagents as acids and alkalies, and by such processes obtaining from these structures ultimates that are definite entities in themselves, usually crystalline, and that can be graphically pictured by means of symbols expressing their atomic composition, and even their molecular arrangement. ...

"A duty of the pharmacist is that of studying *undefined* combinations in which no chemical equivalents are possible. These aggregate masses of materials are, in their vegetable host, dove-tailed together into balanced structures, each possessed of individualities of its own, but united with and interlaced with others, *physical attractions* between groups being a conspicuous factor. Such compounds serve either as nutrients to conserve animal life, or as definite therapeutic agents to be utilized for the correction of abnormal conditions in disease expression. These symbolless structures of "pharmaceutical compounds" are, as a rule, non-crystalline, amorphous and shapeless, in the fresh plant, remaining colloidal when dried, if decomposition does not (create) liberate crystalline products. ...

"As the butcher deals in flesh, not in animals, so the pharmacist deals with vegetable remains, not with the plants themselves. ... The field of a pharmacist's study must be in restricted lines if he hopes to accomplish. He must not attempt to conquer a multitude of problems. ... We are now surely upon the threshold of a proper recognition of *structure-less* pharmacy. We have reached the "breaking dawn" of the pharmacist's opportunities. Contact action, mass action and colloidal qualities of both structureless structures and minute fragments (*not* atoms) of dispersed compounds and elements must be a scientific and recognized part of the most advanced chemico-pharmacal field now looming before us under the name of *colloidal chemistry*.

"III. ... Whilst the ultimates broken out of structures are of value in therapy, the structures yielding the ultimates are possessed of qualities that in many directions make them superior to the artificial products. ... In a time to come will also follow a scientific comprehension of the pharmacist's structures now beyond the eye of the talented men engaged in the study of the products broken out of these, as yet, voidless and formless colloidal bodies. ... With these remarks as a text, it may be well for this writer to extract a few phrases bearing on this subject from past prints from his pen. (See Lloyd Brothers' Drug Treatises, 1904 to 1914).

"JABORANDI (1904). Constituents. —... The alkaloid *pilocarpine* ... is one constituent only, for a number of fortifying or modifying acids and bases are to be obtained from, or are present in, the plants. Practitioners of medicine know from experience that a preparation of true *Pilocarpus microphyllus* carries qualities distinct from those of the alkaloid. ... The so-called active principles of the Jaborandis embrace the alkaloids *jaborine, pilocarpidine, jaboridline, jabonine,* and the acids *jaboric* and *pilocarpic,* as well as other products and educts. ... The chemistry of the Jaborandi bodies is enough, almost, to take the life study of a specialist. ...

"VERATRUM (1904). "*Constituents and Products.* —... Chemistry, as is true of most other plants, destroys, creates and alters, but does not parallel. Structural relationships that exist in the drug may be broken, new substances created, but the natural balance is not maintained by any educt, product or mixture of ultimates. ... No constituent or created product represented *Veratrum.* All the alkaloidal fragments broken out, these so-called derivatives mixed together, are not Veratrum either in structural compositon or in therapeutic value. Separated, they are fallacies; antagonistic are they in their actions. Mixed, they are frauds if viewed as representing the full drug. ... In our opinion, these broken out fragments are chemically made derivatives of Veratrum structure, not natural integral parts. ... The less chemistry Veratrum receives the better. ...

"COLLINSONIA. (1904). *Constituents.* —Collinsonia parallels other vegetable products that as a whole are useful, but in which the isolated structural fragments are not the equivalent of the drug. No definite therapeutical agent has ever been identified in Collinsonia or obtained from it. ... Collinsonia ... is most valuable either as a whole or in preparations carrying its united qualities. No chemistry, no heroic pharmacy can be tolerated in its manipulation.

"MACROTYS (*Cimicifuga*) (1905). *Constituents.* —Macrotys, like other American drugs, has been persistently and repeatedly attacked by chemists, beginning with Mears (1827), passing thence to Tilghman (1834), King (1835), Davis (1861), Conrad (1871), L.S. Beach (1876), Trimble (1878), Falck (1884), Warder (1884), and others, both contemporary with and following those named above. All authorities subsequent to King unite in saying that the most conspicuous product of Macrotys' disintegration is a compound resinous body, which was first discovered by

Dr. John King in 1835. Subsequent studies have been largely devoted to the splitting of this resin into by-products. ... Some of these resinous bodies exist, possibly, in a natural condition in the drug, but the majority are created by drying, chemistry and manipulation. ... Even the touch of the atmosphere, as well as manipulation by means of solvents and subsequent drying, are sufficient to produce great changes and result in newly constructed products. ...

"DIOSCOREA (1905). *Constituents.* —Excepting saponin, obtained in 1885 by Mr. W.C. Kalteyer, there are no representative educts or products of Dioscorea of a definite chemical structure. ... It was a very inferior saponin, and, naturally, did not stand the test of time. ...

"To sum it all up, in our opinion these chemists severally destroyed the plant, and from the products of disintergration obtained certain ultimates that may or may not exist in the plant tissue, and likewise may or may not, singly or collectively, have any decided therapeutical connection with the drug's structural qualities. ... The foregoing excerpts are fairly indicative of the views of this writer concerning the subject of relationships between plant structures and chemical products created therefrom. ...

"The separated dried products broken out of a drug by chemical means or created from drugs by the chemist's art, useful though each might be in its own sphere, did not typify or parallel the therapeutic qualities of the whole drug. ... Fragment or ultimate, broken out of or created from a plant by chemistry, did not represent the therapeutic qualities of the structure from which it was derived. The once prevailing hope that a single, dominating constituent, or ultimate, or a definite substance present in or obtained from a drug, could be taken to standardize the desirable therapeutic qualities of the combined medicinal parts of a plant complexity, also passed away.

"IV. ... "Quality" in a plant pharmaceutical preparation might be defined as a balanced combination of complexities that, in their natural home in the drug, were of such a nature as to require the application of discriminative pharmaceutical methods. ... The present method of standardizing a pharmaceutical preparation by making it carry the greatest possible amount of one dominating agent is not conducive to the highest pharmaceutical thought-standard. ...

"Carrying this line of thought ... the article titled "Standards of Excellence," 1909, ... exemplified as follows: A standard established by one man, or a committee of men, may be correct from their one viewpoint, but need not necessarily be a standard that, under different conditions, may prevail in the thought and action of other men. ... The harmful result of such authorities' rulings, could it be legalized absolutely and irrevocably ... would be to paralyze pharmaceutical research. ... Uncharitable inflexibility as concerns the privilege of others possessed of other viewpoints, such as a belief in the usefulness of nontoxic agents, could do a mighty wrong in preventing pharmaceutical progress. ...

"In accordance with this line of thought, we believe that standardization, through an honest misconception of possibilities and probabilities outside their field, is too often inclined to uncharitable error. We believe that in many cases it would be better if a smaller amount—a *much* smaller amount—of certain dominating drug constituents were present. ... The standard of *pharmaceutical excellence*, in our opinion, ... is to be found in the balanced structure of the preparation's evolution from the crude drug. ... Substances contained in a drug and that are deemed to be inert and inactive, may, under certain conditions, become possessed of exceeding energy. ...

"V. One of the discouraging features connected with pharmaceutical problems has been the systematic attempt, as this writer views the subject, to retard personal investigation by restricting one who is concerned in research to *authoritative* publications that, through the passing of years, become, sooner or later, inadequate. ... The fact is, even the man who follows most carefully formulas recorded in authoritative publications may, by his manipulations, produce a pharmaceutical preparation quite different from that made by some other man, and that, too, even when the ingredients employed by both are identical. ... The quality of a drug depends not alone on the weight of the materials; its physical condition is all-important.

"Indeed, the problems in pharmacy that now most appeal to this writer are not so much in the line of discovering new remedial agents to supplant those now established as to give to the users of medicines the wealth that comes from manipulative pharmacy and balanced research applied directly towards the study of *qualities*. ... Can we not now, in a receptive mental position, move into a higher phase of pharmaceutical research than that based upon mere strength as governed by weight and measure of the materials manipulated? Is not higher pharmacy the art of establishing *quality distinctions*? ... We may become prepared for a receptive argument regarding the action of colloidal bodies, because *the study of colloidal activity is primarily a study of different qualities of a material, and is mainly dependent upon different physical states or conditions of the material.*

"VI. And now, for the first time in this series, is introduced the long neglected (by the majority) subject of what is now known as "*Colloidal Chemistry.*" ... Only by processes that might be called offshoots of colloidal chemistry had I been able to explain, even to myself, the discord that had come into pharmaceutical work under my laboratory care during the past forty years. ... Concerning what colloidal chemistry has in common with plant pharmacy, ... I would reply, 'Everything!' ... The principles of "colloidal activity," now looming up as a mighty factor in the evolution of medicine, ... is liberating from bondage the man who believes that quality is not necessarily dependent on quantity, that the factors that confront the pharmacist cannot be fully explained by symbols, formulae and equations.

"A plea is made for the consideration, it having been time and again argued by me to my classes, as well as in print, that plant structures, as a rule, were inexplicably interlaced, and when normal, usually (if not universally) colloidal. ... Although *destructive* chemistry yields invaluable ultimates, *constructive* pharmacy has a field to itself. ... To dispossess a natural drug-texture of its colloidal qualities is to alter its condition other wise than physically. In this we believe. And in this direction we believe the art of pharmacy will yet evolve until its recognized importance will be established to all concerned in both chemistry and therapy. ... In such as this no reflection is placed on either the analytical or synthetical chemist. Upon the contrary, we believe that the time will come when chemistry will recognize the fact that the *beginning* of this study is the consideration of such problems as may be expressed by the formulae."

Fixed Oils

Oils can be relatively concentrated in the fruit or seeds of some plants. The separated lipid fractions are usually used in cooking but are also important nutritionally for their high content of the essential fatty acids. Certain fatty acid compounds are called essential because they cannot be manufactured in the human body but are necessary for the health of all people. Therefore, they must be consumed in the diet or through the dietary supplements. Since these oils exist in such small amounts in whole foods, to derive therapeutic advantages from their consumption aside from preventing outright deficiency states, they must be supplied in the form of concentrated oil extracts, especially the prostaglandin precursors alpha- and gamma-linolenic acids.

Oils are mostly triglycerides that are compounds made up of three fatty acids bound to glycerol. The types of bound fatty acids differ depending on the plant source. Many vegetable oils are high in the essential polyunsaturated linoleic acid such as commonly consumed corn (60%), sunflower (69%), and soy (50%) oils with the highest content in safflower oil (79%). Therefore, linoleic acid is readily available and often consumed well in excess of need, since these oils are frequently used for cooking. Mono-unsaturated fatty acids such as oleic acid found in olive (*Olea europaea*) oil (82%) are not considered essential but are important in controlling and reducing unhealthy blood lipids. They are less often used in cooking, mostly for light sauteing and sauces.

Oils high in alpha-linolenic acid such as flax (*Linum usitatissimum*) seed oil (57%) or relatively high in gamma-linolenic acid including evening primrose

(*Oenothera biennis*) seed oil (9%), black currant (*Ribes nigrum*) seed oil (16%), and borage (*Borago officinalis*) seed oil (24%) are taken as dietary supplements and not used for cooking. These linolenic fatty acids are referred to by some as nutriceuticals because of their nutritional content, but may also be considered a concentrated medicinal extract due to their therapeutic potential. They are usually dispensed in soft gelatin capsules.

These oils are referred to as fixed oils to distinguish them from volatile oils. The most common fixed oil used in medicine is castor oil from the seed of *Ricinus communis*. In separating the oil from the seed, the toxic principle ricin is left behind in the seed meal. The extraction of a safe medicinal oil fraction from a toxic plant is similar with borage seed oil, in which case the oil does not contain the hepatoxic pyrrolizidine alkaloids found in the borage plant.

Essential Oils

Essential oils are also called volatile or aromatic oils. They are known as essential oils, not because they are essential in the diet, but because they contain the essence of the fragrant aroma of the plants from which they are derived. Any essential oil is made up of dozens of different components in small amounts, usually with one predominant and several in relatively higher amounts than the rest. They are usually prepared by steam distillation in which volatile constituents are extracted from an herb with steam and re-condensed in a cooling coil or column.

A thousand grams of an herb containing 1% volatiles (a relatively large content) would yield only ten milliliters of volatile oil. This demonstrates the high degree of concentration of the volatile components and their greatly heightened activity, in comparison with the whole herb or its native extracts. Taken orally in a vehicle or in soft gelatin capsules, essential oils are sometimes mixed with a powder (excipient), sugar cube, or honey as a vehicle. These concentrated extracts are used in small doses. The local irritant properties of the pure oil and potential organ damage from large doses makes the internal use of essential oil to those thoroughly trained in their applications. In some cases as little as five to fifteen drops, depending on the oil, may be toxic to liver and/or kidneys.

To enhance their safety essential oils are often used only externally and locally as needed. They are often used in oil or cream base topically. They should not be put in bath water without emulsifiers, since the oils will float on the surface and can irritate sensitive tissues. Essential oils can also be placed in boiled water or the medicine cups of steam vaporizers and used as inhalants for sinusitis, bronchitis, or aromatherapy.

Local Use

INHALANTS

Nasal inhalants consist of a medicated wick inside of a plastic tube with an opening at the tip. The wick is impregnated with aromatic oils for use in sinus congestion and nasal catarrh. To treat bacterial infections below the larynx, inhaling certain medications in steam vapor can better provide local mucolytic and antiseptic effects than oral administration of extracts containing the same substances. A vaporizer with a medicine cup for aromatics provides a steady supply of steam to vaporize the volatiles. For short-term exposure a couple of drops of essential oil added to a pot of steaming water removed from the heat can be inhaled under a towel or vapor tent. The aromatics act as a surfactant for the mucus in the respiratory tract. The steam also helps liquify mucus so that it can be more easily expelled. Inhalants can also include balsams.

Sweetened Extracts

Arab medicine was the first to utilize sugar as a pharmaceutical necessity in improving the flavor of noxious tasting medicines. Enhancing the taste of medicines improves compliance with dosing instructions. The improved taste and palatability greatly eases oral administration. In some cases the sweetened tonics of 19th century America were so delicious that they were dispensed with carbonated water at the soda fountain of pharmacies. Thus, a number of modern sodas such as colas and root beer originally were marketed as concentrated extracts for their medicinal qualities and sweetened for dosing compliance. The use of sweeteners in medicinal extracts continues today not only for the attractive taste but as effective vehicles.

Glycerites

The pharmacist WJM Gordon was Lloyd's first employer when he serving as an apprentice in 1863 at the age of 14. Lloyd described how Gordon came to employ and advocate glycerin as an extract solvent (*JAPA* 1925, p. 1120):

"Procter and Gamble, manufacturers of soap and candles, were established between Central Avenue and the Canal, a few squares from Mr. Gordon's pharmacy. As a worthless by-product an immense amount of the "sweet water" refuse in the making of candles was run into the adjacent canal, as the easiest method of its disposal. Mr. Gordon arranged to catch that "sweet water," freely given him without charge. In horse-drawn tanks it was carried to his factory in Deer Creek where it was refined.

Mr. Gordon refined the molasses-like liquid with super-heated steam and charcoal into a pure, odorless form. He was its only manufacturer west of the Allegheny Mountains. Gordon spoke on the use of glycerin as a remedy, adjuvant, and solvent at the American Pharmaceutical Association meeting in Cincinnati in 1864. He utilized glycerin as a substitute for cane sugar in syrups, since it is sweet and not liable to fermentation. Gordon declared that glycerin resembles oil in that it is soothing but also dissolves in alcohol and water at any proportion. Following his presentation, Gordon was made President of the A.P.A. at that meeting. By the time the U.S. Pharmacopoeia of 1870 was published, 33 of the 46 official fluid extracts had glycerin as a constituent. However, glycerin eventually diminished in popularity.

Glycerin is not volatile and does not become hard at the freezing point. It dissolves plant acids, most alkaloids, minerals and their salts. Still, its applications were ultimately more limited that what Gordon had advocated. Lloyd was well informed on the issue of glycerin and its uses (*EMJ*, 1905, pp. 617–9):

"Glycerin was ... to an extent, sacrificed by over-praise in the house of its friends. It was thought to be medicinally nutritive and alterative. ... Its preservative and solvent properties were highly spoken of instead of sugar for the making of syrup of ipecac, senna, etc. Its external use in medicine was not less Utopian. ... It was recommended ... for the making of many medicinal glyceroles. ... It was expected that the whole line of vegetable extracts would be made of glycerin instead of alcohol and water, and in the fluid extracts, then becoming popular, it was freely asserted that it would replace alcohol, sugar and water. ... Not that glycerin does not possess qualities that make it useful, but ... the novelty of its introduction has long since worn off. ...

"The fact is, in some directions glycerin is invaluable. No other menstruum approaches it. It possesses certain qualities equaled by none other. It is neither inflammable under ordinary conditions, nor is it volatile. It possesses neither intoxicating nor narcotic qualities. It neither freezes in the winter nor ferments in the summer. It is an invaluable solvent in the places it is fitted to occupy, but these positions in pharmacy are restricted. In opposition to its good qualities as a menstruum, it is by nature antagonistic to the more universal solvent, alcohol, for a great list of plant constituents soluble in alcohol, and preserved indefinitely by alcohol when in solution, are not only not dissolved by glycerin, but are actually thrown from solution, if glycerin be in excessive amounts. ... Without reason were these preparations made in the day when glycerin was at the height of its glory as a fad.

"It is not a solvent for salts and fats, ... nor, indeed, is it a good extractive agent for the majority of the alkaloidal salts, and the glycosides, and the inorganic compounds that exist in plant structures. Hence, as the majority of drugs embrace in their structures a medley in which such substances as these take an important part, glycerin becomes too often a natural *excluder*, instead of a natural *dissolver*, and glycerin, therefore, should have no part in such preparations.

"But *"a little glycerin"* has a place where the tannates are found. ... The astringent constituents of the roots and barks and seeds partaking thereof for their qualities, are dissolved by glycerin. .... Mangifera indica, stillingia, Iris versicolor, gossypium, geranium, and the like—for these glycerin is invaluable. In some cases just a little glycerin will answer the purpose. With others, as with Mangifera indica, a preparation needs be half glycerin. ...

"Physicians no longer consider glycerin as a medicinal factor, excepting as a carrier of a few external remedies. ...And yet, as we have said, glycerin is now used in enormous amounts, ... as a diluent of remedies where alcohol is inadmissible, or where prejudice prevents the using of alcohol (perhaps to the injury of the preparation), glycerin is employed in quantities that almost stagger one."

Glycerites employed now are herbal extracts that use glycerin (glycerol) as a solvent and preservative. Glycerin remains a suitable solvent for many vitamins, minerals, aromatic oils, organic acids, alkaloids, and polyphenolic compounds. Since its solvent capacity is not as great as water or alcohol, it is not as effective for extraction. Glyerites are usually made by distilling the alcohol from a hydro-alcoholic extract and replacing it with glycerin. Those who are prone to alcohol abuse prefer non-alcoholic extracts, along with others who have parental or religious concerns. Glycerin is a byproduct of alcohol fermentation and is normally present in small amounts in wine and beer. The sweetness and smoothness it gives to extracts often makes their use more pleasant.

Elixirs

Elixirs, also referred to as cordials, hydroalcoholic combination extracts sweetened with sugar or glycerin. Sweetening of herbal extracts began to be popular in 19th century. Prior to that, elixirs described unsweetened medicinal combinations or formulas. The change in taste led also to a change in medicinal quality (*AMM*, 1919, p. 63):

"Originally the term elixir in pharmacy was applied to compound tinctures, and they were destitute of sugar. Thus compound Tincture of Senna (Elixir Salutis) is an example of an original elixir. As a rule elixirs were nasty mixtures and harsh remedies, of which Compound Tincture of Aloes is a good specimen.

"But about half a century ago the compound, "Simms' Cordial Elixir of Calisaya," a sweetened and flavored cordial, was introduced. It was followed by other palatable *cordials* and soon the term "elixir" was used in America in direct opposition to the original meaning. A great list of sweet alcoholic compounds followed, as to the original meaning. A great list of sweet alcoholic compounds folloed, as trade elixirs, and a few are employed yet, but as a rule the elixir is now neglected. Physicians have learned that it is not advisable to give a tablespoonful of flavored syrup and a teaspoonful of alcohol in order to get a trifling amount of medicine."

The elixir craze in late 19ᵗʰ century led to many patent medicine nostrums. This popular movement became noted for fraud associated with 'secret formulas' and recipes. The popularity of some of these elixirs initiated or popularized a number of alcoholic liqueurs as well as sodas. Because of the lack of standard methods and formula, the name attached to a particular elixir could vary widely in content, proportion of ingredients and their quality. Due to the popularity of elixirs in his day and the inconsistency with which they were manufactured by independent pharmacists, Lloyd felt compelled to compile and assess the formula as they had been published in pharmacy journals over several decades. His effort was not due to his belief in the value or necessity of such elixirs but was simply due to the demand by physicians on pharmacists to provide these combinations products. Lloyd addressed this situation by authoring a book, *Elixirs and Flavoring Extracts*, that established reliable standards (*EFE*, 1892, pp. 12–13 and 17–20):

"Combinations, or rather associations, of substances incompatible under all ordinary conditions were advertised under the name elixir, and substances perfectly insoluble in the menstruum employed were represented as being dissolved. ... The burden was too great; elixirs as a class were severely criticized, and many pharmacists and physicians included those which were worthy among those which were indifferent and bad. ...

"Throughout this country the preparation of elixirs is gradually passing from a few wholesale manufacturers into the hands of the many pharmacists. Quantities of elixirs are prescribed. ... Physicians have their favorite elixirs and prescribe them, but these elixirs must, as a rule, be unquestionable."

"We have for many years attempted to systematize the matter, and our efforts have met with some success. ... We believe that, as a rule, under the conditions which confront us in the problem of compound elixirs, physicians desire the associated action of smaller amounts of the several ingredients rather than the full dose of each. ... Where it has been practicable we have endeavored to carry it out. ...

"We vary from the methods employed by the committee appointed by the American Pharmaceutical Association regarding the manner of mixing a tincture or fluid extract with the menstruum. If they are mixed directly together, precipitation results immediately of much of such substances as are insoluble in the resultant menstruum. This produces a preparation which pharmacists and physicians refuse to accept as an elixir. ... This trouble may be overcome to a great extent by following the old process for making medicated waters, that is, by triturating the fluid extract or tincture with magnesium carbonate, or with some other inert powder if this substance is inadmissible, after which the simple elixir is added and the mixture filtered. By this process the insoluble materials are separated at once, which is preferable to having the precipitation extend over days or weeks. ...

"We object to elixirs which contain cinnamon, caraway, coriander, cardamom, or cloves (unless used as aromatic elixirs), for many persons are prejudiced against certain of these substances, and it is not unusual to meet persons with whom the flavor of one of the foregoing is unbearable. The simple elixir should, in our opinion, be as nearly as possible pleasant to the majority of persons, and we have no record of an objection to the flavor of lemon or of orange, separate or combined. ...

"In the pages which follow we find processes for making 271 different elixirs. ... In the large majority of cases, pharmacists are able to extemporize and supply most demands from their stock of standard elixirs, which are those in most common use. Some elixirs may be called permanent, but this term cannot be applied to the larger number. Associations of the alkaloids in acid solution only ... might possibly be claimed as fairly permanent. ... Few organic bodies are permanent in solutions containing far more alcohol than is permissible with the modern elixir, and in consequence many elixirs will alter in appearance, or even precipitate, if they contain the substances which are supposed to be present."

Lloyd's efforts resulted in his first publishing a book on elixirs in 1883. This book, along with the *New York and Brooklyn Formulary* published in 1884, led the pharmacy profession to establish a comprehensive compendium of authoritative formula that were not official in the *United States Pharmacopeia*. Thus was created the *National Formulary* in 1888 by authority of the American Pharmaceutical Association.

Syrups

The evolution of syrups as a form of administering herbal extracts was an attempt to make larger quantities of unpleasant flavors bearable. Lloyd aptly describes this class (*AMM*, 1919, pp. 52 and 54):

"Owing to the unpleasant taste of decoctions and infusions sugar was finally added to them, and thus the class of *syrups* arose. But these preparations are, as a rule, of little strength, or else of uncertain quality, the average dose necessarily being great, even with energetic drugs."

"Such syrups were common in early Eclectic medication, and when derived from several drugs mixed together, were called Compound Syrups. ... The fact began to be apparent that the sugar not only diluted the liquid but weighted the remedy with useless extraneous material, often disturbing the stomach of the afflicted person. Then it was that many far-sighted Eclectics made a crusade against the *syrup craze*, and as a result practically swept these cumbersome substances out of Eclectic practice. While it is true that many syrups made by expert pharmacists are improvements over decoctions and infusions in elegance, the fact remains that as a rule, sugar is worse than useless in medicinal preparations, and is to be viewed as an impurity. Few sick persons relish sweets.

"In a very few cases where sugar is a preservative, a syrup, is, however, for certain reasons, preferable to any other form of the remedy. ... No general formula can be given for making syrups."

Sweet liquid preparations with a mucilaginous or viscous nature can be taken for their demulcent effect for sore or irritated throats in coughs and colds. They also provide a vehicle for other medications, especially for children. Syrups are made with at least half sugar, honey, and/or glycerin often combined with acacia (*Acacia senegal*) or tragacanth (*Astragalus gummifer*) gums. The soothing demulcent effect of the gums (and glycerin) enhances local effects in throat. As for the therapeutic impact that adding sugar had on the efficacy of botanical medicine, Lloyd observed (*EMJ*, 1888, p. 218):

"The majority of the experienced physicians that I recall now, are, as a rule, administering their remedies in accordance with the idea that medicine and water together are the most favorable forms to administer ... not...elixirs or syrups...and it is not unreasonable to suppose that experience has been their teacher. Certainly, they are surrounded by well advertised elixirs, syrups, etc."

Local Use

LOZENGES

Referred to in Europe as troches or pastilles, lozenges are tablets made with herb extracts in a base of about 90% sugar and 7% gums. These hard, sweet tablets are designed to dissolve slowly in the mouth and gradually release the active concentrated herb extracts such as essential oils or other compounds that may be local anesthetics, demulcents, antiseptics, and/or aromatic expectorants. Lloyd gives his assessment (*AMM*, 1919, p. 64):

"*Troches* are ... medicated sugar lozenges, many formulas for them being found in the pages of the U.S. Pharmacopoeia. But they have only a limited use in Eclectic practice, and, indeed, this may also apply to the majority of physicians in other sections of the profession."

Extracts/Fractions In Unsweetened Carriers

Besides combinations with sweet solvents to improve the flavor, extracts and especially concentrated fractions are often combined with vehicles to dilute the active components and disperse them over the absorptive surface for a more gentle and gradual exposure. For internal use, alcohol is often used as a suitable solvent for solid concentrates to be administered in liquid form. These are sometimes referred to as reconstituted tinctures or fluid extracts. More often carrier substances are added to extracts and concentrates used for topical applications. The variety of liquid and semisolid substances that act as solvents and carriers are identified based on their base composition, properties, and intended use.

Medicinal Spirits

The volatile oils distilled from plants can be combined with alcohol to form medicinal spirits such as peppermint spirits. Spirits refer to distillates and products made from them. The word spirit is derived from breath and refers to the ethereal components associated with life forms. Alcoholic spirits are the distilled, volatile components including ethanol and its congeners derived from various fermented beverages made from grain or fruit. This distilled alcohol provides a suitable solvent for the internal use of some aromatice oils. These blends are usually referred to as aromatic spirits. According to Lloyd (*AMM*, 1919, p. 62):

> "This class of preparations embraces the alcoholic solutions of such substances as oils, camphor, glonoine, etc. Among them are to be found ... Whisky, Brandy, Bay Rum, and similar alcoholic liquids. This class is quite voluminous and many of its members are extensively employed in medicine."

Local Use

LINIMENTS

Liniments are usually medicated oils that are applied to the skin with a friction massage and often contain volatile oils or potent medications. They sometimes contain rubbing alcohol or another solvent instead of oil. For example, naturpathic doctors in the mid-20th century utilized an aconite liniment as an analgesic that utilized chloroform as its base. Some doctors preferred a non-oily form in general, as Lloyd indicated of Eclecticism's eminent teachers and practitioners (*AMM*, 1919, p. 60):

> "In this connection I will say that the late Prof. John King used liniments extensively that were *free from oils*, the liquid employed as the medicine carrier being saturated solution of ammonium chloride. He claimed that better effects could be obtained by associating such substances as spirit of camphor, tincture of opium and aconite with this liquid as a carrier than by means of any fat or oil, to all of which he objected on account of their uncleanliness."

LOTIONS

Lotions are similar to liniments but contain usually no oils and are not applied with friction.

SALVES

Also called ointments or ungeants, salves are greasy semisolid applications made with fats (for example, lanolin, lard, or tallow) or white petrolatum that contain substances such as essential oils that dissolve readily in oils. These medicines prepared in a fatty or emulsion base have a consistency thicker than creams and are sometimes firmed with wax but should melt at body temperature. Simple ointment was formerly made by melting one part yellow wax and gradually adding it to four parts lard, stirring the mixture constantly until it cools. Often used over inflammations, ointments serve also as emollients to soften and protect the skin. Preparing ointments for applying nonoily liquid ingredients can be challenging, but lanolin helps this process as described by Lloyd (*AMM*, 1919, p. 61):

> "In some cases aqueous liquids or aqueous extracts are to be incorporated with fats. This is often difficult; but if the physician will prescribe equal parts of hydrous wool fat and simple ointment, large amounts of water or watery liquid will be taken up.

GELS

Hydrocolloid substances consist of carbohydrates that absorb and hold water to form gels. They can be medicated with botanical extracts and used to protect the skin, similar to the effect of demulcents on the mucosa.

CREAMS

Extracts can be added to emulsion bases for application to the skin. These extracts are usually vulneraries that reduce irritation and inflammation and help promote healing. They may include rubefacients to increase local circulation in the skin. Medicated creams can be applied to treat pain, wounds, burns, infections or sores.

CERATES

Cerates are salves that have been hardened with wax. These provide a protective coating to surfaces such as the lips.

SUPPOSITORIES

Typically, suppositories are made by incorporating remedial agents into a fatty base that remains solid at room temperatures. Cocoa butter is the usual base, but up to 10% wax may be added to increase the stability in warm weather. They are preformed in sizes and shapes depending on the oriface in which they are to be used. Rectal suppositories are cone shaped and urethral suppositories are pencil shaped; both weight about one gram. Vaginal suppositories weigh about three grams and are globular.

SHAMPOOS

Herbal shampoos are not only used to cleanse the hair with suds-forming saponins and to provide a pleasing aromatic fragrance. They can also help to nourish the scalp to improve hair quality and to manage the itch of dandruff and inflammation of seborreic dermatitis. Regular shampoo cleansing formulas are used as a base.

Isolated Phytochemicals

The investigations into therapeutic activities of plants usually leads to isolation and identification of a number of active components, known as phytochemicals, from several chemical classes. This is one reason why a single chemical compound or a concentrated extract standardized to one compound or even one chemical class cannot completely describe the activity or range of effects of the whole herb. Pharmacognosy is the science of developing medicine from natural products. It isolates an active compound from plant or animal that can be used or developed into a comparable drug. Research on both types of botanical products (complex extracts and isolated components) is appropriate to assess under what conditions each might be preferable for a particular condition. A familiarity with phytochemical terminology is important to understand pertinent botanical pharmacy, pharmacology, and toxicology. However, there are significant limitations to understanding botanical therapy solely in these terms.

Focusing on individual components can easily be misleading when considering the complex herb. When discussing the effects of whole herbs, their nutrients (e.g., vitamins, minerals, amino acids) are often not addressed, nor are the fibrous components or small quantities of fixed oils or volatile oils normally found in plants, unless they are used specifically for these components. Yet all of these affect how the more potent compounds are digested, absorbed, assimilated, utilized, metabolized, and excreted. Sometimes the inactive compounds can greatly influence the effects delivered by the active ones by increasing, decreasing or in other ways modifying their activity.

When considering the components that are primarily responsible for the therapeutic use of a plant or its extracts, it is important to not fixate exclusively on the knowledge about such compounds. For each active compound in significant quantities, there are similar compounds in lesser amounts with similar yet different pharmacokinetics and pharmacodynamics that yield an overall effect that is distinct from any one of them in isolation. To verify this in your own experience, consider your different perceptions of the effects produced by green tea, black tea, coffee and pure caffeine (given that the amounts of each consumed deliver the same total quantity of caffeine).

Not all generalizations hold true for each class of phytochemical compounds. For example, while the alkaloid berberine in goldenseal is soluble in water, its alkaloid hydrastine is not. Nonetheless, describing the phytochemistry enables a general understanding of the chemical effects, if we are familiar with properties that are common to the phytochemicals of that class. For this reason the major classes will be briefly described with some important distinctions, emphasizing solubility in water and/or alcohol that determine their relative presence in different types of extracts.

Under some classification there are subclasses that indicate greater chemical, and sometimes pharmacological, similarities. Plants covered in the second section of this book will be mentioned when some of their important components serve as examples of that class. These components contribute part of the pharmacological activity for which the plant is used. Certain phytochemicals serve as active biomarkers for extract standardization. At other times standardization is based on an entire chemical class, e.g., flavonoids, when several components in this class appear to provide the major beneficial effects and/or the concentrated extract is primarily composed of this fraction through reducing the more complex native, or crude, extract.

Components Most Soluble in Water or Weak Alcohol

POLYSACCHARIDES

Polysaccharides are high molecular weight carbohydrates that are generally insoluble in alcohol > 30%. Different types of sugar polymers are sometimes linked with uronic acid or other compounds. Hydrocolloidal polysaccharides hold water and are called gums; some are used as bulk laxatives, like psyllium (*Plantago psyllium, P. ovata*) and flax (*Linum usitatissimum*) seeds. Others form highly viscous slippery mucilage when extracted, if molecules are linear, acting as demulcents. Herbs that contain these types of polysaccharides include marshmallow (*Althaea officinalis*) root and slippery elm (*Ulmus rubra*) bark. Still others form gels that are tacky and moist if their molecules are branched, such as comfrey (*Symphytum officinale*) leaves and aloe (*Aloe vera*) inner leaf with its glucomannans and acemannan.

Other branched polysaccharides can be anti-inflammatory or act as immunomodulators. Examples of these herbs are Asian ginseng (*Panax ginseng*) root, astragalus (*Astragalus membranaceus*) root, and calendula (*Calendua officinalis*) flowers. Echinacea (*Echinacea purpurea, E. angustifolia*) arabinogalactans and other polysaccharides in the root and aerial plant are also of this branched type. Polysaccharides have practically no toxicity when taken orally.

TANNINS

Tannins are chains of polyphenolic compounds. They can be polymers of hydrolyzable phenolic acids (gallitannins and ellagitannins) that are antiseptic.

Hydrolyzable tannins are found in uva ursi (*Arctostaphylos uva-ursi*) leaves. Others are polymers containing flavans such as the condensed tannins in black tea (*Camellia sinensis*) leaves. Catechin and epicatechin flavan polymers are sometimes referred to as procyanidins or proanthocyanidins. Short chains of these components are called oligomers and are potent anti-oxidants. Oligomeric procyanidins can be found in grape (*Vitis vinifera*) seeds and skin, cranberry (*Vaccinium macrocarpon*) fruit, cocoa (*Theobroma cacao*) seeds, St. John's wort (*Hypericum perforatum*) tops, and hawthorn (*Crataegus oxyacantha*) fruit, flowers, and leaves.

Tannins are astringent, since they precipitate proteins, creating cross-links and drawing tissues together. Tannins also can precipitate alkaloids. Tannins are not crystalline; they are best extracted by decoction in water. In stored herbal extracts they can be problematic by precipitating compounds out of solution. By using glycerin as a solvent, precipitation can be reduced. Tannins can upset the stomach in large amounts.

PROTEINS

Proteins are precipitated and deactivated in extracts with high alcohol content. Free amino acids occur in higher amounts in alcoholic extracts. Enzymes are proteinaceous and are only active in an aqueous medium. Lectins are other proteins; some are known to be mitogenic in stimulating an immune response. Like some polysaccharides, lectins mimic certain cell surface components of virus and/or bacteria. An active lectin in stinging nettle (*Urtica dioica*) root is called UDA (*Urtica dioica* agglutinin). Proteins can combine with polysaccharides to form glycoproteins or peptidoglycans as occur in echinacea species.

Components Generally Soluble in Both Water and Alcohol

GLYCOSIDES

Glycosides (sometimes called heterosides) are compounds of almost any class attached to a sugar molecule that increases their solubility in water for biological transport. Pharmacology depends on the nature of the aglycon (compound with the sugar removed). Anthocyanin glycosides of peonidin and cyanidin are important contributors to the color and anti-adhesion activity of cranberry (*Vaccinium macrocarpon*). Saw Palmetto (*Serenoa repens*) contains large amounts of beta-sitosterol glucoside, an additional source of sitosterol. The phenolic glycoside arbutin is common in heath family plants such as *Arctostaphylos uva-ursi* and releases the antiseptic hydroquinone.

Anti-inflammatory iridoid glycosides found in devil's claw (*Harpagophytum procumbens*) root and rhizomes are harpagoside, harpagide, and procumbide. Flavonoid glycosides of St. John's wort (*Hypericum perforatum*) such as hyperoside (hyperin), quercitrin, and isoquercitrin appear to contribute to its antidepressant effects. Flavonoid glycosides contribute to the activity of many popular herbs including chamomile (*Matricaria recutita*) flowers, ginkgo (*Ginkgo biloba*) leaves, and hawthorn (*Crataegus oxyacantha*) leaves. Extremely potent types are cardiotonic steroidal glycosides, antitussive cyanogenic glycosides, and laxative anthroquinone glycosides. Triterpene glycosides are widespread, but are usually referred to separately as saponins.

Saponins

Saponins are amorphous, colloidal glycosides that produce foam when agitated in water. This is because they are large molecules with a hydrophilic end having a sugar component and on the other hydrophobic (lipophilic) end having a triterpene or steroid. Aglycones of saponins are called sapogenins; absorption occurs mostly in the form of sapogenins following metabolism of saponins in gut.

Triterpene glycosides such as cimiracemosideA are found in black cohosh (*Cimicifuga* [*Actaea*] *racemosa*), while blue cohosh (*Caulophyllum thalictroides*) has uterine stimulant caulosaponin and caulophyllosaponin. Astragalus (*Astragalus membranaceus*) liver-protective saponins include astragolides I-VIII. Horse chestnut (*Aesculus hippocastinum*) seeds are known for their vasotonic escin, and the sweetness and broad effectiveness of licorice (*Glycyrrhiza glabra*) root for mucosal inflammation is based largely on its glycyrrhizin.

Alkaloids

Alkaloids are nitrogen-containing compounds that react as bases. They are potent pharmacologically, since they often influence nervous system function. Their solubility varies, but they are usually extracted better by either alcohol or water. The natural solubility is opposite that of their salts formed by uniting the alkaloid with an acid. Most form white crystals. The names of alkaloids end in the suffix 'ine'. For example, the alkaloids in goldenseal (*Hydrastis canadensis*) are berberine (uncharacterically yellow), hydrastine, and canadine.

Probably the most used and abused plant derivatives are the alkaloids. Besides caffeine from tea (*Camellia sinensis*), coffee (*Coffea arabica*), and cola (*Cola nitida*), there is nicotine from tobacco (*Nicotiana tabacum*), ephedrine from ephedra (*Ephedra sinensis*), morphine from the opium poppy (*Papaver somniferum*), and cocaine from coca (*Erythroxylon coca*). Historically, plant alkaloids have been, and remain, some of the most popular and effective medications, such as atropine from belladonna (*Atropa belladonna*), quinine and quinidine from cinchona (*Cinchona* spp.), vincristine and vinblastine from Madagascar periwinkle (*Catharanthus roseus*), and many others.

Phenolics

Phenolics are simple molecules containing one phenol component, like caffeic acid, or several, like cichoric acid. Like these, many are phenolic acids or their derivatives and are often mildly astringent or antiviral. Cinnamic acid derivatives found in *Echinacea purpurea* include cichoric acid and caftaric acid, while stinging nettle (*Urtica dioica*) leaves have caffeic malic acid and ferulic acid. Benzoic acid derivatives include gallic acid as found in uva ursi (*Arctostaphylos uva-ursi*) and many other plants. Some herbs contain derivatives of both cinnamic acid and benzoic acid. Examples of these include St. John's wort (*Hypericum perforatum*) with caffeic acid, ferulic acid, isoferulic acid, and chlorogenic acids together with gallic acid, as well as black cohosh (*Cimicifuga* [*Actaea*] *racemosa*) with caffeic acid, ferulic acid, and cimicifugic acid along with salicylic acid. Polyphenols are phenolic complexes.

FLAVONOIDS

Flavonoids are ubiquitous polyphenolic compounds that range from colorless isoflavones to yellow flavonols and flavones to red, blue and violet anthocyanidins. They are largely responsible for colored autumn leaves. The same flavonoid often resides in a plant as both aglycon (without sugars) and glycoside (with sugars). When using water as a solvent, they are best extracted by decoction. They are antioxidants, often interact with enzymes, modulate prostaglandins, and have low toxicity.

Examples of different types of flavonoids include flavones like apigenin and luteolin in chamomile (*Matricaria recutita*), and biflavones in St. John's wort (*Hypericum perforatum*) such as amentoflavone and biapigenin. The unique flavonolignans silibin, silichristin, and silidyanin are components of milk thistle (*Silybum marianum*). On the other hand, ubiquitous flavonols are available in large amounts from St. John's wort including kaempferol, luteolin, myricetin, and quercetin and green tea (*Camellia sinensis*) with quercetin, kaempferol, and myricetin. Isoflavones formononetin and biochanin A are available in red clover (*Trifolium pratense*), while genistein and daidzein are in large quantities in kudzu (*Pueraria lobata*) as well as legumes such as fava bean (*Vicia faba*) and soybean (*Glycine max*).

COUMARINS

Coumarins are derivatives of the prodrug coumarin found in sweet yellow clover (*Melilotus officinalis*) and other herbs. Coumarin, its derivatives in plants, and its human metabolites are not inherently anticoagulant, but coumarin can be converted to an anticoagulant (similar to Dicumarol and Coumadin) when metabolized to 4-hydroxycoumarin by mold or fungus. Some coumarins do have anti-platelet activity, some are spasmolytic, and some are anti-inflammatory. Coumarin derivatives are in St. John's wort (*Hypericum perforatum*) including umbelliferone (7-hydroxycoumarin), the most common human metabolite of coumarin, and scopoletin, a nonspecific spasmolytic compound.

Components Most Soluble in Strong Alcohol

VOLATILES

Volatiles are components of aromatic or essential oils. These odiferous principles are found in almost all plants evaporate readily when exposed to air. They are often antiseptic. Plants like mints that are highly aromatic contain about 1% volatiles, mostly with one or several dominant components along with many minor ones. Some aromatic plants such as thyme have several chemotypes whose content of specific volatiles can vary greatly. All volatile containing plants are mixtures of many aromatic compounds but usually one is dominant. Examples include menthol in peppermint (*Mentha piperita*), terpinen-4-ol in tea tree (*Melaleuca alternifolia*), and eucalyptol (1, 8-cineole) in eucalyptus (*Eucalyptus globules*).

Volatiles are typically soluble in alcohol, though they are partially soluble in hot water. More volatiles will be retained in aqueous solution in a closed container. Volatiles can be separated from plants by steam distillation, expression, or extraction. Many have a potential toxicity to liver and kidneys in high concentrations, especially if consumed as purified compounds or as fractions of plants known as essential oils.

RESINS

Resins are a complex of chemical classes, often including sticky diterpenes, that together are soluble in alcohol but insoluble in cold water. The triterpenes in black cohosh (*Cimicifuga* [*Actaea*] *racemosa*) resin such as actein and 27-deoxyactein are believed to contribute to its hormonal effects. The lactones found in kava (*Piper methysticum*) resin including kavain, dihydrokavain, methysticin, dihydromethysticin, yangonin, and demethoxyyangonin are more soluble in water as components of its extract than as individual isolates.

Resins may be combined with gums (gum resin). Myrrh (*Commiphora myrrha*) is a common gum resin whose resinous components are quite bitter. Some resins are combined with essential oils (oleoresins). Oleoresins can be very pungent to the taste such as ginger (*Zingiber officinale*) with zingerone, shagoals, and gingerols and also act as stong local irritants like cayenne (*Capsicum frutescens*) with capsaicin.

FATTY ACIDS

Fatty acids are nonvolatile lipids that make up fixed oils that are liquid at room temperature. Fixed oils are best extracted by cold pressing, but inexpensive commercial sources may use organic solvents. Polyunsatuated fatty acids are unsaturated and oxidize easily, so they need to be kept refrigerated. Essential fatty acids provide substrates for anti-inflammatory and anti-thrombotic prostaglandin production. Sources for essential fatty acids used therapeutically include evening primrose oil (*Oenothera biennis*) for its gamma-linolenic acid and flax seed oil (*Linum usitatissimum*) for its alpha-linolenic acid. Saw palmetto (*Serenoa repens*) contains a variety capric, caproic, lauric, and myristinic acids that contribute to its activity.

STEROLS

Sterols are ubiquitous steroidal plant compounds found in lipid fractions. These agents are known to lower blood cholesterol. They also act as mild estrogenic agents that are alcohol-soluble and poorly absorbed. Saw palmetto (*Serenoa repens*) contains large amounts of beta-sitosterol along with stigmasterol and campesterol, while stinging nettle root (*Urtica dioica*) also has prostatic effects associated with its beta-sitosterol content.

ALKAMIDES

Alkamides are amines combined by an amide linkage with unsaturated fatty acids. They are sometimes called alkylamides, and alkamides with N-(2-methylpropyl) as the amine portion are isobutylamides. Isobutylamides often produce salivation along with a tingling and numbing sensation of the lips and tongue. Herbs containing isobutylamides are frequently used for toothaches. Echinacea isobutylamide fractions are both anti-inflammatory and increase phagocytosis by leukocytes. Western echinacea (*Echinacea angustifolia*) and purple coneflower (*Echinacea purpurea*) roots contain isomers of dodeca-2E,4E,8Z,10E/Z-tetraenoic acid (or tetracetyl) isobutylamide, as well as many others.

LIGNANS

Lignans contain two phenylpropanoid units. The majority of lignans are most soluble in alcohol, though partially soluble in water. They are known for their antitumor activity, antiviral effect, and enzyme inhibition. Certain lignans decrease natural estrogen effects by inhibiting conversion of androgens to estrogen by the enzyme aromatase and by increasing levels of sex hormone-binding globulin. The major active resin component of chaparral (*Larrea tridentata*) is the lignan nordihydroguairctic acid, or NDGA. Flax seed (*Linum usitatissimum*) is rich in the lignan secoisolariciresinol diglycoside, while stinging nettle root (*Urtica dioica*) contains both secoisolariciresinol and isolariciresinol.

SESQUITERPENE LACTONES

Common in plants of Asteraceae (daisy) family, these have anti-tumor, cytotoxic, and antimicrobial effects. They may cause allergic contact dermatitis in some humans. A well-known example that was long believed to be the major active component in feverfew (*Tanacetum parthenium*) tops is parthenolide.

TRITERPENIC ACIDS

Triterpenic acids possess anti-inflammatory effects including 5-lipoxygenase or cyclooxygenase-2 inhibition. Cranberry (*Vaccinium macrocarpon*) fruit along with leaves and berries of other members of the Ericaceae, or heath, family such as *Arctostaphylos* spp. contain ursolic acid and oleanolic acid, as does hawthorn (*Crataegus oxyacantha*) fruit and leaves. The Ayurvedic herb boswellia (*Boswellia serrata*) is well known for its triterpenic boswellic acids

IRIDOIDS

Iridoids are nonvolatile cyclopentanoid monoterpenes. They are typically bitter, as those in gentian root (*Gentiana lutea*) such as gentiopicrin. Valerian root (*Valeriana officinalis*) contains iridoid valepotriates that are unstable but convert to active metabolites.

3

MODERN ROADS TO THE FUTURE

Where Are We Headed?

The complexity of plant pharmacy, together with the challenge of specific individual prescribing, makes the mechanistic explanation of the biological interactions unfathomable, beyond rocket science. Yet science needs to be employed to allow a fundamental grasp of the principles of complexity, as the empirist Lloyd himself acknowledged (*AMM*, 1919, p. 49):

> "The study of the pharmacy of plant organizations is a problem that needs take the utmost thought of the scientific man, and the utmost care of the manipulative pharmacist. The pharmacy of plant preparations has passed from the hands of the superficial experimenter, into the field of the closest scientific student, the evolution of satisfactory plant preparations being now fully comprehended by those experienced, as among the most difficult of all problems connected with the satisfactory preparation of therapeutic agents. ...
>
> "Only those who do not comprehend the subject of pharmacy, can view it otherwise than as a might work, beyond the power of any one man to grasp in its entirety. Only those who by reason of ignorance bred by inexperience are led to underrate this great art, will presume to encroach on the field, other than as questioners of voices from the past, or as listeners to whispers of the present."

Lloyd believed a thorough understanding of both the science and art of his profession of pharmacy was necessary to begin to grapple with the challenges posed by manipulating medicinal plants. The scientific study of plants as sources of medicine is part of the discipline known as pharmacognosy. However, the art involved in assessing plant materials was an equally important aspect discovered through practical experience only (*AMM*, 1919, p. 51):

"Pharmacognosy ... is that part of pharmacy devoted to consideration of the physical and structural qualities of drugs, but when the term is applied to plants, I must carry the conception higher and further than a microscopic examination of tissues or the simple identification of drugs. While much embraced in this section of pharmacy may be learned by lecture lesson and in book study, a great and important part of the study of pharmacognosy cannot be obtained other than by close attention in practical pharmacy manipulation.

"Taste, odor, physical condition, all that experience in qualities adds to knowledge through our senses, is a part of the work of the phamacognosist. It is not enough that by means of the microscope the fact be demonstrated that the drug is true to name, the qualified pharmacist must be able to establish whether that drug is suitable to make a reliable preparation. It may be correctly named and yet worthless.

"This latter point can only be established with certain drugs by a complete knowledge of chemical methods, with others by the experience that comes with years, yes, a lifetime of scientific work in drugs, and in other cases still by the expertness of experience in which no words and no diagrams are able to convey the knowledge gained by the experienced student. Such knowledge, typical of empiricism lies outside scientific formulae."

The complexity of plant life and the issues surrounding the appropriate medical use of many herbs traditionally employed over the centuries have not been definitively resolved. Over 70 years devoted to exploring botanical challenges and applications did not allow John Uri Lloyd to believe that he had done more than scratch the surface. He expressed this perspective when attempting to answer the query, "Plant drugs—to what do they owe their medicinal value?" (*EMJ*, 1932, pp. 229–31):

"Through an entire lifetime I have studied and written and experimented and recorded, only to find myself each day deeper in the maze of entrancing questioning. ... The longer I work and the more I study, the more I hesitate concerning so-called conclusions. The more light I obtain, the more questionings arise. Changes before unknown introduce problems unexpected. From the depths of every drug, and every fragment of a drug, come questions yet unanswered. Not a plant in nature's entire list but has substances and combinations unknown to us. If these problems were limited to but one drug, our chances for a solution would be better; but they are common to all. ...

"Concerning the chemistry of plant life, I will say that my experience teaches that not one drug has been as yet so fully analyzed, or even partly analyzed, that we can say we *understand* it. ... We know that the term "Chemistry," as applied to life products, is not limited. ... Comes in also the influence of contact action, of capillarity, of endosmosis, of catalysis and colloidal problems embracing physical influences in which there seems to be no known atomic change. ...

"I have spent a lifetime in the study of problems embraced in the topic before us for consideration. Laboratory experimentation has taken the most of ... seventy years of my life. For years I have taught portions of that which I have learned. I have written volumes on details in these directions, but I am now only a humble student of it all."

The recognition that there is more to know than is known about the action of plants and their components in the ecology of the human environment leads one to suspect that by altering the colloidal nature of plant components, the natural living relationships involving energetic exchanges, their kinetic efficiency and/or pharmacological effectiveness may be disrupted or diminished. The truism of the *vis medicina naturae*, the healing power of nature, is that right relationships are hardwired into living systems in ways and by means that we must appreciate and acknowledge even when we don't understand the full mechanisms or implications. In spite of many scientific advances, we still lack the means to adequately assess and effectively explain the inherent significance of many components residing in plants that impact health. Life after all is a mystery to be lived, not merely a problem to be solved. To achieve full health we must be guided by more than limited scientific knowledge.

The significance of the complexity of life forms has to do with their ultimate necessity in maintaining a functional balance. Simplicity in content focuses the effect but limits the scope. Nature and its Creator have provided human and animal life with the vast complexity that exists in the plant world as a means of accessing as essential array of beneficial influences. Determining which is most appropriate for a given set of circumstances is the challenge we face in attempting to understand how best to use these vital tools.

Lloyd had his own biases based on his experience and affiliations as a pharmacist and as an Eclectic. As a pharmacist, he manufactured extracts of plants and so advocated their advantages over the plant itself in regard to its use in medicine. His belief that much of solid, and even soluble, material had no obvious benefit was based on his perception of the crude air-dried plant and teas as weak and his knowledge that simple extracts formed insoluble precipitates on standing. As a latter-day Eclectic, he had little praise for dried, solid, concentrated extracts due to their disruption of natural structures and affinities found in the fresh plant and the claims that strength was equivalent to quality. He recognized in each form some value, but his own emphasis was the development of liquid preparations of fresh plants that were comparable in action to the whole complex plant and maintained a long shelf-life. His preference for liquid over solid medications derived from his belief that the dried whole herb contains therapeutically unnecessary substances and that solid extracted concentrates (fragments) and isolates are too limited in scope. Yet he acknowledged in his final years that each form had its own usefulness and provided certain valuable remedies (*EMJ*, 1934, pp. 443–6):

"I consider vegetable structures ... as intricate structures in which each integral part is related to and united with associated constituents, be they liquid or solid. They are intricate labyrinths of complexities which, taken together, constitute a thing as a whole. The structure, in its entirety, we call the plant, or drug. ... The intricate structure that we call the drug is too cumbersome in form to be used in its entirety. It is made up, largely, of woody matter, of fats that are inert, of coloring matters that have no therapeutic value, and of other extraneous substances that may be excluded, without great injury to the therapeutically valuable structure which, as a rule, seems to be soluble as a whole, in certain appropriate menstruums.

"In the early day, an attempt was made to administer the entire plant in the form of a decoction or infusion, which dissolved parts of the juices, carrying more or less of the medicinal substances of the drug, which could then be given with a fair degree of certainty. But such preparations were open to the objection of fermentation and decomposition by fungus growth. They also carried large quantities of gum and other extractive matters that hindered the action of remedial constituents. Came then the method of distillation in steam, by which the drug structure was broken up, and certain volatile constituents recovered by condensation. This was the day of medicated distilled waters which ... constituted great lists in the Pharmacopeias of Europe.

"Came then (or preceding) the discovery that spirit of wine would abstract from certain drugs many constituents insoluble in water, and that it would preserve these structural solutions in a way that water could not accomplish. As these solutions were usually deeply colored, they were called "tinctures," the word *tincture* referring to the *color* of the preparation. The term "tincture" remains in vogue at the present day, referring to an alcoholic preparation of a drug, regardless of its color, although, be it said, the "tinctures" as a rule are deeply colored.

"The tinctures of the Pharmacopeias of a hundred or more years ago were most artfully and wonderfully complicated. In the making of some of these complicated cure-alls, many ingredients were employed. ... Marvelous were the claims made in behalf of these compounds, called *elixirs*. ...

"Finally, in 1816, came the discovery of morphine. ... It seemed to parallel opium, and to give in a concentrated form the value of opium. It was called an *alkaloid*, from its resemblance to an alkali, in its properties of combining with acids to form salts. A new era was now opened up. Chemistry became more important in plant medicine, the hope being that, as morphine seemed to parallel opium, every plant could be decomposed by chemical means, a something being obtained therefrom that would parallel the value of the whole plant, or its liquid representatives in medicine.

This theory was furthered by the discovery of quinine in cinchona ("Jesuit Bark"), and soon therafter by the discovery of alkaloids in a few other important drugs.

"About this time arose the American schools of medicine, known as the Eclectic and the Thomsonian. Their medicinal preparations were mainly vegetable. They believed in a vegetable *material medica*. ... Professor John King accidentally stumbled upon "podophyllin," which he called, correctly, "resin of podophyllum." Close following, by investigation, he discovered "resin of cimicifuga" and the "oleo-resin of Iris versicolor." These discoveries strengthened the theory that each medicinal plant possessed a *something* that could be separated, and used, in very small amounts, to represent the plant itself. ... Of all the plants they used, less than a meager half-dozen carried any alkaloidal qualities whatever. ...

"The various substances, obtained often by simply drying extracts, which, to make them dry, were often necessarily mixed with such extraneous substances as magnesium carbonate, sugar of milk, and alumina. Then it was that the terms "resinoid" and "concentration" were created, to apply to the powders (misknown as "Eclectic"), that were called by many ignorant people *alkaloids*. ... The entire North American vegetable material medica at the present time furnishes *only two plants* that yield alkaloids having any general use whatever, as alkaloids, in medicine. The two are *sanguinaria* and *hydrastis*. Other plants there are in which the chemist can identify alkaloidal qualities. This also is true. But the alkaloidal feature of such is of no importance whatever, in a therapeutic sense. ... Of the vast majority of vegetable structures, in my opinion, no isolated product comprehends the full qualities of any drug, and hence, in the majority, liquid pharmaceutical preparations stand today supreme, as they have in the past. ...

"I consider the entire line of the so-called alkaloids, glucosides and resins, to be among the most profitable commercial products that can be manufactured. Furthermore, opportunities second to none for their manufacture on a large scale, lie in my direction. But this has never prevented me from expressing my opinion on this subject, or of upholding the cause of the pharmacist who maintains the integrity of his preparations.

"To sum up. The course of medicine from the beginning in the far distant past to the present date, has been a series of faddisms. Each fad has disappeared, to leave a something of utility, which today stands as a useful therapeutic agent in the material medica of the world. The elixir fad, the tincture fad, the medicated distilled water fad, the chemical fad of Glauber, the fluid extract fad of regular medicine, the alkaloidal and concentration fad of early Eclecticism, the synthetic, and coal-tar product fads, are related to each other in that all are fads, and each will leave, probably, a few useful products to mark the enthusiasms of their day."

Standardized Extracts

A great concern in medicine is consistency, to the extent that this can become more emphasized than the quality of the product. A product that meets a certain minimal standard is assumed to be a product of quality, though it may be of minimum quality. The issue of achieving a regular standard of quality in process and content has long been an issue in botanical manufacturing. Those such as Lloyd who sought to achieve excellence as their standard were perceived as at odds with conventional practices described in pharmacopoeias, when in fact they were attempting to advance the art and science of botanical pharmacy. Attempting to merely concentrate the most active components to the neglect of the balanced complexity of the whole was not considered desirable by Lloyd, especially if those compounds had potential for adverse effects (*EMJ*, 1909, pp. 683–5):

"A standard established by one man, or a committee of men, may be correct from their one viewpoint, but need not necessarily be a standard, that, under different conditions, may prevail in the thought and action of other men. To make such an inflexible law would be to paralyze pharmaceutical research. ... A chemist or a committee, thinking only of the conspicuous agent, may ignore the milder entities, and in the glare of this one dominating light establish a very one-sided standard, which may neglect unseen qualities that lie beyond the thing that makes the standard of the man of toxic faith.

"Upon the contrary, the one who considers the drug as the balanced whole ... may get a therapeutic possibility that ... could never have been perceived. From such a view the standard of therapeutic excellence does not necessarily depend upon the ... ultimate, but rather upon its *subjugation* to the associated factors.

"As a result, the person who makes the systematic investigation on these different lines, and finally balances his products in accordance with the evidence at his command, chooses standards peculiarly his own, and very different from the other products. It may even be a better standard of therapeutic excellence than is that based upon the largest possible amount of a conspicuous energetic constituent.

"Nor is it wise to infer that less skill or knowledge is required of him concerned in searching the drug's milder qualities. Upon the contrary, the easiest phase of a standard is that of establishing the one ultimate in a drug. ... The establishing of a balanced drug complexity, that will act as a unit of value, is the one thing needful. ... We believe that standardizers, through an honest misconception of possibilities and probabilities outside their field, are too often inclined to uncharitable error. We believe that in many cases it would be better if a smaller amount—a *much* smaller amount—of certain dominating drug constituents were present in preparations. ...

"This line of thought has, these many years, possessed Eclectic care and dominated

Eclectic experimentation, the intent of Eclectic medication being ever toward kindly medication. ... Let us repeat, the standard of *pharmaceutical excellence*, in our opinion, does not necessarily reside in the one toxic agent, but is to be found in the balanced structure of the preparation's evolution from the crude drug. Nor does *therapeutic excellence* necessarily rest in an overload of a dominating, ever-conspicuous toxic constituent of a drug."

In Lloyd's day the attempt at standardization was largely based on establishing a standard process by which an extract was made. These processes were defined for each official herbal extract in the *United States Pharmacopoeia (USP)* or *National Formulary (NF)*. However, these exacting processes were only adequate in so far as the starting material was of standard quality, and there was no industry-wide assurance of this. For potentially toxic botanical medicines such as digitalis that were commonly used as extracts in those days, the need for establishing predictable potency was considered paramount.

In this regard, an editorial in the *California Eclectic Medical Journal* in 1910 (v. 3, p. 194) emphasized the critical importance of maintaining a consistent potency for often-toxic botanicals they used:

"The only way to secure uniformity in drug products is to standardize them—in other words, to adjust them to definite strength by systematic assay, chemical or physiological. This principle is now pretty well recognized by our leading pharmaceutical manufacturers. In fact, it is to one of the manufacturers, in all probability, that modern medicine owes much of its scientific character. Reference is here made to Messrs. Parke, Davis and Co., who were the first to enter the fields of both chemical and physiological assay and who have practiced and preached standardization for a third of a century."

Developing accurate and relevant biological assays that are readily measurable and consistently reliable proved impractical. The reductionism involved in obtaining standard chemical strength for potentially toxic medicines eventually led to the near abandonment of manufacturing pharmaceutical complex extracts in favor of isolated components or their derivatives. This change was accepted on the premise that science, by measuring and purifying, could improve the precision of the prescribing process and thereby the degree of control over the process. The fallacy of this belief lay in the adverse effects produced by introducing potent chemical compounds into systems known for their complex chemical balance and sensitivity to concentrated chemicals. With the precision of chemical purity comes its unmitigated force. Biochemical individuality still results in different responses due to multiple metabolic parameters. Thus, even for a standard strength medication the safety, efficacy, and proper dosage remain relative concepts based on averages, not individuals.

As a simplified response to the complexity of herbs in their processed forms as dietary supplements, the most widely acclaimed, and commonly misunderstood, is standardized extracts. Unbeknownst to many, the concept of standardization can imply one thing but mean another. The belief that plant products standardized to the content of a particular chemical compound 'marker' ingredient are of equivalent quality and potency is a fallacy. The power of this assumption has led to abuse as standardization claims have become a familiar marketing ploy. However, these claims must at best be taken only at face value. Different standardized products exemplify a wide variation that can occur within this classification.

The different types of standardization have specific implications. The following examples assume accurate, even if misleading, label claims. Standardization based on minimum content claims for components do not assure a specific amount; since greater amounts may be available and can change from batch to batch. This is especially undesirable if the marker compound is a potent active substance such as the alkaloids ephedrine or yohimbine. A higher amount helps to assure a minimum content claim, since the marker may diminish, based on its relative instability and age of the product.

Standardization of extracts based on the content of a chemical marker substance is intended to substantiate the identity of the herb source because of its natural content of that substance. However, in the case of substances that are found in other plants, these spurious plants can be substituted or extracted and added to provide consistent levels of the marker. In cases where the marker can be synthesized it may be added at precise levels to meet label claims. As a simple test for identity, the final product should taste similar to the original plant. If it does not, such a product probably should not be identified by the name of the herb or or claim its traditional uses.

Prefereably, standardization is made to the content of a marker that is believed to be the major, or one of the major, active components. Again, adulteration with other extracted or synthetic sources of this compound is possible. The amount of the active marker, even when described by a standardized weight based on analysis, can vary widely according to the type of analysis used to verify the content. In some cases the standard form of analysis is not the most accurate. When the active marker is a glycoside with an inactive sugar attached, the weight of the glycoside including the inactive sugar is provided rather than weight for only the active component of the chemical standard. Sometimes the weight of the active marker is combined with that of similar compounds found in the plant that are difficult to separate chemically for the assays that analyze the content, so the total weight of similar compounds (with different activities) is given. In any case there is no single component in a complex herb product that represent the total bioactivity of that plant or its complex extract.

A classic example of the unreliability of standardizing to an acknowledged active compound is the use of feverfew (*Tanacetum parthenium*) extract for prevention of migraines. An open clinical study by Johnson and others in 1985 using 50 mg freeze-dried feverfew leaf daily reduced the frequency and severity of these headaches compared to use of placebo. A randomized double-blind study in 1988 by Murphy and others found that 70–114 mg of oven-dried feverfew leaves standardized to parthenolide content (2.2 mcmole) were likewise effective in reducing the number and severity of headaches. A third study by Palevitch and others in 1997 using 100 mg of oven-dried feverfew leaves containing 0.2% parthenolide significantly reduce the pain intensity in another double-blind trial. However, a dried alcoholic extract of feverfew leaf with 0.5 mg parthenolide per capsule failed to reduce the number of attacks in the study by DeWeerdt and others in 1996. Awang in 1998 concluded that the usefulness of feverfew for preventing migraines was not directly dependent on parthenolide, and only whole leaf products should be considered reliable for this condition. A 2002 clinical study by Pfaffenrath and others found a CO_2 extract (MIG-99) used at daily doses containing 0.17, 6.25, or 18.75 mg of parthenolide had no dose-dependent effect or significant migraine prophylaxis in general.

Some cases of standardization list a category of related chemical compounds described by that category, for example, "alkaloids," or as typified by a common measurable active compound, for example, "as ephedrine." Such standards give no true representation of activity or potency. Inevitably, every major active compound in a living plant has similar compounds in the plant associated with its synthesis, breakdown, or modification. These molecular variations are such that they have pharmacological activity somewhat like the major compound and have absorption, metabolism, and excretion properties more or less similar to it. Taken as a total sum of activity, there can be significant variability given the same total quantity of similar yet variable components. This is especially misrepresented when the category of compounds is described as quantified "as the major component" such as ephedrine, since this implies the activity of that component is being represented when actually it is the weight of all similar compounds with different activities.

In a few cases standardized products list several categories of active compounds that are available within a narrow range of concentration in the product. This approach is a measurement method describing what are considered the total bioactive complex. The full representation of all bioactive compounds can best be demonstrated by chromatographic fingerprints that show the relative amounts of important components identified for each medicinal species. This method probably comes closest to trying to assure consistent potency of a given product. Yet based on the limitations described above for each method, there is some variability to be expected. The variation may not be significant if the standardization of process as described for products standardized by herb weight only is also employed. Ultimately, aside from its advantage in product marketing, the value of chemical standards for herbs is greatest for in-house laboratory use by the manufacturer to assure consistency at different steps in the production process. The actual active compound in botanical medicine, as recognized by American herbalists and naturopaths as well as German medical and scientific authorities, is the whole herb.

Standardized Fractions—Phytopharmaceuticals

Standardized products can be complex liquid or solid extracts with consistent designated marker content, but typically they are concentrated fractions developed to contain a predetermined amount of a particular active constituent(s) found in the fresh complex herb. The concentration of the marker compound, whether active or not, is what determines the concentration process, not the therapeutic quality of the extract. Standardized products are usually solid extracts due to need for removal of toxic chemical solvents used in fractionation, eg, hexane, diethyl ether, acetone, methylene chloride, etc. Residues of these toxic solvents remain in trace amounts. Supercritical (liquid) carbon dioxide is a promising new solvent for extracting fat-soluble compounds. While a toxic residue is avoided, this process can be relatively expensive in this application. Also, this fraction does not assure equivalency with those products demonstrating efficacy that were made with other chemical solvents.

Arguments in favor of standardization made by Murray in 1996 address the production process for botanical extracts as pharmaceutical products. By using examples of ginkgo, St. John's wort, and saw palmetto concentrated extracts/fractions in comparison with tinctures, he illustrates the relatively greater strength of the concentrates in terms of percent content of the marker compounds. Of course, that is what makes them concentrates and allows a much smaller dose to deliver the same amount of those markers. The standardized extract of saw palmetto, consisting of 90% fatty acids and 0.2% beta-sitosterol, essentially represents a chemically extracted fraction designated a liposterolic extract. Calling it saw palmetto makes it sound like a herb, though the author makes a point that it does not resemble the tincture or crude herb. It is a phytopharmaceutical drug in Europe where it was developed. Murray argues that less concentrated forms require extremely large doses.

In 2001 Bone distinguished 3 main types of standardized extracts. The first of these could be applied to the extracts of St. John's wort since it involves the Galenical-type extracts which are essentially tinctures with the solvent removed, resulting in a 4:1 to 6:1 strength concentrate. The next two types Bone designates as phytopharmaceutical extracts. He describes semi-purified extracts such as ginkgo as those whose native extracts are further reduced through multiple solvent extraction steps, a process of chemical fractionation, to produce a concentrated extract strength of greater than 10:1. Finally, he defines selective phytochemical extracts as "one particular phytochemical group selectively removed from the herb." As examples of this selective process, he identifies purified essential oils and fixed oils such as evening primrose oil.

Bone also emphasizes the need to look beyond marker label claims to verify equivalence between products. In making a valid comparison between one standardized extract of a herb and another, such claims should be based on phytoequivalence. At the very least this implies not only sharing the same level of marker compounds, but the profile of most measurable compounds in the extract should be at similar levels. Even better is documentation of equivalent levels of components available in the bloodstream or clinical studies indicating equivalent biological potency. Still, variables remain that must be specifically addressed for each individual herb species.

The modern approach of standardizing markers in botanical fractions is a slight modification of the former practice of isolating the major active component. The difference in the modern context is the marketing of the final product as a dietary supplement rather than as a drug. Drug manufacture requires an investment from one third to one half million dollars to prove safety and efficacy to be able to make therapeutic claims for disease. Dietary supplements of concentrated, standardized fractions treated as pharmaceuticals in Europe are able to be sold in the U.S.A. on the same basis as herbs and their traditional extracts, being allowed to make only structure and function claims regarding their influence on normal conditions. This saves the drug companies who manufacture these items a huge investment, while appealing to the public's attraction to so-called natural products. However, the distinction between a phytopharmaceutical drug and the plant from which it was derived remain relevant.

The controversy over standardization is heartfelt among authorities with knowledge and experience using the whole herb or its native extracts. Quoted in an article by Patterson in 1996, there are those like Steven Dentali, Ph.D., who counter the perception of standardization being superior with other rationales: "There is no biological reason why a standardized extract would make a better herb. If it was necessary, we wouldn't be using these herbs already. ... It is foolish to think that one group of compounds will entirely account for an herb's activity. Even inactive compounds play a role in an herb by affecting the distribution and absorption of the active components. When you place an herb in a different medium, you change its effects." Mark Blumenthal, executive director of the American Botanical Council, contributes a remark regarding the implications versus the reality: "Potency is a biological term. Standardization does not always guarantee potency. I do not support standardized extracts to the exclusion of herbs that are nonstandardized." Rob McCaleb, executive director of the Herb Research Foundation, agrees with this nonexclusive approach, though he admits to being biased in favor of standardized extracts.

Tierra in 1999 described his herbalist perspective to standardized extracts, considered as a phytopharmaceutical or herbal drug. The standards used are not industry wide, so products can vary widely between manufacturers. Concentration of an active constituent may lead to the loss of other properties and buffering compounds that may lessen adverse reactions. Their appropriate use becomes limited to treat symptoms or specifically named diseases for which they have been developed and shown to be effective, in contrast to the traditional forms used with the intent of shifting physiological processes that underly pathological conditions. The cost of the technology involved in this process can limit some applications to well-endowed pharmaceutical companies that will pass this cost along to customers. The higher commercial costs are not the only undesirable factor passed onto consumers; the use of toxic solvents can contaminate products with trace residues. These solvents such as hexane, benzene, methyl chloride and acetone may have environmental costs, as well. The concerns about the direction that standardization is heading are many and real.

Differentiating Solvents

Though Lloyd's passing preceeded the modern development of botanical extracts standardized to chemical markers, he anticipated the movement in this direction. By discussing the utilization of different solvents in not only extracting but separating components from the complexity of the whole herb, he initiated the trend toward producing active fractions of plants in distinction of strict isolation of a major active component. This compromise position was a development of his identity as a researcher in pharmaceutical techniques and processes, but also due to his production of liquid extracts. The problems with precipitation in liquids discussed under fluid extracts compelled him to reduce the complexity of his liquid extracts in an attempt to avoid unsightly and unnecessary sediment, or "dirt," in his products.

The issue of effective and efficient extraction of herbs was always a concern of this master in botanical pharmacy. His study on the available solvents in the process moved beyond the content of pharmacy texts of his day. The report of his findings is still pertinent concerning the issues and the limitations of applying and mixing nontraditional solvents as a means of achieving extraction and separation. His legacy is one of ongoing investigation to improve botanical product quality. One of the limitations of the ordinary process of plant extraction recognized by Lloyd is the standard utilization of alcohol as a solvent (*EMJ*, 1889, p. 373–5):

> "There are many exceptions to the employment of an alcoholic menstruum in
> plant extraction. The thrusting of a line of alcoholic fluid extracts (followers of the
> alcoholic tinctures and essences) upon the profession has been conducive of injury as
> well as benefit. Manufacturers and physicians together have broadly accepted in this
> direction without proper discrimination. ... Drugs that cannot properly be extracted

with an alcoholic menstruum are often thrust forward as unquestionably represented in an alcoholic form, and are so demanded by physicians."

In his attempt to develop reduced and selective medicines from the complexity that exists within a whole fresh or dried plant, Lloyd labored for decades to achieve a balance in therapeutic activity. His investigation of each process involved qualitative concerns, and not simply how he could concentrate the more potent components. His methods must be seen in the context of the many potentially toxic plants then in common use in medicine. The selective use of solvents to achieve his end was pharmaceutical manipulation achieved by separation. However, chemical changes resulted in alteration of proportions and components in the products (*JAPA*, 1917, pp. 941–8):

"The selection and adaptation of a suitable menstruum that will first abstract and afterward preserve the abstracted therapeutic constitutents becomes a perplexing problem. ... Galenic pharmacy ... embraces no subject more essential than ... menstrua and connected manipulation, in their own relationships, as well as to materials manipulated. ... Such phases of the problem, as the drug, the menstruum and the product, ... cannot be disregarded, and must not be underrated. ...

"Satisfaction with the inherited processes of the past (involving in pharmacy chiefly alcohol and water as menstrua) is responsible for the neglect of opportunities in outside directions. Surely, in a time to come, very many of the galenical preparations ... must, if pharmacy credits itself, give way to carefully studied natural plant *separates*. Galenical processes, instead of beginning and ending with simple percolation, or infusions and decoctions, will utilize such methods as these merely as a first, or introductory step. ... Discriminative research in the direction of solvents as excluders and abstracters, may be one feature that will yet make the art of pharmacy a recognized science. ...

"Acidulated Solvents. —Concentrated sour acids cannot be used, undiluted, as plant menstrua. Diluted with some of the neutral liquids ... they increase the power of water as a solvent for most alkaloids, and decrease the solvent power of alcohol, with the exception, perhaps, of acetic acid. ... The sour mineral acids, excepting sulphuric acid, when added to water increase its capacity for ... mineral salts generally. ... Salts of many alkaloids may be easily made by passing the vapor of acetic, nitric or muriatic acids through their solutions in appropriate menstruums, most alkaloidal *salts* being insoluble in such as these. ... The artificial alkaloidal salts of the sour acids are, as a rule, much less soluble in alcohol than are either the natural salts, or the free alkaloid. ... Acid solvents are theoretically of no value in abstracting substances from plant tissues other than alkaloids and mineral salts. ...

'If this [acetic] acid menstruum be a part of the final product, the finished preparation will carry the odor of acetic acid. ... It leads many physicians to fancy that the preparation has "soured." ... The "sour smell" problem may be overcome by using an odorless vegetable acid. ... As a plant abstracter, a menstruum made by macerating sliced lemon in an appropriate aqueous or hydro-alcoholic liquid, seems preferable. ...

"Alkaline Solvents.—When an alkaloid-bearing plant is moistened with an alkaline solution, the natural plant alkaloidal texture is broken, the alkaloid being liberated in the vegetable tissue. It can afterward be more easily abstracted by alcohol, but less readily by water. In this manner, the (insoluble in water) alkaloids of plant structures can be washed with water and also freed from other substances, such as gums, many fats and oils, and water-soluble extractives. ... It should be borne in mind, however, that the products obtained represent, *not the drug itself*, nor the alkaloidal *texture of the drug*, but an energetic (alkaloidal) fraction, a product of the drug, more or less modified by the heroic process. The material obtained is a chemically altered, manipulative *product*, and not a naturally abstracted, *textural educt*. ...

"Some vegetable acids are not as soluble in either water or alcohol as are their salts, and in such cases an alkaline menstruum acts kindly. ... Glycyrrhizin is soluble in dilute ammonia, hence an ammoniacal menstruum ... is used in making fluid extract Glycyrrhiza. ... Alkalies render most mineral salts insoluble, or decrease their solubility in alcohol, and if as a preliminary step a drug be percolated with alkaline alcohol, the percolate will be comparatively free from such compounds as calcium sulphate and phosphate. ...

"Sugar and Glucose.—In some cases, syrup acts admirably as a menstruum, and was at one time recognized as an official solvent. ... In many places a little sugar in a menstruum furnishes an exceptional extractor, and it is not unlikely that in a time to come sugar, now practically abandoned, will be used more frequently as part of the menstruum. ...

"Citrate of Potassium.—... Citrate of potassium, or citrate of ammonium, is of value as a component of aqueous or hydro-alcoholic menstrual, in the percolation or maceration of astringent plants, such as Colombo and gentian, such drugs parting more readily with their astringents under this influence, the dissolved product remaining in more permanent solution than is the case with purely hydro-alcoholic menstrua."

Lloyd experimented with fourteen neutral liquid solvents, including water and alcohol. He found these chemical solvents were all necessary if complete extraction was to be attempted (*AMM*, 1919, p. 24):

"...successively applied, most plants, be they green or dry, may be practically abstracted of their soluble content."

In other words, in addition to using water and alcohol it requires a dozen different additional solvents in succession to eventually extract plant material of almost all of the non-fibrous components it contains. This process of successive extraction is analogous to chemical dissection. Selectively removing components from an extract with a different solvent, i.e., fractionation, is used for some concentrated commercial extracts, usually those standardized to a high percentage of active chemical markers. These products are closer to purified constituents than to the herb from which they were initially derived.

The following are the solvents that Lloyd considered useful in separating components through extraction or exclusion (*JAPA*, 1918, pp. 137–40, 143, 147–9):

"The solvents considered ... are (excluding acids and alkalies) those that appeal as being of possible use in plant pharmacy, as solvents or excluders, either alone or mixed. They are ... classified by group solvent relationships. Three classes, then result. ...

"*Class 1*—Glycerin, Water, Alcohol [Ethanol] and Methyl Alcohol [Methanol]. The member of Class 1 mix with each other in all proportions, regardless of order of mixing them. ... The members of Class 1, when pure, are either odorless or possessed of no very marked odor. Excepting glycerin, they evaporate readily and are easily distilled.

"*Class 2*—Acetone, Chloroform, Amylic [Amyl] Alcohol, Acetic Ether [Ethyl Acetate] and Sulphuric Ether. The members of Class 2 mix with each other in all proportions. ... The members of this group are all volatile, and excepting amylic alcohol, ... may be easily distilled. They are all possessed of marked odors, ... sulphuric ether ... unpleasant, that of amylic alcohol being disagreeable.

"*Class 3*—Benzol [Benzene], Carbon Disulphide, Benzin [Petroleum Ether], Turpentine Oil and Liquid Petrolatum [Mineral Oil]. The members of Class 3 mix with each other in all proportions. They are, excepting liquid petrolatum, volatile at ordinary temperatures, some of them being very volatile. Excepting benzol and liquid petrolatum, they are all possessed of disagreeable odors.

"General Remarks on the Three Classes.—Considering these fourteen liquids in the order given, it is found that between the extremes no solvent affinity whatever exists, but as we progress down or up the series, affiliation increases.

"Thus, glycerin ... is practically indifferent to all of Class 2, and will not mix freely with any member or combination that may be made of Class 3. Water is indifferent to all the members of Class 3. Of Class 2 it mixes in all proportions with acetone, takes up of sulphuric ether largely, and is indifferent to the other members. Alcohol mixes freely with all the members of Classes 1 and 2, and is miscible in varying degrees with all but liquid petrolatum of Class 3. Methyl alcohol mixes freely with all members of Class 2, with one member (benzol) of Class 3, and is very friendly towards the other members of the third class. Indeed, the only practically indifferent liquid of the entire list to methyl alcohol is liquid petrolatum. ...

"When we step into Class 2, we find that the first member, acetone, is remarkable in that it mixes freely with all the liquids of the entire list excepting the extremes, glycerin and liquid petrolatum. ... Next, chloroform is possessed of fully as marked affinities, exclusive of the first two members of Class 1, water and glycerin. ... Amylic alcohol ... mixes partially with liquid petrolatum, and freely with all the other liquids excepting water and glycerin. ... Acetic ether will not, in equal amounts, mix with any member of Class 3, and with only two of Class 1, water and glycerin being with it immiscible. Sulphuric ether ... mixes freely with all members of Class 3 excepting liquid petrolatum.

"Passing now to class 3 we strike first benzol. ... It affiliates with two members of class 1 (alcohol and methyl alcohol), with all but one member of Class 2 (acetic ether). ... Carbon disulphide mixes freely with all but one member (acetic ether) of Class 2, and mixes with only one (alcohol) of Class 1. Benzin, turpentine and liquid petrolatum stand practically together in their affinities. None will mix with any member of the first class. All mix freely with the three first members of the second class,—acetone, chloroform and amylic alcohol. They all dissolve in acetic and sulphuric ether. ...

"Liquid petrolatum is separated from the others of this (3rd) class, in that it is odorless, and is not volatile at ordinary temperatures. Thus liquid petrolatum, terminating Class 3, stands isolated as does glycerin heading Class 1. In all respects there two liquids are so antagonistic that it may be said that ... they are the antithesis of each other.

"Solutions of Solvents and Mixtures of Neutral Solvents.—Mix any two miscible solvents, e.g., alcohol and water, and, as has been stated, the solvent action of the resultant liquid is different from that of the original. ... Add to a mixture of water and alcohol, successively, other affiliating liquids, and with each addition the solvent power of the product is altered. ... It becomes possible to make a solution of one liquid in another and then, by adding a third liquid, to throw more or less of one or the other constituent (perhaps both) of the first mixture out of solution. In other words, to precipitate it. (A precipitate, or better, *separate*, may be either a solid or a liquid, and either heavier or lighter than the bulk of the liquid.) ... Each new mixture becomes a new menstruum, each new menstruum is a solvent having distinct affiliating qualities. ... These qualities present great opportunities in manipulative pharmacy.

"It is possible to make combinations that will enable liquids of opposite characters to coalesce. ... Thus, if two parts of acetone be mixed with two parts of glycerin, the mixture will at once separate into two layers, about equally divided. Add now one part of methyl alcohol and agitate;—the liquid immediately becomes transparent, forming a single menstruum. The methyl alcohol acts as a mediator, affiliating the three into one, which, however, has a different solvent action from any of its constituents.

"Neutral Solvent Precipitates.—It is well known that a solvent capable of holding a solid substance in solution need not necessarily be capable of totally redissolving it after it has been precipitated. ... Liquid substances, when isoluble in a menstruum, differ from solid precipitates only in being liquid separates. With them, the rule governing resolution of solids holds good. A precipitated liquid in fine division may be very quickly dissolved in an appropriate menstruum, but, if agglutinated into material drops, or resting in layers, it may dissolve very slowly. Hence it is that the order in which liquids are mixed may become of importance in pharmaceutical manipulation. ...

"It is found that the addition of one solvent to an association of solvents in perfect solution may produce precipitation of one or more of the constituents.

"An Endless Series of Solvents Produced by Neutral Solvents Combined with Plant Constituents.—Whenever we abstract what is apparently a single substance from a plant, by means of water or alcohol, we form at the same time, as the solution progresses, a series of new solvents, having successive powers of abstracting other plant constituents. Thus are formed a continuously changing line of new liquids, that may be of as many different qualitites as it is possible to vary the proportions of the original liquids (resulting from solution of solids), these becoming *new* solvents, in their subsequent action on the soluble plant materials.

"Each solid substance that the menstruum dissolves, becomes in turn a part of a new liquid, which is then a thing in itself, and may itself dissolve another substance, insoluble in the original menstruum, thereby forming a menstruum quite different from either of the preceding, and which is capable of dissolving a third substance, a new liquid spring thus into existene with each successive change. No solid body is present at any time after the solution has formed, and yet the *solution of a solid* produces each new solvent. We have a mixture of liquids possessed of individual solvent qualities, as much so as though we had mixed various liquids such as ether and water.

"Finally, the last liquid formed may not be able to hold in solution a substance that, originally dissolved, constituted a part of the first liquid. This body may then in part be thrown out of solution, resuming the solid form as a precipitate. In so doing, it alters the attributes of the solvent and starts a chain of *backward* reactions and precipitations. Such a "*separate*" may be either liquid or solid. It may rise to the surface, or it may subside. It may be visible (solid), or invisible (liquid). It may be mucilaginous or gelatinous, as transparent as the medium it rests in, but yet not a true liquid or a pronounced solid. As this "backward" reaction follows, chains of alterations and precipitations result, so familiar to persons perplexed by ever-altering plant solutions. Bold must be the man who announces that he comprehends the interchanging rearrangements continuously taking place in a solution of associated plant constituents, seemingly stable and apparently quiescent.

"Our three classes of menstrua, with their fourteen numbers thus afford *in themselves*, as various proportions are used, the possibility of an infinite line of combinations. The successive liquids, produced by means of varying abstractions of the constituents of a single plant, may also dovetail into chains of compound solutions in which lines of separation are lost as these substances coalesce, each into the others. In this field, no recorded experiences govern us. The explorer has not attempted even to systematize the various phases of the problem, as applied to the principal constituents of a single known drug, acted upon as a whole by any compound menstruum, indeed, by any simple liquid."

Lloyd has described in even greater detail than excerpted here, using numerous laboratory examples, how the solvency of fluids is altered one by the other and how this is analogous to any botanical extract. The greater the number of solvents used, as also the greater number of plants combined, the more unpredictable the result becomes. This is true to the extent that even altering the order of the procedure using simple (single) substances changes the degree and type of the reactions and interactions. Therefore, the more complex the procedure in producing a botanical extract, the more likely that alterations in the process will result in different outcomes. Due to the complexity of the components involved, the greater is the simplicity in procedure needed to assure a consistent outcome. The only other method of sustaining a consistent outcome is to develop a process so complex as to produce a simplistic product with minimized components. This complex process is the approach chosen by those who produce concentrated extract fractions with little content complexity.

Confusion in the Ranks—
Standardization Claims for Products of Popular Herbs

Asian Ginseng

Asian ginseng is a herb with thousands of years of chronicled use in the Orient. The root and its extracts have also become some of the most popular herbal products in the West in recent years. Because of the great demand and the value placed on its tonic effects, the cost of ginseng is considerably higher than for most other herbs. As a consequence, the likelihood of substitutions or adulteration is greater in the commercial market. The poor quality of some ginseng products can affect the reputation of the herb and its usefulness, so it is important to identify what standards can be applied to assure the expected quality, content, and results.

An analytical comparison of twenty-five commercial ginseng products in the United States was performed by Harkey and others in 2001. These included several products that were not Asian ginseng (*Panax ginseng*) such as san qi, or sanchi, ginseng (*P. notoginseng*), American ginseng (*P. quinquefolius*), and Siberian ginseng (*Eleutherococcus senticosus*, now referred to as eleuthero rather than a type of ginseng). Some of the products combined several types of ginseng. Only six powders and two liquid products labeled only as *Panax ginseng* were included. Ginseng activity is largely dependent on its ginsenoside content. Using high performance liquid chromatography (HPLC) and HPLC-tandem mass spectrometry, the content of total ginsenosides and seven individual ginsenosides (Rb_1, Rb_2, Rc, Rd, Re, Rf, and Rg_1) was measured by quadruplicate determinations, and the ratio of Rg_1 to $Rb1$ was calculated. The individual ginsenoside content and ratios were used along with eleutheroside content to identify the genera. These phytochemical contents confirmed the label designations for each genera. The ginsenoside content and ratios for all of the individual species powders corresponded to the appropriate range for Asian ginseng root and American ginseng root products. However, both of the ginsenoside ratios for the two liquids labeled Asian ginseng were half of the minimum expected amount, while the liquid American ginseng ratios were appropriately low.

For the six Asian ginseng powder products there was no indication as to whether they were powdered roots or extracts. The total ginsenoside content for five ranged from 2.11% to 3.36%, while the other was only 0.29%. Three of the five were labeled as standardized to ginsenoside concentration. For these three the measured ginsenoside content compare to the amount claimed on the label was 65.7%, 136.8%, and 30.6%. Of the two liquid Asian ginseng products, the total ginsenoside content was 0.44% and 0.69%. Only the latter made a label claim for ginsenoside standardization; it contained 68.4% of the claimed amount.

The American Botanical Council initiated the Ginseng Evaluation Program in 1993 to study the commercial ginseng products available in the United States. By means of phytochemical analysis the label claims were compared to the content and consistency of these products as described by Hall and others in 2001. Ginseng product claims for standardization are based on one of three criteria: (1) the weight per dosing unit of the product (for example, 100 mg of ginseng extract), (2) a product claim based on unspecified characteristics or reference points (for example, 100 mg of standardized ginseng extract), and (3) a specific characteristic and criteria which the product claims (for example, 100 mg of ginseng extract standardized to 5% ginsenosides).

Besides evaluating the consistency of the total ginsenoside content, the ginsenoside Rb_1/Rg_1 ratios were also determined in five lots for thirteen different products. A Rb_1/Rg_1 ratio of 1–3 is indicative of the Asian *Panax ginseng* species, while a higher ratio over 10 is indicative of the American *Panax quinquefolius* species that is very low in Rg_1. The study encountered a problem with one product whose early claims were based on UV spectrophotometric tests that gave an artificially high ginsenoside level compared to the HPLC test that was used in this program and as a standard by other companies for testing products.

Of the 13 root and extract products, 5 extracts did not make total ginsenoside content claims but had the following average ginsenoside content per capsule [and Rb_1/Rg_1 ratio range]: 5.5 mg [1.0–3.1], 6.2 mg [1.0–3.9], 7.8 mg [0.9–3.4], 2.9 mg [0.4–3.2], and 6.9 mg [0.9–2.8]. Overall, these products that claimed no specific ginsenoside levels were, with one exception (2.9 mg per capsule), relatively consistent as a group and contained on average from 5.5–7.8 mg total ginsenosides. All had Rb_1/Rg_1 ratios compatible with true Asian ginseng.

Of the 3 root and 5 extract products claiming standardization to a total ginsenoside content, 3 made Rb_1/Rg_1 ratio claims of 0.5–2.0. All of the lots of these 3, and the lots of 3 of the other 5 were in the Rb_1/Rg_1 1–3 range, while the lots of the other 2 ranged from 2–4 and 3–5. All 8 appeared to provide the appropriate Asian species. As for the total ginsenoside content claims, 7 of 8 products provided at least the minimum content in 80–100% of their five lots where the amounts and claims could be determined and claim was based on the same test (HPLC). One root product had only a quarter to a half of the ginsenoside content claimed in each of the five lots but averaged 9.2 mg per capsule. The average total ginsenoside content per capsule of 6 of the standardized products ranged from 6.9–12.9 mg with one lower (4.0 mg) and one higher (17.7 mg). In general, those claiming to be standardized to specific ginsenoside contents delivered more than those that did not make a content claim. Overall, the product consistency was deemed reasonable.

While this portion of the Ginseng Evaluation Project assessed consistency in only 13 products, a future report will detail results of ginseng content for over 500 commercial products. The greatest discrepancy was in the actual meaning of the term standardized as it appeared on the labels.

EPHEDRA

For certain herbs a phytochemical content that describes a chemical category of active components is sometimes interpreted as representing the activity of a significant component that is a member of that class. A prime example of this scenario is the controversial herb ephedra. This is a concern not only based upon its legimate use but also its commercial and consumer abuse. Chinese ephedra (*Ephedra sinensis*), known as ma huang, has been safely used as a water extract for treatment of colds and asthma for thousands of years in Asia. When one of its major alkaloids called ephedrine was discovered in the late 19th century, it was soon turned into a pharmaceutical isolate for its use in asthma. At that time American ephedra species were shown by Nielsen and others to lack alkaloids and so were unsuitable for comparable use or as a source of ephedrine, although some European species did contain the same alkaloids including the other major alkaloid pseudoephedrine. Since then, pseudoephedrine has become even more popular as a decongestant.

As described by Malchow-Moller and others, the serendipitous discovery in 1972 by a doctor in Elsinore, Denmark, that ephedrine could aid in weight loss occurred from using it for asthma in a products that also contained caffeine. Research showed that caffeine could enhance ephedrine's effects of increasing metabolism and diminishing the appetite. Unfortunately, since both of these plant-derived alkaloids are stimulants, there are a variety of potential adverse effects that may occur with their over-consumption. Cardiovascular toxicity was described by Pentel in 1984 as one problem of abuse for those who consumed excessive amount of pharmaceutical ephedrine and caffeine, alone or in combination, as legal stimulants.

Such herbal combinations products as "Herbal Ecstacy" have this same potential, as described by Zahn and others in a case report in 1999 and have a reputation for use at strenuous dance "raves" according to Brown and others in 1995. In addition, the combination has become popular in energy drinks and supplements used by athletes before exercise. The added stress on the cardiovascular system from intense physical activity apparently increases the risks of ephedrine/caffeine adverse effects, since these mixtures are no longer only consumed in measured amounts, whether isolated or in herbs or extracts that contain them, as previously when designed for use before meals for weight loss or with four to six hour intervals for asthma. The pharmacokinetics of ephedrine that describe its rate and degree of absorption, as studied by Gurley and others in 1998[a], is relatively the same whether it is taken as an encapsulated isolated alkaloid or as capsules or tablets of several different ephedra products.

Complicating the risk is an individualized sensitivity to the stimulant effects of these alkaloids, so that a tolerable dose for some could become unpredictably excessive for others. Besides relatively common indicators of excessive use or overdosage such as palpitations, high blood pressure and insomnia, a number of reports of stroke, heart attack and death have also been associated with its use as reported by Haller and Benowitz in 2000, Samenuk and others in 2002, and Shekelle and others in 2003.

The preparation process is another factor affecting both activity and toxicity. Lee and others in 2000 found that the toxicity of ephedra extracts to several cell lines in test tubes was least after boiling the unground stems for two hours (the traditional method of preparation), even though this resulted in the highest ephedrine content. Preparations made from ground ephedra that was not boiled or briefly boiled were 2–4 times more toxic to the cell cultures, based on the amount for inhibiting half the growth of the cells. The cells most affected by the extracted non-alkaloidal toxins were nerve cells.

The safety concerns surrounding ephedra are further complicated when products labeled as standardized to a particular alkoidal content are not reliably produced. Variations in alkaloid content and in the percentage of label claims were first documented in a preliminary report by Gurley and others in 1998[b]. This was followed by a more in-depth report by Gurley and others in 2000 that specifically focused on ephedra products in regard to their label claims by measuring 15 samples from each product. Using HPLC to determine content of 5 ephedra alkaloids, 20 products were examined; 7 claimed a specific ephedrine content, and 9 others claimed only a total alkaloid content, while 4 made no component claims (including ephedra weight content). Of the 7 making specific ephedrine claims, the actual content ranged from 25–105% of the claim. Of these, 3 were above 80% of claimed ephedrine content, and 2 were below 55%. For all of these 7, the total alkaloid content was from 90-125% of the ephedrine claim, indicating that they considered all of the ephedrine-like alkaloids to be equivalent to ephedrine. This is a pharmacological fallacy. Of the 9 making only total alkaloid content claims, 7 were from 80–110%, while 2 were lower than 70%. Of 4 products with alkaloid content label claims in which samples from two different lots were tested, 3 had significant different ephedrine and/or total alkaloid content in the different lots for the same product. One of these, Herbal Ecstacy, tested low for ephedrine in one lot and high for total alkaloids in both lots. This was due to a higher pseudoephedrine than ephedrine content in samples of both lots.

The lack of consistency in products is ascertained by the variety of proportions in the profile of their alkaloids. An interesting aspect of this 2000 Gurley study was the analytical breakdown of total alkaloids that identified 5 different compounds. Of the 20 brand name products, 1 contained no alkaloids, 3 contained only ephedrine, 6 contained only ephedrine and pseudoephedrine, 4 contained these two plus methylephedrine, 1 contained these three plus norephedrine, and 5 contained these four plus norpseudoephedrine. Reasonable conjecture suggests that the 1 product lacking alkaloids and the 3 with only ephedrine are questionable species. In those 6 species with only ephedrine and pseudoephedrine, ephedrine was always in significantly higher quantities. However, in the 10 products with more than two alkaloids the ratio of ephedrine:pseudoephedrine (E:P) varied greatly. For four products the E:P ratio ranged from 14:1 to 6:1, for 3 products E:P was from 2:1 to 4:3, and for two products it was from 3:4 to 1:3. However, in 1 product in which two lots were studied the differences in the E:P ratio between these two lots of the same product was 5:1 and 1:2.

The significance of these different alkaloid contents and E:P ratios between products is made clear by a study by Moriyasu and others in 1984. They used HPLC to compare individual alkaloid content of sulfuric acid extracts of 9 different ephedra species. The content of four different alkaloids was determined for each species. One (*E. ciliata*) lacked alkaloids. Of the rest all contained both ephedrine and pseudoephedrine in much higher quantities than the norephedrine and norpseudoephedrine that were always very low, indicating that they could have been missed on a less sensitive assay. The E:P ratios varied between species from 10:1 (*E. distachya*) to 1:12 (*E. intermedia*). While their sample of *E. sinensis* showed an unusual E:P ratio of 1: 2.3, the commercial ma huang had a typical ratio of 2.5:1.

Another alkaloidal analysis of 3 Chinese ephedra species by Jian and others in 1988 also used HPLC for extracts made with stronger sulfuric acid. Their finding for *E. sinensis* was an E:P ratio of 2.5:1, while the ratio for *E. intermedia* was 1:5.7. The norpseudoephedrine content of these species was from 9–10% of the total alkaloids. *E. equisetina* had the greatest ephedrine content, an E:P ratio of 2.8:1 and 22% of its total alkaloids was norpseudoephedrine. Even though alkaloid content can vary in each species according to times and processes used for growng, collecting, and drying, it appears that many different species are used as source material for ephedra products. Though Gurley and others failed to identify the species claimed for the 20 products in their 2000 studies, all 9 of these that were featured in their original 1998 study claimed to contain the traditional Chinese species *Ephedra sinensis*. Results indicated otherwise.

ST. JOHN'S WORT

The concept of standardization is intended to give some assurance of consistency, equivalency, and, hopefully, efficacy when clinical use is based upon research utilizing a standardized product. However, research indicates this has not necessarily been the case. In a well-publicized report in 1998 on St. John's wort (*Hypericum perforatum*) products standardized to hypericin as a marker, *The Los Angeles Times* reported its spectrophotometric test of these products. The article claimed to be examining the "potency" of these products, based on label claims, even though the author Monmaney noted: "Scientists say that hypericin is not the only, and probably not even the primary, ingredient of antidepressant activity in St. John's wort." Quality, authenticity, purity, and strength are goals of standardization, though in reality none of these aspects were tested. The findings indicated that 7 of 10 of the products tested had between 75% to 135% of label claims for hypericin, while 3 contained one half or less of the claimed content.

`Permissible ranges for content relative to label claims differs according to experts from 80–120% for a University of Michigan clinical pharmacist to 90–110% for a senior scientist at the *U.S. Pharmacopeia*. However, at least 3 companies complained that their claims were based upon a more accurate method of assay (HPLC) that gave a 20% higher finding. The spectrophotometric test was the standard at that time, so those companies utilizing superior technology than the standard were portrayed as making fraudulent claims. Such a report is not surprising, given the sensationalistic nature of much news reporting. Hopefully, research deemed suitable for publication in peer-reviewed scientific journals would be expected to recognize and address such inequities.

However, an article published in a science journal by Constantine and Karchesy the same year produced a similar analysis of 8 commercial St. John's wort products, 4 of which were from the same companies involved in the *LA Times* report. Again, hypericin content was analyzed with a spectrophotometer as a marker of identification. The UV analysis was performed in spite of at least 2 of the companies using more accurate methods (the same ones identified in the *Times* report). In this study the variation from claimed content was from 47–165% with 4 of the 8 products between 80–120% (2 from 90–110%). Of the 4 companies whose products were analyzed in both studies, the comparative percentages of label claims changed (from the *LA Times* to the from 78.9% to 80.3%, 50.6% to 57.0%, 76.7% to 100.7%, 131.4% to 47.0%, indicative of inherent variation in "standardized" products even for certain companies.

An interesting corollary to the study by Constantine and Karchesy was the examination of specimens of different parts of St. John's wort plants harvested at various sites in Oregon to examine the natural variation in hypericin content. From 4 sites in one county the leaves, stems, and flowers together yielded 0.037–0.097% hypericin. From 6 sites in four other counties the leaves and flowers contained 0.011-0.138%, but the combined flowers only from these 6 sites yielded 0.387%. This clearly demonstrates the advantage of harvesting the reproductive parts of the plants to maximize hypericin, and the need to concentrate extracts of the whole plant to achieve the same levels that occur naturally in the flowers. Unfortunately, the dates of collection were not noted, a factor that causes great variation in the content of plant organs and hypericin as documented by Tekel'ova and others in 2000.

Recently it has been recognized that hyperforin is likely the major contributor to St. John's wort antidepressant effect. However, many commercial products fail to make standardization claims for this compound rather than hypericin due to its rapid degradation from light and oxygen. Two studies compared contents of flavonoids, hypericins, and hyperforin in different unnamed commercial products. A report by Liu and others in 2000 used HPLC to measure phytochemical contents in five products purchased in Arkansas. Another report by Ganzera and others in 2002 utilized HPLC to analyze five products purchased in 1998 and twelve products in 2000 from Mississippi and California. Individually, the 5–6 flavonoids, pseudohypericin, hypericin, and hyperforin varied greatly between the products within both studies. The findings by Ganzera showed the content of total flavonoids and hypericins were similar from both years, but hyperforin was much lower on average in the older products due to its instability.

Unfortunately, neither of these two reports specified which of the products were herbs or extracts nor which claimed to be standardized. Ganzera and others noted that their products were capsule and tablets containing extract or plant material. Of these, most were only standardized to "hypericins," and none of those with label claims of 0.3% hypericin or 4.0% hyperforin could be confirmed. In the 1998 products they measured 0.05–0.12% hypericins and 0–0.25% hyperforin, while in the 2000 products they found from 0.03-0.15% hypericins and 0.07–1.30% hyperforin in the products. They noted that verifying label claims was difficult because standardization methods were not noted on the label (for example, unspecific photometry or selective HPLC). Also, standardized extracts contain not only the extract but up to 8 other ingredients such as excipients as well. Liu and others determined the percentage of total hypericins of their 5 brands of capsules ranged from 0.05–0.26%, while hyperforin was from 0.19–1.00% of the entire capsular content.

A study by De los Reyes and Koda in 2002 used HPLC to determine the content of both hyperforin and hypericin in 6 brands (5 American, 1 German) of extract powder, capsules or caplets and one brand of the encapsulated whole herb that made label claims only for hypericin. Hypericin content claims were 0.3% for 4 extracts, 0.2% for 2 extracts, and 0.15% for the herb. The variation of hypericin content from the claimed level of standardization was from 56.6% to 130.0% for the extracts, while the herb capsule had 80.9%. It was not noted whether the capsules or caplets contained other ingredients besides the extracts or herb.

The potency based on percentage of hyperforin contained in the products (for which no label content claims were being made) was from 0.05–1.89%, while the encapsulated herb had 0.20%. For the extracts there was no obvious correlation between percentage content of label claim for hypericin and potency based on hyperforin content. For example, the extract with the highest percentage of the hypericin claim (130.0%) had the lowest hyperforin content (0.05%). Nonetheless, there were a couple of products (1 German, 1 American) that had both accurate hypericin claims (98% and 110%, respectively) and significant hyperforin content (1.89% and 1.16%, respectively).

Another comparison of products in 2002 was accomplished by Ang and others who utilized liquid chromatography (LC) with UV detection, confirmed by photodiode array spectra and LC/mass spectrometry. They analyzed 3 St. John's wort extracts "standardized to 0.3% hypericin," St. John's wort cut and sifted leaves/flowers, a tea bag, a multiple herb tea bag, and a number of functional foods for hyperforin, adhyperforin, hypericin, and pseudohypericin. One of the extracts was "extra strength," one also contained the herb and millet, and the third had a number of excipients added. Therefore, product content percentages of hypericins were variable: 0.25%, 0.20%, and 0.15%. The nonstandardized contents of hyperforins were 0.80%, 1.28%, and 0.45%. The 3 described products were not identified with the particular contents.

The cut and sifted herb and St. John's wort tea bag contents had 0.13% and 0.21% hypericins and 1.06% and 0.51% hyperforins, respectively. The tea bag herb mixture containing St. John's wort and 7 other herbs had very low amounts of hypericins and hyperforins. The functional foods included "puffs," a snack bar, and 3 noncarbonated drinks. These combination ingredient products all had extremely low or undetectable amounts of hypericins and no detectable hyperforins.

As Constantine and Karchesy demonstrated, St. John's wort herb hypericin content reflects not only the plant part, but as indicated by Tekel'ova and others, a consistently high hypericin and hyperforin content depends on the date the flowers are harvested. Hypericin rises from 0.10% as the buds open into flowers with 0.45% (around the end of June at the time of the Catholic feast day for the birth of St. John the Baptist) and then rapidly diminishes to 0.04% as the unripe fruit develop in early July, whereas hyperforin continually increases from 2.47% as young buds grow and form flowers with 6.68% that change into unripe fruit with 8.48%. Pseudohypericin follows the same changing content pattern as hypericin. (These two together are typically measured in standardized extracts as "total hypericins.") The flavonoids also follow the same pattern of increasing and diminishing with flower and fruit formation, respectively. So, on the basis of content of significant hyperforin and maximum flavonoids, documented standardization to relatively high levels of hypericin could serve as one quality indicator for the unextracted flowers.

BLACK COHOSH

The concept of standardization is intended to provide some assurance of consistency in a product, especially when applied to some of the best researched brand name extracts. In considering one of the most advertised botanical products for the aging baby-boomer generation, the perception of consistency lacking. According to Blumenthal and Malone in 1998, "all of the scientific research" is based on "one" proprietary black cohosh (*Cimicifuga [Actaea] racemosa*) product, Remifemin®. They describe the solid extract, manufactured by Schaper and Brümmer, as standardized on the basis of 1 mg triterpene glycosides per tablet, calculated as 27-deoxyacteine. This was re-iterated in 2001 by McKenna and others in describing the product as a 20 mg tablet of plant extract standardized to 1 mg of triterpene glycosides calculated as 27-deoxyactein.

However, both of these review articles note that most studies were done using a liquid extract, while McKenna and others quoted the company's scientific brochure as describing this product strength of 40 drops as equivalent to 40 mg of the herbal drug and containing a total of 2 mg of triterpene glycosides, "equal" to 2 tablets. So the scientific studies of one named product are actually two separate extracts and forms. The doses used in the studies on these two forms range from 2–8 tablets to 40 drops of the ethanolic liquid extract daily.

In an article in1998 by Liske of the company Schaper and Brümmer, he reviews the literature on Remifemin® and describes the two Remifemin® products. One is a 60% ethanol/40% aqueous liquid preparation, and the other is a 40% isopropanol/60% aqueous extract converted into a solid tablet. The different solvent capabilities of 60% ethyl alcohol versus 40% isopropyl alcohol make the solute content of these extracts distinct, while the process of removing the toxic isopropanol solvent to make a solid extract likewise would lead to chemical alterations. At this date Liske did not make any claims about product standardization to triterpene glycosides, though in reference to the rootstock he claims that they "are considered its decisive components" without explaining what this means. While the root was noted as containing a variety of compounds, no distinctions were made between the content of components found in the traditional ethanolic extract and the solid extract made with isopropyl alcohol (rubbing alcohol) as a solvent except to say that both lacked estrogenic isoflavones. He also noted the lack of estrogenic effects for both ethanolic and isopropanolic-aqueous extracts.

The description of Remifemin® based on a translation of German scientific brochure from Schaper and Brümmer in 1997 is that each tablet is equivalent to 0.018–0.026 ml liquid extract of the rootstock; the extract is 0.78–1.14 : 1 strength, corresponding to 20 mg dried root. Other ingredients include cellulose powder, lactose monohydrate, potato starch, magnesium stearate, and peppermint oil.

The first scientific study on this product published in English by Düker and others in 1991 described the Remifemin® tablets used as each containing 2 mg of a dried aqueous-ethanolic extract of the rhizome of *Cimicifuga racemosa*, 2 tablets yielding 8 mg of extract daily. The math in this description is obviously erroneous. The product description is likewise questionable, based on Liske's description of the tablet as an aqueous-isopropanolic extract. Duker and others described a separate methanolic extract (not Remifemin®) with 3 chloroform fractions that showed estrogenic effects. Liske noted that research showed ethanolic and isopropanolic extracts do not have estrogenic effects. This demonstrates the solvent differences for extracting bioactive compounds when using different types of alcohol (ethanol and isopropenol versus methanol).

A difference between the ethanolic and isopropanolic extracts was elicited in hormonal assays using yeast cells with human estrogen alpha-receptors to test estrogen-dependent gene transcription. Only the isopropanolic extract was shown to have an anti-estrogenic effect in this system utilized by Zierau and others in 2002.

In 2003 the American Botanical Council published *The ABC Clinical Guide to Herbs* (senior editor Mark Blumenthal) that included a description of the Remifemin® isopropanolic solid extract stating: "One tablet contains black cohosh extract corresponding to 20 mg of the drug standardized to 1% 27-deoxyacteine." An errata to the book was published on April 15, 2003, indicated that the correct description should be: "One tablet contains black cohosh extract with monitoring of active compounds (triterpene glycosides) corresponding to 20 mg of crude drug." According to this, the overt quantitative standard now appears to be the 20 mg of the crude drug (whole root) from which the extract is made. Likewise, the description for the liquid (ethanolic) extract states: "Twenty drops correspond to 20 mg of crude drug." A label claim of specific phytochemical content is no longer made for either preparation, though the triterpenes are still assumed to be active and their content monitored in the tablet form. The changing descriptions of these two "standardized" products with the same name have become, as Alice said in Wonderland, "curiouser and curiouser."

According to Remington's *Practice of Pharmacy* 6th ed. in 1917, one ml of *Cimicifuga* fluid extract (1 gm root :1 ml extract) is 37 drops. Using comparative proportions, liquid Remifemin® is 1/27 fluid extract strength. The dried rubbing alcohol extract tablets, meanwhile, apparently contain fillers, binders and flavoring with 20 mg of an extract made from 20 mg of rhizome. Of course, comparing proportional amounts of a weak to a concentrated liquid extract and a solid extract to the intact herb does not suggest equivalency between these forms. However, it does demonstrate the unusually dilute nature of this modern standardized product.

ECHINACEA

A final example of standardization illustrates how its use can be misconstrued in attempting to evaluated the quality, and even the identity, of products. In an attempt to assess the validity of label claims, in 2003 Gilroy and others obtained 59 preparations sold as echinacea in the Denver metropolitan area. The investigators decided to use thin layer chromatography (TLC) as a means of determining the legitimacy of content claims for these products. They based the interpretation of their findings on the assumption that the relative content of *Echinacea purpurea* could be determined by the cichoric acid yield. They also assayed echinacoside as the marker for *E. angustifolia* to differentiate these two species.

The third commercial echinacea species, *E. pallida,* also contains echinacoside, therefore this marker could not be used as a means of distinguishing this species from *E. angustifolia.* Five of the 59 samples were identified on their labels as *E. pallida,* but the authors states that differentiating between it and *E. angustifolia* "was never a concern." Unfortunately, the authors failed to note claims about the part of the plant used. Normally, *E. pallida* and *E. angustifolia* roots are the parts used for such products. If this is true for these samples, species identification can be made by the caffeoyl phenolic compound cynarin present in *E. angustifolia* roots but absent in *E. pallida* roots (and *E. purpurea* as well), as shown by Perry and others in 2001.

The roots can also be easily distinguished due to *E. pallida* root's lack of the tongue-tingling isobutylamides that typify *E. angustifolia* (and *E. purpurea*). Isobutylamides and the polyacetylene or 2-ketoalkenes and 2-ketoalkyne components found in *E. pallida* are readily demonstrable by TLC. The authors referenced the research by Bauer and Remiger in 1989 that describe these differences with TLC, but surprisingly use this means to only identify the phenolic markers. In addition, Cheminat and others determined in 1988 that cichoric acid was the main phenolic product in *E. pallida* flowers and leaves, with some was present in the root as well. Likewise, Perry and others in 2001 found cichoric acid in *E. angustifolia* roots, making this a nonspecific marker for absolutely identifying *E. purpurea.*

The inadequacy of using the phenolics, cichoric acid and echinacoside, as suitable echinacea markers, as well as not characterizing the processed forms of the samples, come to bear on the issue of evaluating *E. purpurea* products. The juice of the aerial plant preserved with 22% ethanol is an established remedy, and the most researched echinacea product on the market. In 1999 both Bauer and Kreuter indicated that the enzyme polyphenol oxidase rapidly breaks down cichoric acid in the cold-pressed fresh juice. Kreuter pointed out that clinical research had employed the cold-pressed and unheated *E. purpurea* plant juice, so only this juice with little or no cichoric acid has been proven clinically effective. When the juice is heated to destroy the enzyme, cichoric acid will be consistently retained. However, in 1999 Bauer found that heat-stabilized juice products had much lower isobutylamide content on average. The isobutylamide components are believed to be more therapeutically active as immune enhancers than the cichoric acid.

Arnason reported that in 1998 Bauer observed that cichoric acid declines in tinctures in six days. Livesey and others indicated in 1999 that cichoric acid diminished in tinctures with 55% alcohol at room temperature after 7 months but was stable in powder during this time even at higher temperatures. Nusslein and others in 2000 showed cichoric acid could be preserved in aqueous extracts over four weeks by adding 50 mM ascorbic acid or 40% ethanol. Thus, it is obviously necessary to characterize the form of the product when assessing relative cichoric acid content, rather than generalizing average content to all forms.

In their evaluation Gilroy and others did not identify these products as powdered root/plant or extracts, but simply reported that 9 were tablets, 32 were capsules, 4 were softgels, and 14 were liquids. Only 21 of the products were standardized, but their forms were not specified. The standardized products had much lower recommended doses, suggesting that these were solid extracts rather than the root. It is obvious that the softgels and liquids were extracts, as were likely some of the tablets and capsules. Whether these were processed as pressed plant juice, its dried powder, or as liquid or solid solvent extracts of fresh or dried roots cannot be deduced. Nonetheless, not all extracts are standardized, so we don't know from the information given what the forms of the standardized products were. Calling all of the products simply echinacea is inherently misleading, since they represent many possible identities: root, aerial plant, juice, or their solvent extracts and concentrates. (See accompanying chart on echinacea formulations.)

The authors' premise in assessing the content of the particular caffeoyl phenolic markers is understandable, since these compounds are typically used to "standardize" products of these species. They addressed those products that claimed to be standardized to specific polyphenols. Of the nine samples that identified either echinacoside or cichoric acid as markers, none matched the label claim. Rather, seven had on average only 26% of the label claims, and the other two contained no measurable amounts. Ten product labels made claims to be standardized to total phenolics, but this fails to distinguish between particular species markers. In his talk at an international echinacea conference in 1999 Arnason noted that even though the total phenolic content had been the common echinacea standard for years, it was a "completely, utterly useless measure, in the opinion of all the phytochemists in the room, as to the quality of echinacea products."

Gilroy and others assayed phenolic marker content of standardized products as well as those whose identifying label claim was simply the species used in the product. It is interesting to note that, based on their phenolic evaluation approach, 21 of 30 (70%) of the nonstandardized products matched the label species claim, while only 10 of 19 (53%) of the standardized products were the appropriate species. For those products containing cichoric acid, the nonstandardized yielded on average about 2.5 times more than the standardized samples. In the products with echinacoside, the content of nonstandardized samples averaged more than 3 times the yield of those that were standardized. The doses of nonstandardized products were about twice those of standardized.

Finally, Gilroy and others claim that only four of the products (7%) met the four FDA labeling requirements. They observe that the better compliance score for standardized than nonstandardized products was due to the presence of the "Supplements Facts" box. However, products that do not make standardization or structure/function activity claims and companies that have less than 100 employees are exempt from this label requirement. The authors' conclusion that the "claim of "standardization" does not mean the preparation is accurately labeled, nor does it indicate less variability in concentration of constituents of the herb," is an appropriate assessement of these echinacea products. One could accurately state that standardization claims provide no basis for determination of quality of these products in terms of therapeutic efficacy. Trying to evaluate echinacea products on the basis of phenolic markers without specifying the plant part and form of each preparation being assessed is meaningless. Even knowing those features is of little value beyond limited characterization of the product. Quality is a function of effect, not just identity.

As for their effects, a study of ethanolic extracts of the roots by Bauer and others in 1988 of the three major *Echinacea* species looked at the immunological activity in mice of these extracts and their fractions when given orally. All three extracts significantly enhanced phagocytosis, the consumption by immune cells of unwanted particles. The lipophilic fractions containing isobutylamides (*E. angustifolia* and *E. purpurea*) or polyacetylenes (*E. pallida*) were more active than the polar fractions with echinacoside and cynarin (*E. angustifolia*), cichoric acid (*E. purpurea*), or echinacoside (*E. pallida*). For stimulating phagocytosis, a high isobutylamide (a type of alkamide or alkylamide) content in *E. angustifolia* and *E. purpurea* appears most desirable.

Though standardizaton by isobutylamide might seem appropriate, it is uncommon and does not assure the entire beneficial effect of products from these *Echinacea* species.. In 1998 Wills and Stuart assessed the levels of both alkamides and phenolics in 32 brands of manufactured echinacea products. No claims of standardization were noted. The results were individually reported for the different types of preparations. All contained *E. purpurea* and in 6 products this was combined with *E. angustifolia* root or its extracts (3 tablets, 1 capsule, 2 liquid extracts). Tablets included 6 root products, 2 whole herb or tops, and 2 combinations of root and herb. Capsule products analyzed involved 2 from roots, 1 of the herb, and 1 of the combination. Liquid extracts were prepared from the roots (6), herb (6), or their combination (3).

Two samples of each product were analyzed. Although at least one sample of each form had no detectable alkamides, their range and average in liquid extracts was higher than in dried products. For phenolics, the opposite pattern held true;

dry products had a higher range and average phenolic content than liquid extracts. This concurs with the observation by Arnason that cichoric acid appears stable in powdered form, while alkamides are stable in the alcohol extracts, but decline greatly in the powder. In both the dry and liquid products, those with the highest and lowest alkamide or phenolic contents were products of roots, tops, or both. So in attempting to maximize either of these components, the plant part utilized is not as important as the liquid or dry form of the product.

In 2000 Wills and Stuart studied *E. purpurea* storage and showed that undamaged fresh plant material could be kept at room temperature and 60% relative humidity for 30 days with no significant loss of alkamides or cichoric acid. However, storage of the dried and crushed plant led to alkamide degradation at room temperature and above, especially in the light, but not at low temperatures in the dark. Cichoric acid was stable as long as the moisture was low, and enzymes were de-activated by blanching. Perry and others determined in 2000 that storage of oven-dried *E. purpurea* roots for 64 weeks at room temperature led to an 80% reduction in alkamides. Even when stored well below freezing the roots lost a significant amount of alkamides during this time.

Kim and others looked at different drying methods in 2000 and found that for preserving alkamide content in *E. purpurea* roots or leaves, freeze-drying was the best method to employ. In another study with *E. purpurea* flowers the same year Kim and others determined that freeze-drying was much more effective than air-drying for preserving the caffeoyl phenolics cichoric acid and caftaric acid. So, while standardization of echinacea to its multiple active components is improbable, stablization and preservation of both the important alkamides and phenolics appears to be best achieved through freeze-drying.

Table 3   Echinacea Products of Different Types*
         (X = Commercially Available Product)

WHOLE HERB					
Common name	Echinacea	Echinacea	Echinacea	Echinacea	Echinacea
Scientific names	*Echinacea angustifolia*	*Echinacea pallida*	*Echinacea purpurea*	*Echinacea purpurea*	*Echinacea purpurea*
Plant part	Root	Root	Whole plant	Aerial plant	Root
Fresh, living			x		
Freeze-dried	x			x	x
Air/oven dried: bulk	x	x			x
cut/sifted	x	x		x	x
powdered	x			x	x
COMPLEX FRACTIONS					
Fresh herb extracts: Freeze-dried juice				x	
Juice in alcohol				x	
Green tincture	x		x		x
Dried herb extracts: Tea (bag)	x		x	x	x
Tincture	x	x	x		x
Fluid extract	x				x
Solid extracts	x		x	x	x
Standardized concentrates: echinacoside	x	x			
cichoric acid				x	x
total phenolics	x	x	x	x	x
fructofuranosides				x	
SUBFRACTIONS					
Cell culture medium: Polysaccharides				x	
Arabinogalactans				x	

*See Table 1 and Glossary of Terms from Table 1 on pp. 52–54.

Issues of Quality Versus Quantity

Where standardization is concerned, the question arises: what is the appropriate standard? If the product is herbal, the standard is the proper herb and its medicinal portion. Appropriating a subfraction or single component of this herb as the basis for standardization of an herbal product is to establish a substandard. The herb and its therapeutic activities are not limited to the effects of the compound(s) used as the means of phytochemical standardization. If a single chemical compound is used as the standard by which a product is assessed, it then must be perceived as a chemical product, and the herbal complexity in which it is based can best be described as suprastandard, going beyond the standard. To the extent that the chemical product's herbal complexity is most complete, that is, the medicinal part of the plant rather than its extract, this form can rightly be considered the superstandard.

It is clear, as discussed by Awang in 1999, that standardization by identifying and quantifying active components is often not possible. Herbs with unique characterizing active compounds like the ginkgolides in ginkgo prove to be the exception. More commonly, herbs like echinacea, St. John's wort, and ginseng defy simple characterization based on standardizable compounds due to the complexity of their bioactivity and multiple active components. Now, taken in a larger sense as defined by the American Herbal Products Association (Eisner, managing editor) in 2001, "Standardization refers to the body of information and controls necessary to produce material of reasonable consistency. This is achieved through minimizing the inherent variation of natural product composition through quality assurance practices applied to agricultural and manufacturing processes."

In 2001 McGuffin describes how the assessment of quality cannot be accomplished purely on a quantitative basis. He explained how in large part even quantification may not be reliable if the appropriate analytical methods have not been employed. The methods require research and scientific consensus for each type of chemical to achieve validation for use with herbs containing those compounds. The precision and accuracy varies and depends greatly on scrupulously following appropriate protocols. For many botanical compounds no validated methodologies are currently available. Compendia such as the *American Herbal Pharmacopoeia* and the *United States Pharmacopeia* along with the Institute for Nutraceutical Advancement have established some analytical methods utilizing microsopy, high performance liquid chromatography, gas chromatography, thin-layer chromatography, and spectrophotometric analysis for about three dozen herbs with others under development.

As a minimum, identity and quantity that conform to label claims must be assured, and procedures to determine these must be required. When claims go beyond weight of the herb or extract in each dosing unit, standardized assay processes should provide phytochemical profiles of a product that illustrate the appropriate levels of designated markers. They should also indicate the relative presence or absence of the important associated compounds in the same chemical classes. The methodology for this process should follow validated procedures and protocols. More than the measure of a single, possibly added, compound must be required. The process must have established means of documentation to validate claims and ensure public trust and confidence.

After the Council for Responsible Nutrition, in cooperation with the National Nutritional Foods Association (NNFA), the American Herbal Products Association, and the Utah Natural Products Alliance, submitted proposed guidelines to the FDA to address issues of quality concern, the FDA released a draft of proposed Good Manufacturing Practices in 1997. As reported by Boswell in 1998, these company guidelines for extracts include a quality control unit for materials, procedures and tests, along with adequate lab facilities and records. Written procedures must cover identifying and handling of raw materials, lot identification, and rejected materials. Oldest stock must be used first, and expiration dates should be supported by data. Records must be kept for master and batch production and control. Written procedures for testing purity, composition and quality of the product and correct labeling and packaging must be followed. Complaint files must be kept. Distribution records must be adequate for a recall if necessary, and records and samples must be retained. Finally, procedures must be in place for salvaged and returned products. Implementation of these standards by NNFA member companies was to be phased in by 2002, with compliance determined by third-party inspection of manufacturing facilities.

Unfortunately, in a separate ruling on labeling guidelines also described by Boswell, the FDA eliminated the requirement that dried extracts list the name of the solvent used for extraction. This reduces consumers' ability to assess the desirability of the product based on prior chemical treatment of the herb. In this ruling they also made optional for liquid extracts the listing of the ratio of starting material to final volume, which typically serve as a relative indication of strength for otherwise nonstandardized extracts. The FDA also provided that the quantity could be specified by either volume or weight, and the solvents could be listed either on the ingredient list or nutrition label.

In 1999 Landes and Campbell proposed that functional testing may be the ultimate means of establishing biological activity beyond measuring and manipulating content. The effect of an herb is, after all, the reason people use it. However, the appropriate activity, the best means of measuring it, and relative value of this assay compared to those measuring content have not been determined, and these would vary for each herb. Yet products could be designed to pass such assays with flying colors without necessarily producing the desired therapeutic effect better than others that failed the test. In 2001 Miller advocated using functional tests in combination with phytochemical fingerprinting as the best means of assuring quality. Phytochemical assays, even with all of the inherent drawbacks, would not be completely replaced, but assurance of identity and therapeutic efficacy would be enhanced. Ultimately, clinical research to demonstrate efficacy and batch to batch testing to establish and document consistency would still be necessary.

On March 7, 2003 the FDA issued proposals for labeling and manufacturing standards for herbal products and other dietary supplements to establish current good manufacturing practices (GMPs). These include "requirements on design and construction of physical plants that facilitate maintenance, cleaning, and proper manufacturing operations, for quality control procedures, for testing final product or incoming and inprocess materials, for handling consumer complaints, and for maintaining records." According to the FDA press release, "manufacturers of dietary supplements will have to compete based on the quantity of their product, not through potentially misleading labels. ... The proposal includes flexible standards that can evolve with improvements in the state of science, such as in validating tests for identity, purity, quality, strength, and composition of dietary ingredients." We shall see.

References—Standardization

Ang, CYW et al. Determination of St. John's wort components in dietary supplements and functional foods by liquid chromatography. *J. AOAC Internat.*,85(6):1360-9, 2002.

Arnason, JT. North American raw materials: the case for an isobutylamide standardized product. *Echin. Past, Present Future Internat. Conf. 1999 Proc.*, Session Three, pp. 4-5 and slide 40, Skamania, Wash., June 10-12, 1999.

Awang, DVC. Prescribing therapeutic feverfew (Tanacetum parthenium (L.) Schultz Bip., syn. Chrysanthemum parthenium (L.) Bernh.). *Intergrat. Med.*, 1(1):11-13, 1998.

Awang, DVC. Standardization of herbal medicines. *Alt. Ther. Wom. Health,* 1(7):57-9, 1999.

Bauer, R et al. Immunological in vivo and in vitro examinations of echincea extracts. *Arzneim.-Forsch./Drug Res.*, 38(2):276-81, 1988.

Bauer, R and Remiger, P. TLC and HPLC analysis of alkamides in echinacea drugs. *Planta Med.*, 55: 367-71, 1989.

Bauer, R. Standardization of Echinacea purpurea expressed juice with reference to cichoric acid and alkamides. *J. Herbs, Spices Med Plants*, 6(3):51-62, 1999.

Blumenthal, M and Malone, D. Black cohosh – foreign research documents health benefits of a Native American botanical. *Whole Foods,* pp. 32-4, Apr., 1998.

Bone, K. Standardized extracts neither poison nor panacea. *HerbalGram,* 53:50-5, 2001.

Boswell, C. Setting quality standards for dietary supplements. *Chem. Market Reporter Focus Report,* pp. FR13-4, July 13, 1998.

Brown, ERS and others. Use of drugs at 'raves.' *Scot. Med. J.,* 40:168-71, 1995.

Cheminat, A et al. Caffeoyl conjugates from Echinacea species: structures and biological activity. *Phytochem.,* 27(9):2787-94, 1988.

Constantine, GH and Karchesy, J. Variations in hypericin concentrations in Hypericum perforatum L. and commercial products. *Pharmaceut. Biol.,* 36(5):365-7, 1998.

De los Reyes, GC and Koda, RT. Determining hyperforin and hypericin content in eight brands of St. John's wort. *Am. J. Health-Syst. Pharm.,* 59:545-7, 2002.

De Weerdt, CJ et al. Herbal medicines in migraine prevention. *Phytomed.,* 3:225-30, 1996.

Duker, E-M et al. Effects of extracts from Cimicifuga racemosa on gonadotropin release in menopausal women and ovariectomized rats. *Planta Med.,* 57:420-4, 1991.

Eisner, S (man. ed.). *Guidance for Manufacture and Sale of Bulk Botanical Extracts.* Botanical Extracts Comm., Am. Herbal Products Assoc., Silver Spring, MD, 2001.

Ganzera, M et al. Hypericum perforatum – Chemical profiling and quantitative results of St. John's wort products by an improved high-performance liquid chromatography method. *J. Pharm. Sci.,* 91(3):623-30, 2002.

Gilroy, CM et al. Echinacea and truth in labeling. *Arch. Int. Med.,* 163:699-704, 2003.

Gurley, BJ et al. Ephedrine pharmacokinetics after the ingestion of nutritional supplements containing Ephedra sinica (ma huang). *Ther. Drug Monitor.,* 20:439-445, 1998[a].

Gurley, BJ et al. Ephedrine-type alkaloid content of nutritional supplements containing Ephedra sinica (ma-huang) as determined by high performance liquid chromatography. *J. Pharm. Sci.,* 87(12):1547-53, 1998[b].

Gurley, BJ et al. Content versus label claims in ephedra-containing dietary supplements. *Am. J. Health-Syst. Pharm.,* 57:963-9, 2000.

Hall, T et al. Evaluation of consistency of standardized Asian ginseng products in the Ginseng Evaluation Program. *HerbalGram,* 52:31-46, 2001.

Haller, CA and Benowitz, NL. Adverse cardiovascular and central nervous system events associated with dietary supplements containing ephedra alkaloids. *NEJM,* 343:1833-8, 2000.

Harkey, MR et al. Variability in commercial ginseng products: an analysis of 25 preparations. *Am. J. Clin. Nutr.,* 73:1101-6, 2001.

Jian Z, et al. Simultaneous determination of six alkaloids in Ephedrae Herba by high performance liquid chromatography. *Planta med.,* 54(1):69-70, 1988.

Johnson, ES et al. Efficacy of feverfew as prophylactic treatment of migraine. *Br. Med. J.,* 291:569-73, 1985.

Kim, H-O et al. Retention of caffeic acid derivatives in dried Echinacea purpurea. *J. Agric. Food Chem.,* 48:4182-6, 2000.

Kim, H-O et al. Retention of alkamides in dried Echinacea purpurea. *J. Agric. Food Chem.,* 48: 4187-92, 2000.

Kreuter, M. Echinacea purpurea substances, characteristics and immunological active principles. *Echin. Past, Present Future Internat. Conf. 1999 Proc.,* Session Two, p. 3 and slide 7, Skamania, Wash., June 10-12, 1999.

Landes, B and Campbell, TC. Functional testing – could this be the future of herbal quality assurance? *AHPA Report,* pp. 1, 10–2, 1999.

Lee, MK et al. Cytotoxicity assessment of ma-huang (Ephedra) under different conditions of preparation. *Toxicol. Sci.,* 56:424–30, 2000.

Liske, E. Therapeutic efficacy and safety of Cimicifuga racemosa for gynecologic disorders. *Adv. Ther.,* 15(1):45–53, 1998.

Liu, FF et al. Evaluation of major active components in St. John's wort dietary supplements by high-peformance liquid chromatography with photodiode array detection and electrospray mass spectrometric confirmation. *J. Chromatogr.,* 888:85–92, 2000.

Livesey, J et al. Effect of temperature on stability of marker constituents in Echinacea purpurea root formulations. *Phytomed.,* 6(5):347–9, 1999.

Malchow-Moller, A et al. Ephedrine as an anorectic: the story of the 'Elsinore pill'. *Internat. J. Obes.,* 5:183–7, 1981.

McGuffin, M. Issues of quality: analyzing herbal materials and the current status of methods validation. *HerbalGram,* 53:44–9, 2001.

McKenna, DJ et al. Black cohosh: efficacy, safety, and use in clinical and preclinical applications. *Alternat. Ther.,*7(3):93–100, 2001.

Miller, MJS. Herbal medicine standardization: problems and possibilities. *JANA,* 3(4):1–2, 2001.

Monmany, T. Labels'potency claims often inaccurate, analysis finds. *The Los Angeles Times,* p. A10, Aug. 31, 1998.

Moriyasu, M et al. High-performance liquid chromatographic determination of organic substances by metal chelate derivatization. III. Analysis of Ephedra bases. *Chem. Pharm. Bull.,* 32(2):744–7, 1984.

Murphy, JJ et al. Randomised double-blind placebo-controlled trial of feverfew in migraine prevention. *Lancet,* pp. 189–92, July 23, 1988.

Murray, MT. Understanding the benefits of standardized botanical extracts. *Am. J. Nat. Med.,* 3(8):6–12, 1996.

Nusslein, B et al. Enzymatic degradation of cichoric acid in Echinacea purpurea preparations. *J. Nat. Prod.,* 63:1615–1618, 2000.

Nielsen, C et al. The occurrence and alkaloidal content of various Ephedra species. *J. Am. Pharm. Assoc.,* 16(4):288–94, 1927.

Palevitch, D et al. Feverfew (Tanacetum parthenium) as a prophylactic treatment for migraine: a double-blind placebo-controlled study. *Phtyother. Res.,* 11:508–11, 1997.

Patterson, E. Standardized extracts: herbal medicine of the future? *Herb Market Review,* pp. 37–8, 1996.

Pentel, P. Toxicity of over-the-counter stimulants. *JAMA,* 252(14):1898–1903, 1984.

Perry, NB et al. Alkamide levels in Echinacea purpurea: Effects of processing, drying and storage. *Planta Med.,* 66:54–6, 2000.

Perry, NB et al. Echinacea standardization: Analytical methods for phenolic compounds and typical levels in medicinal species. *J. Agric. Food Chem.,* 49:1702–6, 2001.

Pfaffenrath, V et al. The efficacy and safety of Tanacetum parthenium (feverfew) in migraine prophylaxis—a double-blind, multicentre, randomized placebo-controlled dose-response study. *Cephalg.*, 22:523–32, 2002.

Samenuk, D et al. Adverse cardiovascular events temporally associated with ma huang, an herbal source of ephedrine. *Mayo Clin. Proc.*, 77:12–6, 2002.

Shekelle, PG et al. Efficacy and safety of ephedra and ephedrine for weight loss and athletic performance. *JAMA*, 289(12):1537–1545, 2003.

Tekel'ova, D et al. Quantitative changes of dianthrones, hyperforin and flavonoids content in the flower ontogenesis of Hypericum perforatorum. *Planta Med.*, 66:778–89, 2000.

Tierra, M. Standardized herb extracts: an herbalist's perspective. *Natural Foods Merchandiser*, pp. 54–5, Feb., 1999.

Wills, RBH and Stuart, DL. Evels of active constituents in manufactured Echinacea products. *Chem. Austral.*, 17–19, Sept., 1998.

Wills, RBH and Stuart, DL. Effect of handling and storage on alkylamides and cichoric acid in Echinacea purpurea. *J. Sci. Food Agric.*, 80(9):1402–6, 2000

Zahn, KA et al. Cardiovascular toxicity after ingestion of "Herbal Ecstacy." *J. Emerg. Med.*, 17(2):289–291, 1999.

Zierau, O et al. Antiestrogenic activities of Cimicifuga racemosa extracts. *J. Ster. Biochem. Mol. Biol.*, 80:125–130, 2002.

Freeze-Drying

The drying of fresh flash-frozen herbs by converting and removing ice as water vapor under reduced pressure is technically known as lyophilization. Its industrial application was developed in the 1930s, and the widespread use and isolation of penicillin only became possible as a result of freeze-drying. Its application to several pharmaceutical plant drugs was extensively researched and discussed in the *Journal of the American Pharmaceutical Association* in the 1950s. This process both preserves the components found in the fresh plant and concentrates juices or aqueous extracts. This is done by means of physics, not chemistry. Concentration occurs by reducing the volume through removal of only water. When applied to herbs, freeze-drying prevents most enzymatic conversions of active constituents. By avoiding common causes of component degradation, the content and activity of the fresh herbs are better preserved with indefinite shelflife under optimal conditions.

It is the simplicity of the process that allows for the retention of the inherent complexity and integrity of the components that determines the activity available in the fresh plant. By minimizing enzymatic and solvent influences, chemical changes are also reduced. Freezing, the lowering of temperature to produce a solid from a liquid, is by nature the means of reducing and practically stopping change, primarily chemical alterations, from occurring. Heat is increased molecular activity, and when the temperature is raised to change ice crystals into water in the solid matrix of plant tissue, it is instantly vaporized and removed in the negative pressure (vacuum) in the chamber, so that when the water crystals are fully removed the formerly frozen material is stabilized. Lack of water or other fluid environment is another means of assuring minimal chemical change. The frozen-dehydrated plant material, unlike air or oven-dried herbs, is porous and easily crumbles so the powdering process generates practically no heat from the friction of grinding.

The powdered plant is then encapsulated and bottled to prevent the influence of oxygen, moisture, and light from changing and deactivating the components responsible for the medicinal effects. The capsules provide a simple means of consuming appropriate amounts of what might otherwise be considered distasteful fresh herbs. The microscopic structures of the powder resulting from the freeze-drying process reveal compartmental separation with adjacent spacing that allows the solids to become readily re-hydrated when exposed to fluids or taken internally. This enables rapid dissolution and better digestion in the gut that can thereby improve assimilation through increasing the rate and amount of absorption of active components.

As described by Kern, the application of freeze-drying in pharmaceutical manufacturing has several major advantages: properties of labile substances remain unchanged, preservaton is prolonged, and the solubility of lyophilized products is fast and complete.

Preserving Nutrients—Fresh Fruits/Vegetables/Mushrooms

Most of the research with freeze-drying plants has been done with foods. Since part of the value of whole medicinal herbs is their content of nutrient components that provide adjunctive health benefits, it is important to see how the freeze-drying process helps preserve these contributors as well.

One advantage of freeze-drying whole vegetables and fruit is their ability to rapidly regain their fresh structure. Freeze-dried green beans had a size, shape and color similar to when fresh and reconstituted more rapidly in either hot or cold water than those that were dehydrated by other methods, according to Hamed in 1966 and Foda and others in 1967. Hamed showed the vitamin C and beta-carotene were preserved 3.5 and 4.5 times better, respectively, for freeze-dried than air-dried green beans. For green beans, garden peas and spinach Weits and others in 1970 found the retention of vitamins and minerals was best when freeze-drying compared to air-drying, canning, or deep-freezing.

Constituent preservation depends somewhat on the type of plant and its other components. Peaches and apricots that were freeze-dried were compared with fresh for their beta-carotene and vitamins B1, B2, and C content by Popovskii and Sarukhanyan in 1974. Freeze-drying provided good taste qualities and shape retention, as well as easy rehydration, but some loss of vitamin C occurred in most varieties. Fonseca and others in 1972 found the loss of vitamin C in papaya and passion fruit was 0-7% during freeze-drying and storage for up to 7 months, but strawberries lost 37–42% during dehydration in this study. Beta-carotene was very well preserved except for yellow papaya that lost 5% during drying and passion fruit that lost 75% during the first month of storage.

Freeze-dried whole strawberries and raspberries, 11 varieties each, retained their original aroma, had a good taste and appearance, and could easily be powdered in the research by Lempka and Prominski in 1966. That year Lempka and others determined vitamin C losses during lyophilization were from 15–44% for the 22 varieties of these berries. However, Kyzlink and Curdova in 1966 found that vitamin C in strawberries was 90–96% of the initial value after freeze-drying and after 15 weeks of storage, along with 80-90% preservation of anthocyanin. In 1970 Zhukova determined that freeze-dried strawberries and raspberries had greater vitamin C content than these berries dried by other methods. In 1972 he showed that both vitamin C and anthocyanin were preserved better by lyophilization than by sublimation without pre-freezing. Sulc and others in 1980 compared raspberry pulp concentrates that had been freeze-dried or spray dried at 50–60 degrees C. The color (anthocyanin) loss was 11% for freeze-drying and 16% for spray drying, while the aroma loss was 17% and 24%, respectively. Higher spray-drying temperatures led to a 70% color loss and 58% aroma loss.

A study by Asami and others in 2003 comparing organic versus conventional growing methods on total phenolic content also evaluated air-drying versus freeze-drying for the preservation of these mostly flavonol constituents. While organic growing produced significantly greater phenolic content in corn and marionberries, freeze-drying preserved phenolics as well as freezing and significantly better than air-drying. For strawberries, freeze-drying was significantly better for preserving both total phenolics and vitamin C. Comparisons for preserving vitamin C in corn and marionberries were not made.

Though freeze-drying is superior to other drying methods, retention of nutrient components by lyophilization is not entirely complete, and their preservation has much to do with storage conditions such as temperature. In 1975 Do and others found freeze-dried sour cherries (*Prunus cerasus*) retained the color and flavor of the fresh fruit and when rehydrated were firm and plump. When stored at 70 degrees F (21 C) for six months they retained an acceptable color, flavor, and shape, but vitamin C was reduced by 90%. However, at 100 degrees F (38 C) the anthocyanin color began turning brown after two months, the flavor degraded after 4 months, and vitamin C completely disappeared after six months. In 1976 they determined that total anthocyanin for 100 grams hydrated weight decreased from 13.2 mg for fresh sour cherries to 9.28 mg for freeze-dried compressed samples, and then to 5.04 mg and 1.10 mg when the freeze-dried cherries were stored for six months at 21 degrees C and 38 degrees C, respectively. Three of the seven anthocyanins disappeared completely at 21 degrees C after six months and at 38 degrees C after two months.

A study of 3 types of Polish mushrooms by Lempka and others in 1970 found that lyophilization preserved vitamin B2 better than other drying methods. For freeze-dried fresh edible button mushrooms (*Agaricus bisporus*) Fang and others found in 1971 that flash-freezing led to better quality and firmer texture than slow freezing. Based on comparisons of color, flavor, and rehydration capacity, vacuum freeze-drying of these same cultivated mushrooms was proved by LeLoch-Bonazzi and others in 1992 to be clearly superior to hot air drying or simply vacuum drying.

However, the volatile substances compared in fresh and freeze-dried boletus mushrooms (*Boletus edulis* and *B. vesipellis*) by Dudareva in 1975 were somewhat less in the dried form and also had different proportions. In 1974 he had found the amino acid loss in these edible mushrooms was slight with freeze-drying but amounted to 30% when dried at 45-60 degrees C. Another study indicated freeze-dried shiitake (*Lentinus edodes*) mushrooms were similar to the fresh in volatiles and amino acid composition and had more vitamin B1 than the air-dried shiitake, as analyzed by Tanaka and others in 1976. In contrast, air-dried shiitake mushrooms had a composition that was significantly different than the fresh shiitake, but retained a fairly large quantity of vitamin B1. The advantages of freeze-dried shiitake as a food suggests the use of lyophilization for its medicinal use as well.

Preserving Fresh Herb Components

Herbs have been shown to retain their aroma much better when freeze-dried than air-dried. For example, dill (*Anethum graveolens*) was shown by Huopalahti and Kesalahti in 1985 to retain four times more of the absolute amount of 70 volatile compounds when freeze-dried compared to air-dried. Air-dried dill contained only 10% of the total volatiles found in fresh dill. For thyme (*h Thymus vulgaris*) and sage (*Salvia officinalis*) Bendl and others demonstrated in 1988 that freeze-drying resulted in higher essential oil content than drying at 40 degrees C. The characteric thyme components thymol and carvacrol were also higher with lyophilization, though after storage for eighty days the levels were similar to the oven-dried. The thujone, eucalyptol, and beta-pinene in the sage were higher with lyophilization, and loss with storage was low even though the thujone in the oven-dried sage was markedly decreased during storage.

Volatiles including the characteristic phthalides from fresh celery (*Apium graveolens*) tubers were drastically reduced by drum-drying, according to Berger and others in 1983. In contrast, freeze-drying preserved about half of the phthalides, and other aromatics were also present at much higher concentrations. In 1984 Mazza found the volatile essence of freeze-dried horseradish (*Armoracia lapathifolia*) was slightly greater than for its air-dried (50 degrees C) roots. Since the volatiles are largely generated enzymatically from slicing the roots for processing, both dried forms contained greater volatile content than fresh roots but in different proportions.

The flavor is greatly affected as well, as Freeman and Whenman showed in 1974 with onions (*Allium cepa*). Freeze-dried onion had a stronger and more characteristic flavor than hot-air dried onion. Likewise, flash-freezing with liquid nitrogen preserved the onion flavor much better than slow freezing. In 1992 Leino discovered that freeze-dried chives (*Allium schoenoprasum*) had a more fresh-green and onionlike aroma and less of a haylike odor than air-dried chives. Garlic (*Allium sativum*) flavor and its attendant activity was also shown by Yu and others in 1988 to benefit from this method. Freeze-dried garlic powder retained more allicin and flavor compounds in general than air-dried garlic.

In 1989 Kirsi and others discovered that the total aroma of dried raspberry (*Rubus idaeus*) leaves was better for green leaves when oven-dried with a 35 degree C temperature, though pleasant aroma content was equilavent, while freeze-drying preserved the total aroma better for rolled leaves and fermented leaves with greater pleasant aroma content in the fermented leaves.

Debelmas and Herisset in 1966 found the odor of freeze-dried Roman chamomile (*Chamaemelum nobile = Anthemis nobilis*) was more pronounced than controls, and water extractables increased. The paper chromatogram of the aqueous extracts produced more flavonoid spots for the lyophilized flowers, but thin layer chromatograms (TLCs) of the ether extracts did not show regular differences. That year when Debelmas and others studied Roman chamomile flowers that were freeze-dried, dried at room temperature, or dried at 37 degrees C, the organoleptic (sensory) characteristics were better for lyophilization, though the essential oil yield was somewhat lower.

Likewise, in 1967 Herisset and Besson found the lyophilized peppermint (*Mentha piperita*) leaves had a slightly lower essential oil content, while of comparable composition to the volatile oils of air-dried leaves. In the least favorable study, Paris and others in 1966 found the petals of red roses (*Rosa gallica*) had a better color when freeze-dried but lost their perfume, confirmed on thin-layer chromatograms by a different composition of essential oils compared to petals dried at room temperature. The tannin content of lyophilized petals was also lower. However, in 1975 DePasquale and Silvestri indicated that the essential oil in fresh freeze-dried chamomile (*Matricaria recutita = M. chamomilla*) flower heads had a higher essential oil content than the air-dried flowers.

Aside from typical volatile losses, chemical conversions occur during normal drying procedures that introduce changes to other components found in the fresh herbs. Dandelion (*Taraxacum officinale*) root studied by Ali and Guth in 1962 had more myristic, stearic and oleic acids when freeze-dried, whereas oven-drying resulted in more unsaturated fatty acids that oxidize more easily. Carotene and xanthophylls levels were higher in freeze-dried alfalfa (*Medicago sativa*) than in other dehydrated alfalfa tested by Livingston and others in 1980.

In 1987 Kartnig and others compared the content of known active components of hawthorn (*Crataegus monogyna*) leaves dried by different methods. The total flavonoid, hyperoside, catechin, polymeric procyanidin, oligomeric procyanidin, and total procyanidin content by percentage in the dry leaves was greatest for nitrogen-shock freeze-drying when compared with drying at room temperature for eight days, 40 degrees C for fourteen hours, or 60 degrees C for fourteen hours. A high-performance liquid chromatography (HPLC) assay was utilized by Ancharski in 1986 to illustrate the difference between air-dried and freeze-dried Western echinacea (*Echinacea angustifolia*) roots from the same fresh batch. It is obvious from a simple viewing that not only are more of the components preserved with freeze-drying, but most are present in larger quanities than in the air-dried sample.

Herbs also have different appearances based on drying techniques. Better preserved of color in lyophilized herbs was first shown by Mary and others in 1954. Oven-drying leaves of spearmint (*Mentha spicata*), podophyllum (*Podophyllum peltatum*), and castor (*Ricinus communis*) plants resulted in dark green samples, while freeze-drying retained the fresh bright green appearance, and chlorophyll was more readily extracted.

Pharmaceutical drug plants were subjected to lyophilization studies in the 1950s to compare the outcome to other drying methods. Rubin and Harris discovered datura (*Datura stamonium*) gave essentially the same alkaloid yield when dried at room temperature, in an oven at 40 degrees C and under high vacuum-low temperature lyophilization. However, the freeze-dried sample was bright green rather than the brown appearance of the other samples. Similar results were found by Chambers and Nelson, in that belladonna (*Atropa belladonna*) leaves that were dark olive green when dried in an oven for 45–65 degrees C or at room temperature and bright green when lyophilized. Oven drying caused more proteolysis, and the freeze-dried leaves have a slightly higher alkaloid content. Bioassays showed no pharmacological differences. Sommers and Guth showed the percentage of chlorophyll was higher in belladonna leaves with lyophilization.

In 1954 Cosgrove and Guth showed the same increase in chlorophyll in freeze-dried digitalis (*Digitalis purpurea* and *D. lutea*) leaves compared to oven-drying. That same year they found that even though the average total glycosides from the freeze-dried leaves and tinctures made from them were less than for oven-dried leaves and associated tincture, the potency was equivalent for the two tinctures. They believed the higher glycoside measurement may have been due to the greater optical density of the secondary glycosides and aglycons associated with component breakdown due to heat and enzymatic action associated with oven-drying. Paris and Herisset in 1967 confirmed that the lyophilized digitalis (*D. purpurea*) leaves, when compared to the air-dried leaves, had more primary glycosides and fewer secondary glycosides such as digitoxin and gitoxin that are produced by hydrolysis.

Some compounds are more extractable from freeze-dried plants. The extraction of condensed tannins and total phenolics was increased up to 17% (avg. 3%) when fresh eucalyptus (*Eucalyptus* spp.) leaves were freeze-dried, as reported by Cork and Krockenberger in 1991, whereas oven-drying at 70 degrees C reduced the amount extracted by 2–21% (avg. 11%). Terril and others who identified this phenomena in 1990 in lespedeza (*Sericea lespedeza*) forage believed that oven drying and sun drying, unlike freeze-drying, increase polymerization of tannins or formation of complexes with other constituents that leads to their reduced extractability. However, Hagerman noted in 1988 that only early in the growing season was more tannin extracted from lyophilized than fresh or oven-dried leaves of burr oak (*Quercus macrocarpa*), sugar maple (*Acer saccharum*), or shagbark hickory (*Carya ovata*) trees.

Certain active compounds available in the fresh plant appear to be preserved in significant quantities only by freeze-drying. One example of such components is the biologically active agents found in the stinging hairs of nettle (*Urtica* spp.) leaves. According to Maitai and others in 1980, the histamine and acetylcholine in the stinging hairs are destroyed by conventional air-drying and are broken down in solution after extraction. Freezing was the most effective means of adequately preserving the activity that these compounds contribute to the effects of the leaves. Mittman found in 1990 that in 31 patients using freeze-dried stinging nettle for hay fever 58% found it moderately or highly effective while 42% indicated that it was infective. Approximately half believed it was as effective as previously used medications, a view shared by only 1 in 5 of the 38 subjects using placebo.

Appropriate dosage for freeze-dried herbs compared to others is necessarily a consideration when the bioactive components are better preserved by freeze-drying. In the first clinical study with feverfew (*Tanacetum parthenium*) by Johnson and others in 1985 to prevent migraine headaches, fresh freeze-dried leaves in capsules were used in an open trial at an effective dose of 50 mg daily. The following double blind study by Murphy and others in 1988 replicated the efficacy results but used from 70–114 mg (avg. 82 mg) daily of leaves that were oven-dried at 37 degrees C and then powdered and encapsulated.

Application to Aqueous Solutions, Extracts, Juices

When traditional preparations utilize water extracts in place of the fresh or dried plant, this may be assumed to be a consequence of a particular benefit to be derived from processing the whole herb. Typically, the advantage consists of removing the material bulk for ease of consumption. Ease of assimilation of compounds from a fluid medium during illness is another consideraton. In some cases stomach or intestinal irritation or other side effects associated with resinous components or other compounds less soluble in water can be avoided. The problem with aqueous based extracts has been previously described as a vulnerability to microbial fermentation and degradation when kept at room temperature for a short time. Even refrigeration will only preserve water-based extracts for several days. Freeze-drying is the method of choice where solutions contain substances that are unstable or are easily oxidized. The shelf-life of an aqueous solution of superoxide dismutase (SOD) was 14 days, or 12 days when 2.5% lactose was added, but freeze-drying the SOD-lactose solution extended the shelf-life of the SOD to 1160 days, according to research by Li and others in 1987.

The advantage of freeze-drying water-based extracts goes beyond the convenience of not having to constantly prepare the material for consumption. Larger doses can be taken without having to consume large quantities of fluids. Water should of course be used in sufficient quantities along with the encapsulated freeze-dried powder, but this is much easier on the palate when the taste may be less than pleasant. Both the convenience and palatability support regular dosing compliance.

Flink and Karel determined in 1970 that the volatile components in freeze-dried solutions containing carbohydrate are retained in microregions that form as a result of separation from ice crystals during the freezing process. Volatile retention percentage when freeze-drying an aqueous solution increases with water solubility and with increased initial concentration of solids, especially water-soluble polymeric gum fiber, according to Smyrl and LeMaguer in 1978. Ironically, gums were considered by Lloyd to be an undesirable feature of water extracts. In freeze-dried extracts their properties lead to the retention not only of flavor but activity due to volatile components.

One of the advantageous features of freeze-drying is the increased rate of dissolving back into solution for most materials compared to other means of drying. For instance, Lachman and Chavkin showed in 1957 that even botanical gums and hydrocolloidal fibers such as acacia, tragacanth, alginate, agar, and pectin that are not readily soluble but, rather, notoriously difficult to disperse in water, dissolve at a much greater rate with no significant change in viscosity or pH when freeze-dried.

Kern's 1960 study of lyophilized methyl xanthine alkaloids was very revealing. The rate of solubility was 22 times faster for freeze-dried caffeine than its nonlyophilized form, while the total solubility of freeze-dried caffeine was 50% greater in distilled water. Likewise, the solubility of theophylline in distilled water was increased by 44% when freeze-dried. The lyophilized materials needed to be kept in dry, air-tight containers to maintain these properties.

The popular South African rooibos tea (*Aspalathus linearis*) was found by Joubert in 1990 to reconstitute immediately in water when freeze-dried, but formed lumps when the spray-dried tea was added to water. This rapid reconstitution facilitates the rehydration in the gut of encapsulated freeze-dried powders when taken with water, so that they mimic the original fluid forms. A study by Piscoya and others in 2001 with freeze-dried extracts of cat's claw (*Uncaria tomentosa* and *U. guianensis*) showed this form was effectively soluble in water so as to produce antioxicant and anti-inflammatory effects in test tubes. Their clinical study using freeze-dried decoction of *Uncaria guianensis* found that formulating this powder with an excipeint to produce tablets resulted in an effective product for treating osteoarthritis of the knee.

In applying freeze-drying to drug plant extracts in the 1954, lyophilization of aqueous extracts of digitalis (*Digitalis lutea* and *D. purpurea*) were shown by bioassay to be potent and instantaneously soluble in water by Cosgrove and Guth. Kern found the lyophilized infusions prepared from digitalis leaves was of greater bulk, finer texture, and fluffier than the solids remaining when the extracts were dried on a steam plate. The total glycosidal content of the freeze-dried infusions was equivalent to the standardized official tincture of *USP XIV* when made from the same amount of powdered leaf with less toxicity and a cardiotonic activity not apparent in the tincture.

When cabbage (*Brassica oleracea. v. capitata*) juice was studied by Omarov with others in 1976 and Omarov alone in 1985, he found that no amino acid loss occurred after freeze-drying and storage of fresh cabbage juice, and the S-methylmethionine (vitamin U) content remained the same though ascorbic acid decreased by 44%. As for fruit juices, amino acid content as measured by Ivasyu and Deryabina in 1980 was the same in the freeze-dried juice and purees as in fresh for cherries, black currant, apricot, apple, and plum-grape juices. In 1983 they found the mineral composition remained unchanged from fresh after freeze-drying for strawberry puree and only slightly changed in apricot, apple, cherry and grape-plum purees.

When the anthocyanin colorants were extracted with an acid solution from elderberries (*Sambucus nigra*) and freeze-dried by Bronnum-Hansen and Flink in 1985, for a 94% recovery of these compounds addition of 2.5% malto-dextrin was needed to help stabilize the product due to its hygroscopic (moisture attracting) property. While light intensity and the presence of oxygen did not significantly affect the stability of the anthocyanin, high temperature or water activity significantly increased the rate of degradation. With the dry extract stored at ambient temperature and low water activity, the freeze-dried anthocyanin half-life was greater than five years.

As concerns common medicinal herbs, freeze-drying the juice avoids the addition of ethanol as a preservative that introduces chemical alterations to the fresh extract. An example of this application is the popular echinacea juice product. Lyophilized fresh expressed juice from the aerial parts of purple coneflower (*Echinacea purpurea*) was administered orally by Munder in 1986 to mice for ten days at doses of 1 or 10 mg/kg. One day after the last dose the total splenic cell count was raised due to granulocytes and T, but not B, lymphocytes. In laboratory cell cultures this freeze-dried purple coneflower echinacea juice enhanced splenic cell proliferation and had an inhibitory effect on the growth of tumor cells.

References—Freeze-drying

Ali, SEF and Guth, EP. Study of the lipid fraction of freez-dried dandelion root. *J. Pharm. Sci.*, 51:924–8, 1962.

Ancharski, M. Fresh freeze-dried botanical medicine. *Complem. Med.*, July/Aug., 1986.

Asami, DK et al. Comparison of the total phenolic and ascorbic acid content of freeze-dried and air-dried marionberyy, strawberry, and corn grown using conventional, organic, and sustainable agricultural practices. *J. Agric. Food Chem.*, 51(5):1237–41, 2003.

Bendl, E et al. Investigation on the freez-drying of thyme and sage. *Ernaehrung (Vienna)*, 12(12):793–5, 1988 (*Chem. Abs.* 110:133871w).

Berger, RG et al. Quantitative composition of natural and technologically changed aromas of plants. X. Changes of aroma substances during processing of dry products from celery tubers. *Z. Lebensm.-Unters. Forsch.*, 177(5):328–32, 1983 (*Chem. Abs.* 100:66794b).

Bronnum-Hansen, K and Flink, JM. Anthocyanin colorants from elderberry (Sambucus nigra L.). 2. Process considerations for production of a freeze dried product. *J. Food Technol.*, 20:713–23, 1985.

Bronnum-Hansen, K and Flink, JM. Anthocyanin colourants from elderberry (Sambucus nigra L.). 3. Storage stability of the freeze dried product. *J. Food Technol.*, 20:725–33, 1985.

Chambers, MA and Nelson, JW. An investigation of high-vacuum freeze drying as a means of drug preservation. I. *J. Am. Pharm. Assoc.*, 39:323–6, 1950.

Cork, SJ and Krockenberger, AK. Methods and pitfalls of extracting condensed tannins and other phenolics from plants: insights from investigations on Eucalyptus leaves. *J. Chem. Ecol.*, 17(1):123–34, 1991.

Cosgrove, FP and Guth, EP. The effect of freeze-drying on the glycosidal content of Digitalis purpurea and Digitalis lutea L. *J. Am. Pharm. Assoc.*, 43(2):90–2, 1954.

Cosgrove, FP and Guth, EP. Preliminary studies concerning the lyophilized water-soluble extracts of Digitalis purpurea and Digitalis lutea L. *J. Am. Pharm. Assoc.*, 43(5):266–8, 1954.

Cosgrove, FP and Guth, EP. Carbohydrate and chlorophyll content of leaves of Digitalis purpurea L. and Digitalis lutea L. after freeze-drying and oven-drying. *J. Am. Pharm. Assoc.*, 43(5):268–9, 1954.

Debelmas, J and Herisset, A. Preservation of chamomile romaine (Anthemis nobilis) flowers by lyophilization. I. Preliminary studies. *Ann. Pharm. Franc.*, 24(2):93–9, 1966 (*Chem. Abs.* 66:49232d).

Debelmas, J et al. Industrial lyophilization of medicinal plants. II. Roman chamomile, Anthemis nobilis—Comparative effects of lyophilization and various drying methods on capitulum quality. *Ann. Pharm. Franc.*, 24(9–10):587–92, 1966 (*Chem. Abs.* 66:79511m).

DePasquale, A and Silvestri, R. The contents of active principles in the various parts of matricaria chamomilla L. *Essenze Deriv. Agrum.*, 45(3–4):292–8, 1975 (*Chem. Abs.* 85:166551k).

Deryabina, OA and Ivasyuk, NT. Mineral content of freeze-dried fruit-berry puree and juice with pulp. *Konservn. Ovoshchesush. Prom-st.*, (2):36, 1983 (*Chem. Abs.*, 98:142129w).

Do, JY et al. Freeze-dehydrated and compressed sour cherries I. Production and general quality evaluation. *J. Fd. Technol.*, 10:191–201, 1975.

Do, JY et al. Freeze dehydrated compressed sour cherries II. Stability of anthocyanins during storage. *J. Fd. Technol.*, 11:25–72, 1976.

Dudareva, NT. Effect of drying methods on free amino acids in mushrooms. *Prikl. Biokhim. Mikrobiol.*, 10(2):326–7, 1974 (*Chem. Abs.* 81:62330p).

Dudarevea, NT. Aromatic substances of fresh and sublimation-dried mushrooms. *Prikl. Biokhim.Mikrobiol.*, 11(1):147–8, 1975 (*Chem. Abs.* 82:137967h).

Fang, TT et al. Effects of blanching, chemical treatments and freezing methods on quality of freeze-dried mushrooms. *J. Food Sci.*, 36:1044–8, 1971.

Flink, J and Karel, M. Retention of organic volatiles in freeze-dried solutions of carbohydrates. *J. Agr. Food Chem.*, 18(2):295–7, 1970.

Foda, YH et al. Effect of dehydration, freeze-drying and packaging on the quality of green beans. *Food Technol.*, 21(7):1021–4, 1967.

Fonseca, H et al. Change in the levels of ascorbic acid and beta-carotene in freeze-dried fruit. *Solo*, 64(2):53–9, 1972 (*Chem. Abs.* 79:4007m).

Freeman, GG and Whenham, RJ. Changes in onion (Allium cepa L.) flavor components resulting from some post-harvest processes. *J. Sci. Fd. Agric.*, 25:499–515, 1974.

Hagerman, AE. Extraction of tannin from fresh and preserved leaves. *J. Chem. Ecol.*, 14(2):453–61, 1988.

Hamed, MGE. Freeze-drying of green beans. *Z. Lebensm.-Unters. Forsch.*, 131(3):144–9, 1966 (*Chem. Abs.* 66:18073z).

Herisset, A and Besson, P. Industrial lyophilization of medicinal plants. V. Peppermint, Mentha piperita. *Ann. Pharm Fr.*, 25(6):459–62, 1967 (*Chem. Abs.* 67:102706k).

Huopalahti, R and Kesalahti, E. Effect of drying and freeze-drying on the aroma of dill. *Essent. Oils Aromat. Plants*, pp. 179–84, 1984.

Ivasyu, N and Deryabina, OA. Free amino acid content of fruit and berry purees and juices with pulp after freeze drying. *Vopr. Pitan.*, (4):74–5, 1980 (*Chem. Abs.* 93:166310w).

Johnson, ES et al. Efficacy of feverfew as prophylactic treatment of migraine. *Br. Med. J.*, 291:569-73, 1985.

Joubert, E. Chemical and sensory analyses of spray- and freeze-dried extracts of rooibos tea (Aspalathus linearis). *Int. J. Food. Sci. Technol.*, 25:344–9, 1990.

Kartnig, T et al. Investigations on the procyanidin and flavonoid contents of Crataegus monogyna-drugs. *Sci. Pharm.*, 55:95–100, 1987.

Kern, JH. Freeze drying as a method of processing some pharmaceutical products. *Dissert. Abs.*, 20:3328–30, 1960.

Kirsi, M et al. The effects of drying-methods on the aroma of the herbal tea plant (Rubus idaeus). *Flav. Off-Flav.*, pp. 205–11, 1989.

Kyzlink, V and Curdova, M. Comparison of the preservation of L-ascorbic acid and anthocyanins in strawberries preserved by freeze-drying and heat sterilization. *Sb.Vys. Sk. Chem.-Technol Praze., Potraviny.*, 9:41–53, 1966 (*Chem. Abs.* 72:99352n).

Lachman, L and Chavkin, L. A study of the lyophilization of several pharmaceutical gums and suspending agents. *J. Am. Pharm. Assoc.*, 46(7):412–6, 1957.

Leino, M. Effect of freezing, freeze-drying, and air-drying on odor of chive characterized by headspace gas chromatography and sensory analyses. *J. Agric. Food Chem.*, 40:1379–84, 1992.

LeLoch-Bonazzi, C et al. Quality of dehydrated cultivated mushrooms (Agaricus bisporus): a comparison between different drying and freeze-drying processes. *Food Sci. Technol. (London)*, 25(4):334–9, 1992.

Lempka, A and Prominski, W. L-Ascorbic acid in freeze-dried berries. *Przem. Spozyw.*, 20(6):402–4, 1966 (*Chem. Abs.* 66:104072d).

Lempka, A et al. Losses of L-ascorbic acid during lyophilization of selected berries. *Pr. Zakresu Towarozn. Chem., Wyzsza Szk. Ekon. Poznaniu Zesz. Nauk., Ser. I*, (26):23–37, 1966 (*Chem. Abs.* 66:45592y).

Lempka, A et al. Effect of technological factors and conditions of storage on the level of riboflavin in lyophilized mushrooms. *Pr. Zakresu Towarozn. Chem., Wyzzsza Szk. Ekon. Posnaniu, Zesz. Nauk., Ser. 1*, (36):35–42, 1970 (*Chem. Abs.* 75:1395555b).

Livingston, AL et al. Comparison of carotenoid storage stability in alfalfa leaf protein (Pro-Xan) and dehydrated meals. *J. Agric. Food Chem.*, 28:652–6, 1980.

Maitai, CK et al. Effect of extract of hairs from the herb Urtica massaica on smooth muscle. *Toxicon*, 18:225–9, 1980.

Mary, NY et al. The effect of freeze-drying on chlorophyll in the leaves of some selected drug plants. *J. Am. Pharm. Assoc.*, 43(9):554–7, 1954.

Mazza, G. Volatiles in distillates of fresh, dehydrated and freeze dried horseradish. *Can. Inst. Food Sci. Technol. J.*, 17(1):18–23, 1984.

Mittman, P. Randomized, double-blind study of freeze-dried Urtica dioica in the treatment of allergic rhinitis. *Planta Med.*, 56:44–7, 1990.

Munder, PG. Immunological experiments to evaluate the activities of orally administered echinacin. Unpublished. Max-Planck-Institut fuer Immunbiologie, March, 1986.

Murphy, JJ et al. Randomized double-blind placebo-controlled trial of feverfew in migraine prevention. *Lancet*, 2:189–92, 1988.

Omarov, MM. Amino acid composition of cabbage juice. *Izv. Sev.Kavk. Nauchn. Tsentra Vyssh. Shk., Tekh. Nauki*, (2):93–4, 1985 *(Chem. Abs. 107:22196y)*.

Omarov, MM et al. Drying cabbage juice by sublimation. *Konservn. Ovoshchesush. Prom-st.*, (2):41–3, 1976 *(Chem. Abs. 84:149516q)*.

Paris, RR and Herisset, A. Industrial lyophilization of medicinal plants. VI. Folia digitalis (Digitalis purpurea). *Ann. Pharm. Fr.*, 25(11):669–72, 1967 *(Chem. Abs. 70:22867k)*.

Paris, RR et al. Industrial lyophiliaztion of medicinal plants. IV. Red rose, Rosa gallica. *Ann. Pharm. Fr.*, 25(6):453–7, 1967 *(Chem. Abs. 67:102705j)*.

Piscoya, J et al. Efficacy and safety of freeze-dried cat's claw in osteoarthritis of the knee: mechanisms of action of the species Uncaria guianensis. *Inflamm. Res.*, 50:442–8, 2001.

Popovskii, VG and Sarukhanyan, BE. Change in the biochemical composition of peaches and apricots during freeze drying. *Promst. Arm.*, (7):74–5, 1974 *(Chem. Abs. 81:150579g)*.

Rubin, M and Harris, LE. Comparative methods of drying and assay of Datura stramonium Linne. *J. Pharm. Sci.*, 39:477–8, 1950.

Smyrl, TG and LeMaguer, M. Retention of sparingly soluble volatile compounds during the freeze drying of model solutions. *J. Food Process Engineer.*, 2:151–70, 1978.

Sommers, EB and Guth, EP. Extraction of constituents of lyophilized Atropa belladonna. *J. Am. Pharm. Assoc.*, 46(1):55–7, 1957.

Sulc, D et al. Color and flavor changes of raspberry pulp concentrates during spray and freeze drying. *Ber.-Int. fruchtsaft-Union, Wiss.-Tech. Komm.*, 16:113–26, 1980 *(Chem. Abs. 95: 78733x)*.

Tanaka, F et al. On the differences in the quality and composition of shii-take according to different processing methods. *Mushroom Sci.*, 9(1):521–9, 1974/76 *(Chem. Abs. 86:119470u)*.

Terrill, TH et al. Condensed tannin concentration in sericca lespedeza as influenced by preservation method. *Crop Sci.*, 30:219–24, 1990.

Weits, J et al. Nutritive value and organoleptic properties of three vegetables, fresh and preserved I six different ways. *Int. Z. Vitaminforsch.*, 40(5):648–58, 1970 *(Chem. Abs. 74:52259p)*.

Yu, TH et al. Flavor retention of garlic powders. *Shi'h P'inK'o Hsueh (Taipei)*, 15(3):296–303, 1988 *(Chem. Abs. 112:137738x)*.

Zhukova, LA. Vitamin C content in variously dried strawberries and raspberries during storage. *Sb. Nauch. Tr. Leningrad. Inst. Sov. Torg.*, 38(2):145–9, 1970 *(Chem. Abs. 77:3918f)*.

Zhukova, LA. Vitamin levels in strawberries and raspberries dried by sublimation. *Vop. Pitan.*, 30(1):77–81, 1972 *(Chem. Abs. 76:152155m)*.

The Best of Both Worlds

There is much talk about the need for standardization in quality herb products. Most people consider this a chemical process and a feature unique to extracts of herbs. However, there are foundational means by which whole herbs, the source material for all extracts, should also be standardized. These are biological and physical processes.

First, total quality consistency can best be assured when the preparation process is also standardized. This means that consistent growing, harvesting, handling, and manufacturing steps are employed for this product, whether the plant is cultivated or wild crafted. Optimum consistency requires not only the same species but the same seed stock grown by the same methods at the same locale (or minimally, the same variety with the same methods on similar soil in the same climate), the same time of harvest, and the same separation of plant parts. This is standardization by part. When leaves are indicated on the label as the herb content provided, these must be free from appreciable quantities of stems or other extraneous material. Then follows the same type of drying, powdering, and/or extraction procedures, and the same encapsulation or tableting. Standardization by weight of the herb usually describes the quantity of whole, complex herb part or its powder provided per dosing unit. This unit is typically a capsule, though two or more capsules may be recommended per dose. In the case of tablets, the total weight of the tablet is not the same as the herb weight if binders, fillers, coating, or other additives are used. The bottling technique, storage, and shipping practices are to remain the same. Variations in these processes can affect the potency of the final product. The botanical source and processing information may be provided on the label, but it is not yet legally required.

Finally, it is possible on the basis of standardizing the plant stock, process, part, and weight to obtain a finished whole herb product with relative consistency in its chemical make-up. On this basis, depending on the herb and the state of knowledge about its components and their concentrations and activities, specific quantities or ranges of content can be specified. This may involve documented levels of marker substances, active components, or chemical classes of active component as one means to indicate that the herb is identifiable, consistent, and/or reliable/potent. Since the content cannot be specifically manipulated in whole herbs to the extent possible with extracts, the biomarker content is best described in terms of a range of concentration. For these quantities to be meaningful, the analytical testing method by which they determined should also be identified.

An established means of addressing most of the post-agricultural issues is the officially designated standardization as described in the *USP* and *NF* for about two dozen herbs that are used to make official drug extracts and dietary supplements, respectively. It is well understood by those in pharmacy that to establish a standardized extract from a plant, one must begin by setting standards for the plant material from which the extract is made. These specifications are listed in the updated editions and revisions of these texts that are now published together in one volume. Peculiarly, the standards set for dietary supplement plants in the *NF* are more extensive than those for the official drug plants in the *USP*. The *NF* standards and procedures specified include a description of the species, its part, and often its powder; packaging and storage, labeling, reference standards, botanic characteristics; identification, ash content, water content, extractable matter, volatile oil, specific phytochemical content; pesticide residues, foreign organic matter, heavy metals, and microbial limits. Herb products meeting these requirements may designate this by an indicatation on the label.

Preferable to single phytochemical standardization is proof of content for multiple active components as documented by chromatographic fingerprinting. As seen with extracts and herbs, standardization to single marker compounds or chemical categories does not necessarily assure identity, consistency, or reliability/potency. The chemical content information may be provided on the label as one means of assessing the product, but it is neither legally required nor entirely adequate by itself.

Comparing Chromatographic Assays—
Popular Juice and Extracts Versus Freeze-dried Fresh Herbs or Juice

Recognizing that fresh freeze-dried botanicals contain greater bioactive complexity than any form apart from the fresh plant, their preference for uses ranging from dietary supplements to botanical medicines can best be demonstrated not by simple standardization to one or several marker compounds but by chromatographic displays of the phytochemical array. This phytochemical assay is most convincing when chromatographic comparisons are made between the freeze-dried herb and other product forms. The high-performance liquid chromatography (HPLC) assay is often the best method to employ for these comparisons.

A series of pamphlets developed by David Lytle and based on his phytochemical assays describing freeze-dried botanicals were published by Eclectic Institute, Inc., (EI) beginning in 2001 to make similar comparisons between the freeze-dried fresh herbs and other commercial products. The revealing results described in these brochures follow.

BLACK COHOSH

The first EI brochure in May, 2001, for black cohosh (*Cimicifuga [Actaea] racemosa*) utilized an HP-TLC for comparison of a 185 mg capsule of freeze-dried whole root with 2 tablets of an uncharacterized brand name standardized extract made from the root of this plant. The whole root is richer in the triterpene glycoside used as the standard marker (27-deoxyactein) and in associated triterpene glycosides (including cimicifugoside), along with additional compounds that are visually undetectable in the TLC of the extract.

A later version of this EI pamphlet for black cohosh from September, 2002, uses HPLC-ELSD chromatogram to further demonstrate that two 370 mg capsules of the whole root (assayed to contain on average 1%, or 7.4 mg, total triterpene glycosides) have much higher quantities of each of the triterpene glycosides A, B, and C as well as cimiracmoside A, 27-deoxyactein, and actein than 10 tablets (a 5-day dose) of the leading European extract. In a comparison with a different product, two 120 mg extract tablets standardized to 2.5% total triterpene glycosides (6 mg) not only failed to provide as much of these compounds as the freeze-dried root capsules, but the extract was not even derived from true American *Cimicifuga racemosa*. Rather, this standardized extract was made from a Chinese species, based upon the chromatographic profile that showed it lacked 27-deoxyactein and cimiracmoside A. Likewise, an HPLC of the organic acids found in freeze-dried black cohosh capsules (including caffeic acid, ferulic acid, salicylic acid, and cimicifugic acids) shows their content in the given quantities is both greater than the European standardized extract and distinctively different from the product apparently made from Chinese species. For example, the Chinese species lacks salicylic acid. Even more than the triterpene glycosides to which black cohosh products are commonly standardized, these organic acids are known to contribute to the anti-inflammatory and hormonal effects.

CRANBERRY

(*Vaccinium macrocarpon*) is most often consumed as a juice, and it is in this form that most of the studies have been done on its usefulness for urinary tract infections. A cranberry beverage must be sweetened to allow for its consumption on a regular basis. An assay of the sugars by HPLC in June, 2002, of 8 fluid ounces of a typical cranberry beverage compared with those naturally occurring in the freeze-dried berry showed extremely high amounts in the drink with greater amounts of fructose than glucose due to the addition of high fructose corn syrup. In contrast 12 capsules of the berry (3.6 grams) has a minor amount of sugar with more glucose than fructose.

Compared by HPLC to a capsule of cranberry extract (400 mg), a capsule (300 mg) of the freeze-dried cranberry has much greater amounts of anthocyanosides (red anthocyanin pigments, 0.5%-1% by vis spectroscopy pH differential assay method) that include arabinosides, glucosides, and galactosides of cyanidin and peonidin. Unlike some cranberry extracts, there are no added colorants such as beet root extract used to improve the appearance, and no reasons or need to use such additives. It is known that the cranberry tannins called procyanidins (also called proanthocyanidins) are largely responsible for the mucosal anti-adherence effect of this fruit on bacteria. Bioactive procyanidins are concentrated in the skin and seeds of cranberry. So, procyanidins are very high in the whole freeze-dried berry (0.75%–1.5% by HPLC) that retains both of these, whereas the extract has relatively small amounts of these components.

GOLDENSEAL

The EI goldenseal (*Hydrastis canadensis*) brochure from January, 2002, describes its freeze-dried root product produced from its own cultivated plants. The issue of goldenseal endangerment in its wild state has led to a number of prominent herbalists to recommend the therapeutic substitution of other berberine-containing plants such as the bark of the plentiful Oregon grape (*Mahonia* spp.) or barberry (*Berberis vulgaris*). With a completely different non-berberine phytochemical profile, rather than rationalize substitution of the Oregon grape that grows extensively around the EI farm, the company committed itself to cultivating goldenseal plots that provide the "real deal." It is unfortunate that some companies now market berberine-source substitutes without identifying their true identity, but instead pass off herbs such as Chinese *Coptis* species as goldenseal. The differences can be readily demonstrated with HP-TLC profiles of the herbs, since *Coptis*, *Berberis* and *Mahonia* species all lack the alkaloid hydrastine. Therefore, instead of standardizing the total alkaloid content of such products "as berberine," hydrastine should be a specific marker for all legitimate standardized goldenseal products.

Assaying with HPLC makes the differences between the fresh freeze-dried goldenseal root (containing 6.5%–8.5% total alkaloids calculated as berberine and hydrastine by HPLC) and a spray-dried extract obvious. The high temperature spray-drying apparently leads to increased breakdown of hydrastine and berberine found in lower quantities in the extract, along with higher amounts of hydrastinine and canadine (tetrahydroberberine). This creates chromatographic alkaloid profiles of the spray-dried product that are disproportionate to those found in the fresh freeze-dried root.

KAVA

Even when a whole herb is not used, based on long-standing tradition in the region where the plant is native, a traditional water-based extract preserves important distinctions by comparison to modern forms made with nonpolar chemical solvent extracts. The perfect example of this difference is kava (*Piper methysticum*), a plant of the South Pacific where for millennia the fresh root has been pulverized in cold water to obtain a water-based extract of the fresh juice. The natives of Vanuatu, the islands where the "nakamal" kava culture originated and where its regular consumption is an integral part of the local lifestyle, not only demand fresh kava be used but prize certain cultivars that are renowned for their pleasant psychotropic effects. These are now known to be high in kavain and dihydrokavain and low in dihydromethysticin. For medicinal use cultivars high in kavain and methisticin are preferred there. Dried kava and cultivars that are more pronounced in their physical and mental effects, based on the high content of dihydrokavain and dihydromethysticin, are not consumed on a regular basis in these islands. In this country of kava connoisseurs the total kavalactone content is not relevant, if either the preparation or the cultivar (and *ipso facto*, the chemotype) is inappropriate.

The EI March, 2002, kava brochure illustrates with HPLC how the freeze-dried "nakamal" juice of the kava has the most desirable chemotype for regular use. High in kavain and methysticin, moderate in dihydrokavain, and low in dihydromethysticin, this water-based extract contains the components pressed fresh from kava. The content of such a product has been time-tested for ages by being used on a regular basis without any evidence of liver toxicity that has recently been associated with concentrated solid extracts having 30–70% of unspecified total kavalactones. Dried kava root, its bark, stem or leaves, nonpolar solvents such as acetone, and inappropriate cultivars or their mixtures can be used to manufacture these artificially high kavalactone concentrates. For effective doses with human consumption, this is unnecessary. The content provided by freeze-drying fresh kava juice is still in the range of 15–20% total kavalactones, and a 425 mg capsule provides as much of these as a 140 mg tablet of a concentrated extract delivering 55% kavalactones.

Milk Thistle

Most standardized products advertised as milk thistle (*Silybum marianum*) or milk thistle extract are actually a 75%–80% concentrate of the extract fraction called silymarin. The medicinal herb called milk thistle is actually the fruit of the plant, but it is commonly called a seed due to its appearance. Silymarin is a mixture of flavonolignans consisting mostly of silybin, silydianin, and silychristin that are obtained by successive extraction and reduction. Initially chemical solvents such as hexane and petroleum ether are used to reduce the lipid content from up to 30% down to 3%–4% to prevent rancidity from occurring. In the freeze-dried seed meal this is accomplished by cold pressing the fruit to reduce the oil to an equivalent content without chemical solvents that persist as residues.

The seed meal consists of about 4% silymarin when assayed using the spectroscopic method in July, 2002. In comparing the flavonolignan content between six 600 mg capsules of the seed meal (144 mg silymarin) and one 175 mg capsule of the 80% silymarin fraction (140 mg silymarin), the seed meal capsules contain approximately equivalent amounts of silybin, silydianin, and isosilibinin. The seed meal contains significantly more silychristin, the flavonoid taxifolin, and other components as well as ten times the protein. In addition, while the fiber content of the seed meal is 28.8%, the silymarin fraction consists of about 0.1% fiber. Clearly, more whole meal content needs to be consumed to obtain equivalent silymarin as available in the extract fraction, but the full spectrum of bioactive components and no solvent residues result in a more complete source of the bioactive flavanolignans, flavonoids, and other components.

ST. JOHN'S WORT

In May, 2002, the EI brochure on fresh freeze-dried St. John's wort (*Hypericum perforatum*) revealed that more total hyperforins are obtained than the same weight of a standardized European extract. This is accomplished when care is taken to utilize only the top two inches of the plant with its leaves and the reproductive tops that concentrates this component. Higher levels of total hypericins are also retained with lyophilizing this portion compared to the standardized extract. What is most impressive is the retention of flavonoids including biflavones that have been credited with providing additional antidepressant activity by mechanisms different from hyperforin. Together with the standardized 0.2–0.4% hypericins, the 2–4% hyperforins, and the associated flavonoids, procyanidins and essential oils in the fresh plant are also delivered by freeze-drying.

Achievable Quality Standards for All Products

Herbal complexity makes attempts at standardizing products necessarily challenging. Feasibility demands manageable features. What is most required is accurate characterization of important features for each product. The first step must be accurate identification of the plant. This is more easily accomplished when the herbs are cultivated. A commercial exchange of raw materials for product manufacture requires that the purchases take necessary measures to assure correct plant and plant part has been obtained. This is especially important when the herbs have been collected from the wild. Even intact specimens require expert assessment by a variety of techniques to determine their specific identity.

Identification requires a name, and common names often include other species of the same genus (or other genera), so the standard common identifiers as designated in the American Herbal Products Association *Herbs of Commerce* (2nd ed.) should be used in the United States, along with the appropriate italicized scientific binomial designating the genus and species of plant. Starting with this means for describing the correct plant, assurance of consistency at a minimum involves using this species. For some plants like kava it is further helpful to specify the appropriate variety, cultivar, or chemotype. This is the first standard of consistency and purity, and must be correct and clear on a product label. [Common name; *Genus species*]

Optimally, for plant consistency there should be continuity in germ plasm, that is, maintaining a plant community by preserving its seed stock for replanting annual crops on similar land. This presumes the need for cultivation modifications, including organic farming practices for biological renewal of the soil such as crop rotation, adjusted to annual changes in climate. Timely management as applied to smaller farms provides the most effective agricultural adjustments. Precise refinements in crop management practices can be achieved on a large agribusiness scale only with great difficulty. At the other extreme some high intensity commercial growing processes involve environments such as greenhouses and hydropon,iaside from pharmaceutical organ-tissue cultures housed in vats with nutrient broth. Maintaining growing techniques consistent with recognized quality control issues is a necessary means of achieving Good Agricultural Practices. However, only 50–100 medicinal species are widely cultivated, so Good Harvesting Practices must be employed in the wild in addition. When herbs are conscientiously obtained from private or public property, the suitability of particular locations according to environmental purity, ecological safety, sustainability, and proper respect of property ownership must be priorities. The pattern of growing conditions as far as chemical or organic cultivation or wildcrafted herbs is the second important distinction that needs to be made. [Common name; *Genus species*—growing conditions]

Harvesting the proper parts of the plant that are known to naturally demonstrate the desired therapeutic activity is necessary for "whole herb" products. Extracts that concentrate small amounts of active components from less potent parts or from parts containing additional undesirable compounds should be recognized as utilizing what would otherwise be construed as waste. While not representing the most desirable and potent parts necessary when using the complex herb approach to botanical therapy, utilizing these parts as raw materials for fractions or isolates is not uncommon. Designating the precise plant organ is the third standard for characterization of herbal products. [Common name; *Genus species*—growing conditions, plant part]

The means by which this part is converted from being picked fresh from the plant to its form in the bottle needs to be clearly identified and maintained. Whether it is freeze-dried, air-dried, oven-dried, or sun-dried and/or aged marks differences in the final dried form. This conversion of the fresh plant part to its dried form (whole or powdered) should clearly be made the fourth part of its standard identity. [Common name; *Genus species*—growing conditions, plant part, drying method]

Herbs in their entirety or cut and sifted forms are generally sold for brewing loose tea, while powdered herbs are typically supplied in teabags and capsules. Each step progressively exposes more surface area to oxygen, humity, light, and/or other destructive influences. The process used for size reduction can further affect herb quality, depending on whether difficult grinding produces destructive heat from friction, or whether chopping or crushing is adequate to effectively reduce the form. Pressing into tablets typically involves additives, heat, and pressure. When sold in opaque boxes or bottles that prevent inspection of the herb appearance, it is important to describe whether it is still physically intact and entire, or whether the structure has been reduced to forms that make it more readily consumable. The description should include whether it is loose or in bags, capsules, or tablets. [Common name; *Genus species*—growing conditions, plant part, drying method, physical form]

When the whole herb is not consumed, its extract content will vary based upon the solvent(s) used to produce the extract. Legal requirements are restricted to designating the percentage alcohol (ethanol) content, but consumers should be informed of the nature of the solvent agents involved in the production of liquid extracts. If it is ethanol, was it produced from organic fruit or grain? Is the water distilled or from a spring, private well, or tap delivered by a public utility company? If the extract is solid rather than liquid, was another form of alcohol substituted to reduce cost and avoid the regulations associated with ethanol? If so, what toxic variety was employed, methanol, isopropanol, or other? If alcohol was not used, were other toxic nonpolar solvents such as acetone or hexane utilized? For all extracts, the solvents should be consistent in a product sold under the same name and be clearly disclosed on the label. The final aspect of describing the use of solvents to extract an herb is the relative strength of the final extract. For liquid extracts a ratio (weight of herb extracted to volume of final extract in metric equivalents) between 1:10 and 1:1 would be expected, whereas for solid native extract ratios (weight of herb extracted to final weight of solid extract) from 1:1 to 10:1 are possible. [Common name; *Genus species*—growing conditions, plant part, drying method, physical form, solvent/strength]

A native/crude extracts may be reduced by fractionatation to remove much of the complexity that characterized the product as herbal. This reduction is accomplished by using a different solvent to extract the native extract, producing a smaller fraction of the whole plant. What is lost from the native extract in this process is unmentioned. Whereas the fraction is considered a concentrate, in terms of the rest of the content present in the whole plant or native extract it is a dilution or a reduction, since less or none of these components is available. Some highly concentrated fractions are extracts of fractions, each step using a different solvent. Since each step removes more complexity as the fraction becomes more pure, the different solvents that lead to the final commercial fraction must be consistent and should be identified as a part of the standard methodology. Additionally, it is necessary to denote the degree of concentration. For fractionated extracts a ratio of product strength between 10:1

and 50:1 is likley. [Common name; *Genus species*—growing conditions, plant part, drying method, physical form, solvents/concentration]

The last aspect for characterization of a standard manufacturing process is the one most often considered when describing "standardization" of a product in quantitative terms. This is the percentage or total content of a chemical identification marker and/or class of active compounds. Concentration of a particular marker or chemical category of compounds not only reduces the inherent phytochemical complexity but disrupts the natural balance. Seldom if ever is a single marker in an herb or its native extract adequate for representing the activity of a herbal product, but in extract fractions that is sometimes about all that is left. In concentrated fractions it should be imperitive to identify and to standardize the major bioactive marker(s) when known, or to designate within a chemical class the relative contents of the most significant components of that class. As a part of the complete standardization of process and product, this information should ultimately be backed up by a phytochemical profile of the product that demonstrates not only the relative levels of the designated markers but the presence or absense of significant congeners. The methodology for this process should follow validated procedures and protocols. Assays for pesticide and/or solvent residues, heavy metals, and microbial contamination are final steps to assess inappropriate contamination of the final product. [Common name; *Genus species* —growing conditions, plant part, drying method, physical form, solvent(s)/strength, chemical profile]

Each of these phases of characterization is important. However, they are presented in the order of diminishing necessity for whole botanical foods or remedies, including native aqueous and/or alcoholic liquid extracts. In contrast, the order of these phases becomes increasingly important for concentrated solvent extracts, fractions, and near isolates. Whether whole herbs or phytochemical fractions are considered, quality products are manufactured with due compliance given to these issues. Each individual's own personal approach to health determines their preference for a particular type of product. Compliance with accurate characterization can contribute to making appropriate choices to achieve the healthful goal for which everyone strives.

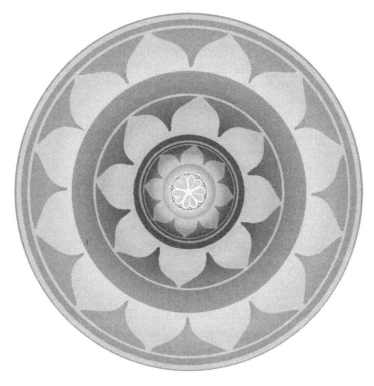

PART TWO

CHANGING PERCEPTIONS
AND PREFERENCES—
POPULAR HERBS IN AMERICAN TRADITIONS

Broad Traditional Uses Contrast with Modern Applications

In most discussions of the uses of a particular herb, it is often mistakenly assumed that it is appropriate to utilize any form of that herb. This flies in the face of empirical and scientific knowledge that recognizes that each form has distinct differences, advantages and limitations that make one or several forms more proper than the rest for treating a particular individual's condition. The proper choice depends not only on the individual but on a variety of factors affecting the availability of the active components. The relative solubility of the desirable compounds will depend on the solvent and temperature used in cases of extraction that determine the initial presence and preservation of these constituents. Internally, their availability depends on alterations by digestion, metabolism by the intestinal bacterial flora, assimilation from the GI tract, and the interactions with other components that affect their absorption, metabolism and excretion on both organ and cellular levels. These are the features that impact the pharmacokinetics of the active components. The pharmacodynamic interactions of components are likewise affected and reflect the changes in multiple component bioavailability due to these factors. Every variance produces changes of greater or lesser significance on the efficacy of the product consumed.

For this reason, the emphasis in the following chapters will be on evidence that distinguishes one form from another. Sometimes there is a great similarity between some, or even many, forms pertaining to their use for a particular condition. In other cases it is easier to perceive which forms are more appropriate to obtain the desired outcome. Since such distinctions have often been neglected in the literature, there are many types of conditions for which the proper form has not been specifically identified in articles and books referenced here. For each form that is discussed, the uses listed are limited to those directly attributed to that form in the listed references. Certainly, the applications of traditional forms of products for each herb go beyond these listed uses. Attention has not been given to reported uses for which the form of the herb used was not specified. An attempt has been made to recognize different traditions that use an herb in different manners to illustrate diverse applications proper to that form. For conditions in which several forms are effective, factors that may take precedence include availability, cost, and patient or prescriber preference.

In most cases traditional uses of unspecified forms apply to the fresh or dried herb and its infusion or decoction. Such assumptions are not always certain, so the listings for the whole herb and water extracts frequently do not represent the full scope of their traditional application. The whole herb and more complex (native or galenic) extracts generally have a much broader scope of application, compared to those products that are reduced to concentrated fractions of specific types of compounds. The narrowing of therapeutic uses is most typical for isolated components that have become the standard of conventional medical practice. The fact that the whole herb contains all of the active fractions and components suggests that it provides the complete medicinal effects when appropriate doses are utilized. It has been observed that, like nutrients available in whole foods, the therapeutic advantage can be equivalent when less of an active component is available in the complexity of a complete herb, due to its additive and synergistic activities. On the other hand, sometimes a high dose provided by a concentrated extract or isolate is necessary to deliver the desired therapeutic effect. Each form deserves consideration when making a complete assessment and therapeutic judgement.

The nine representative herbs covered here demonstrate the diversity of potential choices for each herb depending on the intended use, documented evidence, and preferred form. This limited number of herbs is used simply as an illustration of the immense differences in applications for any single herb and how the perceptions of its use have changed, and in some cases remained the same, over time. As the emphasis in preferred forms or applications has changed between plant parts, from one culture to another, from traditional to modern practice, or from a food to a medicine, the inherent potential remains the same. The validation of any form depends on its appropriateness for the intended use, not simply its efficacy for a single isolated condition currently associated with a particular form.

Liberties have been taken with some of the common names used for the following herbs. While acknowledging the need to establish consistent identifiers for product labeling, the tendency to reduce the identification of herbs to standard limited forms tends to deplete some of the rich heritage that has accrued in association with its use over thousands of years. For this reason various select names applied to each herb over time are mentioned and in some cases discussed. These all reveal something about the nature of the plant or its relationship to humans and their perceptions. Oftentimes friends acknowledge one another by names that are peculiar to their own relationship, using nicknames that appeal particularly to them. The fact that people can have personal affinities with particular plant species calls for the freedom to relate to them in their own preferred ways, including use of a name that has its own unique appeal.

Note: In identifying the year associated with a published study, the year of publication of the study will often be referred to as if it were the year the study was performed. This should not be taken literally; the actual dates the study was performed is usually not available, whereas the study's publication date is pertinent to identify the appropriate reference citation.

4
CLASSIC NATIVE AMERICAN HERBS

The Eclectic profession in general and Lloyd Brothers Pharmacists in particular were adamant about developing the native American medicinal plants, that is, expanding their utilization through adapted medical applications. Important uses were known as part of the traditional practices of native Americans. These typically involved applying or consuming the fresh plant part in season, the dried herb or root, or a water extract. When employed regularly, the consumption of dried herbs or the preparations of teas was sometimes considered distasteful or inconvenient by Anglos. So, doctors looked for other effective forms of employing American botanical remedies.

Influenced by homeopathy and advanced by by John Scudder, Eclectics began utilizing fresh plant tinctures to optimize the retention of the living herbs' vitality and potency. Eclectic doctors required easily stored and administered forms of medicines for clinical and home therapy. However, these alcoholic extracts were new forms with different content than the whole fresh herb (all components), dried herbs (altered phytochemistry), or the teas (water-soluble compounds) and tinctures (mostly alcohol-soluble constituents) made from dried herbs. Since native American herbs had not been used in this form before, ingenuity and scrupulous clinical observations were required to delineate the appropriate indications for their use.

Through pharmaceutical and clinical innovations, as well as honest communication of clinical observations, Eclectic doctors established specific indications for these green tinctures that they then called specific medicines. A large number of native American botanicals became standards in medical practice by the early 20th century. A survey by the Lloyd Brothers at this time to assess the frequency of use of medicinal plants among American doctors solicited responses from over 30,000 physicians of all types of practice throughout the country. The more than 10,000 responses were summarized by Lloyd [*JAPA*, 1912, pp.1235–1241] and among the top herbs rated by popularity were goldenseal (#2) and Western echinacea (#11).

Goldenseal was a mainstay in early Physiomedical and Eclectic practice. Also valued as a concentrated source of the alkaloid berberine in regular medicine, it suffered from overharvesting in its native habitat. Goldenseal was valued not only for the contributions of berberine, but its other alkaloids and components made its properties unique. In fact, one of the Lloyd Brothers most popular goldenseal products was "Colorless Hydrastis," lacking the yellow berberine. The traditional uses of goldenseal have always been distinct from those of other species from around the world that contained berberine together with different alkaloids than those found in goldenseal. Yet these are now being recommended as substitutes to avoid threatening goldenseal's survival in its natural habitat. To supply the ongoing demand, increasing cultivation of this valuable herb is a necessary solution that allows goldenseal to continue its prominent contribution to the practice botanical medicine.

Introduced through the Eclectics by the Lloyd Bros. Pharmacists, Western echinacea root rapidly grew to become the most popular herb in American medicine early in the 20th century. Though its use was condemned in the pages of the *Journal of the American Medical Association* at that time, those who used it in practice knew its great value and broad scope of effective application. It later came to be the established means of treating infections by naturopathic doctors who eschewed the antibiotics-only approach to fighting infections. Only after German studies of its American cousin, the purple coneflower (*Echinacea purpurea*) plant, demonstrated an impact on the immune system was the significance of its wide application appreciated. While difficult to grow outside of its natural range, Western echinacea has not enjoyed the international popularity of its easily cultivated cousin. Yet continuing high demand that threatens localized communities of wild sources suggest it is time to develop adequate commercial supplies by cultivating this important herb in its native habitat as well.

Cranberry was a late arrival on the Americal botanical medicine scene. The longstanding use of cranberry as a seasonal food led to its development also as a popular beverage. Like other plants of its family, those who were chronically bothered with bladder infections observed that cranberry could help reduce the incidence and severity of these problems with regular consumption. The flavor of the unsweetened berries or juice, the loss of bioactive components with juice extraction, and the use of many deleterious chemicals in its production make the use of a low-caloric organic form an attractive preventive measure and complement or alternative to antimicrobial treatment. Study of its antioxidant activity and other protective effects suggests a broader application of the berries' potential as a functional food. The similarities and differences between cranberry and other members of its genus and family illustrate how some properties are shared with related plants, yet each species remains unique in its contributions.

Goldenseal, Western echinacea, and cranberry have maintained their popular use in America, yet never gained this same acclaim in Europe outside of Great Britain. The two roots are recognized as the most popular herb combination in America, but it was as individual remedies that they were initially adopted and popularized by the Eclectics. Cranberry is consumed in much larger quantities in America that either of these herbs, yet it remains relatively unappreciated elsewhere. These plants demonstrate that to enjoy the bounty of botanical medicines from the New World garden, it is unnecessary to focus on the exotic tropics when such useful roots and berries grow in our own temperate forests, plains, and marshes.

GOLDENSEAL—Digging for Rare Herbal Treasure
Hydrastis canadensis L. —rhizome and roots

Summary

Goldenseal root has been used effectively by doctors in America since the early 19th century. With the discovery and identification of berberine, the yellow alkaloid which gives hydrastis roots and rhizome their characteristic color, some doctor's believed that they had obtained the component responsible for the therapeutic effects of this plant. However, subsequent research and clinical applications indicated that berberine was only one of a number of active alkaloids along with other components that contribute to the overall activity of the whole root.

Clinical applications of goldenseal mainly treat gastrointestinal problems associated with inadequate digestive and biliary secretions. Infections of the ears, eyes, or mucous membranes also respond to its local application. Infectious diarrhea has responded to goldenseal and berberine not only because of their antimicrobial activity, including immune effects, but also due to the prevention of bacterial adhesion and the antisecretory activity of berberine. Other alkaloids contribute in ways that are similar to, yet distinct from, the prominent berberine influence. For example, the effects of the alkaloid hydrastine help reduce congestion and diminish uterine blood loss. The activities of goldenseal, such as its effects on the uterus, do not always correlate with those of berberine. Not only should the effects of goldenseal not be equated with any one of its components, but the combined effects of all of its alkaloids do not adequately describe the influence of the entire root or its traditional extracts. Substituting other herbs for goldenseal simply because they contain berberine, along with a distinctively different profiles of other active components, is not clinically equivalent. The legitimate concerns about over-harvesting wild goldenseal must be addressed by relying on cultivation for commercial supplies, if the current popularity and future of this herb can be expected to sustain its historical success.

Names

Goldenseal root is actually the rhizome of the plant *Hydrastis canadensis* with its attached rootlets. According to the Lloyds, the term "golden seal" was first applied to it by the Thomsonians in reference to the yellow seal-like scars on the fresh rhizome. It was also called yellow root and yellow puccoon. Based on its use as an eye wash, the names eye-balm and eye-root were sometimes employed. The association of the root with liver problems led to its being called jaundice root and yellow eye. Its application as a dye due to its yellow alkaloid berberine led to a number of designations signifying this use, including Indian paint.

Root Description and Plant Distribution

Goldenseal root is either collected in the spring after the plant begins to grow or in late summer before it loses its leaves. Internally, it is bright yellow when fresh. The dried powder has a dull yellowish hue. The goldenseal powder releases a characteristic odor that has been described as peculiar and persistent. The taste is powerfully bitter and causes an abundant flow of saliva.

Benjamin Smith Barton in 1798 was the first medical author to attend to its properties, crediting the Cherokees for its applications, including for cancer. He reported that the plant's original distribution centered around the Ohio River valley. In smaller quantities its territory extended to the Great Lakes, east to the Appalachians, west into the Ozarks, and through Tennessee. The plant grows on hillsides in rich, open woods with abundant leaf mould.

Native Medicinal Uses

Those to first use goldenseal for medicinal purposes were eastern Native Americans. Moerman noted the Cherokees used it mostly as a digestive aid to improve the appetite and treat dyspepsia. It was also taken as a general tonic, as well as being applied as a wash locally for inflammations. The Cherokees also reportedly used it as a cure for cancer. The Iroquois seem to have utilized it more extensively. They used the infusion of the root for dyspepsia, but they also took it as an emetic (presumably in large quantities) to treat biliousness. The infusion was generally employed for liver and gall bladder troubles. The root decoction was taken for diarrhea and also for whooping cough. Either the infusion or decoction was taken for fever and pneumonia.

Moerman indicated the Iroquois combined it with other remedies in the treatment of earaches, scrofula, and as drops for sore eyes. The Micmac, meanwhile, applied the root to treat cut or chapped lips.

Early Anglo Medical Recognition

In 1804 Barton described the extract as a bitter tonic in use in western Pennsylvania. An infusion in cold water was given for eye inflammations. The second edition of the *Pharmacopoeia of the United States* included hydrastis in 1830. In 1833 the *Thomsonian Recorder* identified it as a remedy for eye, stomach and bowel problems. Wooster Beach, founder of Eclectic medicine, included hydrastis in his *American Practice of Medicine* in 1833, noting both its bitter tonic and mild laxative properties. The *United States Dispensatory* included it in the appendix of its second edition in 1834.

However, it was *The Eclectic Dispensatory of the United States of America* of 1852 by Drs. John King and Robert Newton that firmly established hydrastis as an important medicine. King's use of the article since 1833 allowed him to speak authoritatively and advocate its use as a remedy for urethral discharges and chronic gonorrhea. In 1856 Dr. Edwin M. Hale introduced it into homeopathic practice. Prof. Roberts Bartholow included it in his Materia Medica for the doctors of regular medicine. After its re-inclusion in the 1860 *USP*, it again attracted the attention of the entire medical profession. However, it was a favorite of both the Eclectics and the Thomsonian medical doctors known as Physiomedicalists. Physiomedicalists treated only with nontoxic herbs to support and enhance function to achieve a physiological balance.

Isolated Alkaloids

The Lloyds documented how the naming of hydrastis constituents caused much confusion. Rafinesque applied the name hydrastine to the yellow pigment (berberine) in 1828. In 1862 this main alkaloid was identified by Mahla as identical to the berberine from *Berberis* species. Eclectic physicians were reluctant to accept the "renaming" of this yellow component. Commercially, hydrastine remained the preferred term for berberine, even though Durand had discovered a white alkaloid insoluble in water from hydrastis in 1851 that he had named hydrastine. The Eclectic pharmacist William Merrell described an extract in 1862 that he produced commercially and named Hydrastine that contained "all the medicinal elements of the root together." According to Lloyd, after 1880 the Eclectics finally relinquished the use of this term when referring to the alkaloid berberine. A third alkaloid was separated from hydrastis in 1873 by A.K. Hale. After 1891 the name canadine was given to this other white alkaloid. It is also sometimes referred to as tetrahydroberberine. Another alkaloid was only recently identified in 1998 by Gentry and others as 8-oxotetrahyd rothalifendine.

Commercial Preparations, Doses, Alkaloid Content

ROOT POWDER

From 130 mg to 1.3 gm of the powder was given every 4–6 hours by Physiomedicalists and 65 mg to 2.0 gm by Eclectics. The 1946 *NF* gave an average dose of 2 gm, while Kuts-Cheraux indicated the naturopathic dose was from 640 mg to 2.6 gm. The old estimated amount of alkaloids in this dose of powder was 50 mg. The best amount of goldenseal root to use depends on its intended application.

Powdered hydrastis rhizome and roots were required to yield not less than 2.5% alkaloids. In a 1931 study by Gillis and Langerhan of plants grown in Washington state, using the *USP* assay method, the average percentage dry weight of ether-soluble alkaloids from 6-year-old plants harvested in late fall and mid-spring was 4.20–4.29% for the rhizome and 2.88–3.38% for the roots. The *USP* assay for the average alkaloid content of the leaf was 1.65%.

A thin-layer chromatogram of the alkaloids of goldenseal provides an effective means of determining possible adulteration with *Berberis* or other species containing berberine but no hydrastine. In a comparative study of ten powdered or coarsely chopped goldenseal root products by Govindan and Govindan in 2000, five contained both hystrastine and berberine, four contained berberine, and one contained neither. In the five goldenseal products the range of hydrastine content as measured by high performance liquid chromatography was 0.60–3.22%, while the berberine content was 0.56–4.54%.

INFUSION

Infusions were made with one ounce of powdered root per pint water and given in doses of 0.5–2.0 fluid ounces by Eclectics. Physiomedicalist and naturopathic doctors used half this strength. Water extracts were not considered as effective for internal use as hydro-alcoholic preparations. The white alkaloid hydrastine is not soluble in water, so its contribution is lost when using this form.

HYDROALCOHOLIC EXTRACTS

Three different types were in common use from about 1870 to 1950; tinctures were the most common form before and after these dates.

TINCTURE

The 1880 *USP* tincture was 1:5 strength, made with 50% alcohol. The average dose of the 1946 1:5 *NF* tincture was 8 ml, while Kuts-Cheraux gave the dosage range as from 4-16 ml. The old estimated amount of alkaloids per dose was 40 mg for the tincture. A nonofficial 1:12 tincture made by Physiomedicalists with 50% alcohol was given in doses of from 4–12 ml. The 1946 *National Formulary* 8th ed. specified for a 1:5 tincture from 0.45–0.55 gm% (gm% = grams per 100 ml) ether-soluble alkaloidsm, using old methods of measurement. A modern HPLC analysis of hydrastis 1:5 alcoholic extract by Leone and others in 1996 described the alkaloid yields as 1.0 gm% berberine, 0.5 gm% hydrastine, 0.02 gm% canadine, and 0.02 gm% canadaline (1.54 gm% total alkaloids).

Fluid Extract

This concentrate (1:1, 75% alcohol) of hydrastis rhizome was official in the 1880 *USP*. From 1/3–1 ml were administered in syrup by Physiomedicalists. A 2 ml average dose was given in the 1946 *NF*, and Kuts-Cheraux indicated naturopathic dosage ranging from 0.3–3.3 ml. The *NF* fluid extract (1:1) yielded 2.25–2.75 gm% ether-soluble alkaloids. The old estimated amount of alkaloids per dose was 50 mg for the fluid extract.

Specific Medicine

An alcoholic preparation called Specific Hydrastis made by Lloyd with rhizome and roots contained the full complement of goldenseal alkaloids but lacked most water-soluble components. The two main alkaloids of goldenseal were both considered important contributors to its different effects; the bitter yellow berberine as a stomachic, and the non-bitter white hydrastine as a mucosal tonic. Canadine was also present along with oily and resinous principles. The typical dosage range was 0.07–0.70 ml, but sometimes larger or smaller amounts were used.

Liquid Hydrastis

Since precipitation of almost 20% of the berberine in the fluid extract would occur within three weeks, in 1874 John Uri Lloyd prepared a 1:1 extract with official alcohol, afterward replacing the alcohol with 1/3 glycerine and 2/3 water. This process removed the gums, oils and resins but left the berberine and other alkaloids. This product was made with the intent of diluting it for use as an orificial or topical wash.

Alkaloids

When reduced medicinal activity was desired, isolated berberine was given. According to Felter and Ellingwood, berberine was rarely employed among the Eclectics. Berberine and hydrastine were identified as individual medicinal agents, but canadine was not used alone, in spite of its demonstrable activity. The Eclectic dose for berberin sulfate or hydrochorate was 65–325 mg. The alkaloid hydrastine hydrochloride was official in the 1946 *NF* with an average dose of 10 mg.

Early Physiomedicalist and Eclectic Applications

Experimental studies and clinical experience led to the observation that the various hydrastis products each had their own sphere of activity and appropriate utilization. The Eclectics in the late 19th century even utilized a product by Lloyd, known as Colorless Hydrastis or Lloydrastis, from which the berberine had been removed to treat local conditions of the skin and mucous membranes.

Root Powder

Small doses were used by Physiomedicalists for bowel and subacute bladder and uterine conditions; large doses could aggravate the symptoms. This remedy was especially useful in diminishing excessive mucus discharges of the GI tract. Its action was best for mucosal congestion with excessive secretions. At the same time it promoted healing of ulcerations. Large doses were necessary for depressed and atonic conditions.

Physiomedicalist Dr. William Cook claimed goldenseal to be a pure tonic. While he taught that it influenced the entire system, goldenseal root was largely used as an appetite stimulant and digestive tonic. It improved bile secretion and thereby aided in elimination through the bowels.

The Eclectic Ellingwood found that 350 mg of the powder was effective for stomach atonicity that resulted in indigestion. He also reported that Prof. Farnum claimed success in treating a number of gall stone cases with the powder when the symptoms are mild to moderate and short lived. Biliary colic due to catarrh was likewise helped as long as stones were not impacted in the gall bladder or bile ducts.

John Scudder, Eclectic originator and author of Specific Medication, reported in 1870 that he preferred using goldenseal powder or its infusion. In 1897 Bloyer concurred that older Eclectic doctors preferred the root powder or its aqueous extracts. These often proved effective but were disagreeable to patients. They believed goldenseal contracted blood vessels but not large muscles. Though a feeble oxytoxic, it effectively reduced uterine bleeding and congestion in fibromas, subinvolution and hemorrhagic endometritis. Hydrastis, given for reducing hemorrhage in the females, was reported by Drs. Harvey Felter and Finley Ellingwood as among the most valued remedies for menorrhagia and metrorrhagia when caused by a lack of uterine tone in the months after giving birth. Later, Grieve mentioned the powder being used for habitual constipation, combined with any aromatic. Both she and Lust acknowledge its use as a nasal snuff for congestion and mucus discharge.

Infusion

The water extract was used as a wash topically and on mucous membranes, such as for oral ulcerations as an antiseptic mouthwash. It can be applied with a toothbrush for pyorrhea and sore gums. Its local use by doctors in nasal, pharyngeal and vaginal conditions with discharges were quite successful. In purulent conditions of the eye and corneal ulceration it led to rapid healing. For topical use on the skin Physiomedicalists usually combined it with other herbs appropriate for healing the specific malady. They especially included it for skin ulcers and wounds. Lust recommended it as a wash for erysipelas and ringworm, followed by sprinkling with the dry powdered root. Internally, they used goldenseal tea in combinations for urinary tract infections and various other conditions.

HYDROALCOHOLIC EXTRACTS

The uses were similar but the forms varied, often depending upon the professional affiliation.

TINCTURE VERSUS FLUID EXTRACT

Physiomedicalists preferred the more concentrated fluid extract over the tincture. The Eclectic Scudder found the tincture to be a good preparation. The tincture was intended for poor appetite, indigestion and constipation due to torpid liver but not for active mucosal inflammation with poor secretion. Felter reported the use of hydrastis tincture or fluid extract for chronic alcoholism was considered by Bartholow very beneficial for abandoning strong drink and improving nutrition when combined with capsicum.

SPECIFIC MEDICINE

A condition identified prior to 1900 that responded well to Specific Hydrastis was the American malady termed "ice-water dyspepsia." Felter described this as digestive atony from ingestion of large quantities of cold fluids and undue consumption of ice cream and sherbets. He advised using 0.7 ml (10 drops) before meals and at bedtime. Dyspepsia with excessive belching and a sense of weakness with irritability just below the sternum was effectively treated with small doses, around 1-2 drops Specific Hydrastis according to Ellingwood. This liquid form was preferred to the powder or isolated alkaloids that could further irritate the stomach. With atonic dyspepsia involving both the stomach and liver, the required dose might be 1 ml. As reported by Felter and Lloyd, a 1 drop dose was used by Webster for myalgia associated with visceral causes.

LIQUID HYDRASTIS

According to John Fearn, M.D., 2 drops of Lloyd's non-alcoholic Liquid Hydrastis glycerite given every three hours in a teaspoon of the vehicle Glyconda with Specific Medicine *Mangifera indica* helped stop the bleeding of a large uterine fibroid tumor before its surgical removal. Dr. Pitts Howes believed large fibroids complicated by hemorrhage could be controlled by his method. He would make a tampon of absorbent cotton saturated with a solution composed of equal parts hydrastis and glycerin and pack it against the posterior aspect of the uterine cervix, filling the vagina fairly well. These tampons were used at night and in the morning following a warm water douche. The hydrastis seemed to work through the blood vessels to tone the uterus and reduce the fibroid, while the glycerin caused a drawing of fluid from the fibroid tissues.

ALKALOIDS

Berberine was given by Physiomedicalists in doses of from 65–325 mg as a tonic and from 650–975 mg for malaria. So-called "hydrastine" (berberine) sulfate was used by Scudder as a local wash for conjunctivitis and for gonorrhea. The therapeutic benefits of hydrastis upon the mucous membrane and conjunctiva were considered by Dr. John King to be superior to berberine. Felter reported in 1906 that physiological experiments by conventional medical doctors showed the alkaloids exerted control over the female genital tract blood vessels. Felter acknowledged that dyspepsia without irritability could be treated with berberine salts, for which Ellingwood recommended from 5–16 mg of true hydrastine sulfate or its hydrochlorate.

Laboratory Research—Extracts and Alkaloids

Vasoactivity

HYDROALCOHOLIC EXTRACTS

Opposing outcomes based on relative concentration was observed by Palmery and others in 1993. While hydrastis extract at low doses inhibits contraction of rabbit aorta induced by histamine, a higher dose caused a dose-dependent vasoconstriction. Berberine and hydrastine content of this extract were 0.433 and 0.405 gm%, respectively. In 1996 they again showed hydrastis extract inhibited adrenaline-induced contraction on rabbit aorta *in vitro* in low doses. The total extract made with 70% ethanol was active in a lower concentration than the isolated alkaloids. Likewise, in 1997 they showed the anti-serotoninergic activity of the total extract on isolated rabbit aorta was more potent than individual alkaloids or their additive effects.

ALKALOIDS

Berberine, canadine and canadaline alone and in combination were shown by Palmery and others in 1996 to inhibit adrenaline-induced contraction on rabbit aorta *in vitro* in low doses. Palmery and others in 1996 also found hydrastine may be antagonistic to the adrenolytic activity of the other alkaloids. In 1997 they found the relative anti-serotonin effect of the individual alkaloids was: canadaline > canadine > berberine > hydrastine.

Smooth Muscle Relaxant and Cholinergic

HYDROALCOHOLIC EXTRACTS

The effects of hydrastis extract on rabbit bladder strips as shown by Bolle and others in 1998 included relaxation that was partially blocked by the β-adrenergic receptor blocker, propranolol. Also in 1998 Baldazzi and others showed hydrastis extract inhibited the contractions of rabbit prostate strips stimulated by norepinephrine and especially by phenylephrine. The same year Cometa and others found hydrastis alcoholic extract also inhibited tracheal contractions of strips from the guinea-pig by both β-adrenoceptor-dependent and—independent mechanisms. In 2000 Abdel-Haq and others potentiated the relaxant effect of isoprenaline with the alcoholic extract.

ALKALOIDS

The contractile effect on isolated guinea-pig ileum can be explained by berberine and canadine having a similar dose-dependent indirect cholinergic effect. Shin and others researched berberine in 1993, and it seemed to act by increasing acetylcholine release, inhibiting cholinesterase, and blocking α_2-adrenoceptors. Cometa and others showed in 1996 that canadaline was only slightly cholinergic.

In examing effects on strips of rabbit bladder muscle, Bolle and others tested the four major hydrastis alkaloids alone in concentrations several times higher than found in the extract produced no relaxation. Combined in concentrations similar to the extract (berberine 1.0 gm%, hydrastine 0.5 gm%, canadine 0.02 gm%, and canadaline 0.02 gm%), the alkaloids produced a mild synergistic relaxing effect. Other components are apparently responsible for the most of this effect through several mechanisms.

When rabbit prostate strips contractions induced by norepinephrine or phenylephrine were inhibited by berberine, it appeared as though berberine affected α_2-adrenergic receptors more than α_1-recptors. All of the alkaloids increased the relaxant effect of isoprenaline. The greatest potency found by Abdel-Haq and others was with canadaline and then canadine, followed by berberine and hydrastine.

Uterine Relaxant or Stimulant

HYDROALCOHOLIC EXTRACTS

Cometa and others in 1998 demonstrated that a 70% ethanol extract of goldenseal root relaxed rat uterine preparations in the lab. Haginiwa and Harada in 1962 found extracts of hydrastis show anticonvulsive activity on a mouse uterus. On the rat uterus hydrastis liquid extract produced a decrease in uterine tone and amplitude, according to Gibbs in 1947.

ALKALOIDS

Using isolated guinea-pig and cat uteri, Supek found in 1946 that berberine had a stimulant effect similar to hydrastine's action. On the other hand in 1944 Gibbs noted using the rat uterus that berberine caused a slow reduction of rate, tone, amplitude, and response to acetylcholine. Hydrastine increased the rate of uterine contractions and speed of contractile response to acetylcholine in rats. However, he found hydrastine and hydrastine together with berberine produced a decrease in uterine tone and amplitude. To further complicate the confusion, Imaseki and others showed in 1961 on the mouse uterus that berberine produced a marked contraction, but canadine (tetrahydroberberine) caused a transitory relaxation.

The variable reactions of animal uteri to the same stimulant was recognized and documented by Kulz in 1925. He concluded that applying the results of isolated animal studies to humans was unreliable and impractical. Therapeutic effects should be based on clinical findings, rather than laboratory animal responses.

Antimicrobial Activity

HYDROALCOHOLIC EXTRACTS

Scazzocchio and others in 1998 and in 2001 tested the 1:5 strength alcoholic extract against strains of *Staphylococcus aureus, Streptococcus sanguis, Escherichia coli, Pseudomonas aeruginosa* and *Candida albicans*. They found it was bactericidal in one half hour or less, whether undiluted or diluted by one half. Exceptions were *Candida* yeast that required one hour when diluted and *E. coli* that required two hours. The extract was more potent than the isolated alkaloids, except for canadaline. An antimicrobial effect against *C. albicans* or *E. coli* was not potent for the individual alkaloids. The same year Gentry and others showed hydrastis root ethanolic extract at high concentrations inhibited the growth of *S. aureus, Klebsiella pneumoniae, Mycobacterium smegmatis*, and *C. albicans*. The activity was greater against the more clinically relevant *Mycobacterium tuberculosis* and *M. avium* complex.

ALKALOIDS

Berberine was shown in 1952 by Johnson and others to be an effective antibacterial agent, about 100 times stronger than hydrastine against gram negative microbes according to Poe and Johnson in 1954. Recently, Scazzocchio and others found that hydrastine has little antimicrobial activity, but the other alkaloids have significant potency. Against *Escherischia coli*, only canadaline and berberine were effectively antibacterial. Canadine and canadaline, but not berberine, are effective inhibitors of *Pseudomonas aeruginosa*. *Candida albicans* was not effectively inhibited by the individual alkaoids. However, in 1982 Mahajan and others showed berberine's inhibitory effects on fungi that were isolated from the eyes of humans with various ocular conditions.

Testing by Gentry and others of individual components for inhibiting *Mycobacterium* showed that this was due to berberine; hydrastine and canadine were inactive, as were two quinic acid esters. Studies by Amin, Sabir, Mahajan, Ghosh, and their fellow researchers have shown the laboratory antimicrobial effects of berberine sulfate, hydrochloride, tannate, or chloride against Gram-positive and Gram-negative bacteria, fungi, and protozoa. In 1991 Kaneda and others determined the mechanism of berberine sulfate's antiprotozoal effects against *Entamoeba histolytica*, *Giardia lamblia*, and *Trichomonas vaginalis* was by disrupting the growth and intracellular composition. Subbaiah and Amin found berberine sulfate also effectively prevented intestinal and hepatic amoebiasis in rats and golden hamsters, respectively, when three doses of 3 mg/kg were given orally in 4-hour intervals.

Immune Modulation

LIQUID HYDRASTIS

In 1999 the total extract as a 1:1 non-alcoholic glycerine product of the root given orally by Rehman and others to rats was shown to significantly increase primary IgM response in the first two weeks following antigen exposure.

ALKALOID: BERBERINE

Berberine hydrochloride and berberine sulfate were identified by Kumazawa and others in 1984 as potent macrophage activators against tumor cells in the lab. Two studies in 1988 by Sun and others found berberine sulfate also blocks adherence of *Streptococcus pyogenes* and *Escherichia coli* to epithelial cells.

Antisecretory

NONALKALOIDAL EXTRACT

In 1886 Dr. Jeancon tested a colorless, nonalcoholic goldenseal extract after the removal of its alkaloids. When given internally to healthy animals it produced constipation, since its action was astringent.

ALKALOID: BERBERINE

Though not a potent bactericidal agent against *E. coli*, Sack and Tai and their fellow researchers showed berberine inhibits the secretions caused by its enterotoxin in lab tissue and in living animals. It had the same anti-secretory effect against cholera toxin. Though 10 mg/kg reduced intestinal motility in mice, the anti-secretory effect of berberine's impact on diarrhea is selective. Akhter and others showed the results depend upon the initiating agent.

Choleretic

ALKALOID: BERBERINE

Berberine tripled the excretion of bile after 90 minutes in a 1958 study by Velluda and others. In a study in cats in 1962 by Turova and others berberine caused a 14–30% increase of bile secretion in the first hour. The second hour was normal. Chan showed in 1977 that berberine hydrochloride increases the bilirubin excretion by the liver and bile flow for 90 minutes in rats when given intragastrically. However, after eight days there was no significant difference from controls.

COX-2 Inhibition

ALKALOID: BERBERINE

Due to its cyclooxygenase-2 (COX-2) inhibitory properties in human colon cancer cells, as shown by Fukuda and others in 1999, berberine may have a preventive effect for colon cancer. COX-2 inhibition also produces anti-inflammatory effects.

Human Studies—Extracts and Berberine

Digestive Effects

HYDROALCOHOLIC EXTRACTS

According to Wolf and Mack in 1956, when given internally, a 54% alcoholic extract of hydrastis increased gastric acidity in 10 out of 15 trials. It was as effective when taken directly into the stomach as when tasted in the mouth before entering the stomach. This was superior to five other herbal bitter stomachics tested. By comparison, 50% alcohol in water significantly reduced gastric acidity in this subject in all four trials.

ALKALOID: BERBERINE

A clinical study by Turova and others in 1964 with 225 patients suffering from chronic cholecystitis used 5–20 mg berberine hydrochloride and sulfate orally three times daily before meals for two days. It helped eliminate symptoms, increase bile bilirubin levels and decrease gallbladder bile volume.

Antimicrobial

ALKALOID: BERBERINE

A 0.2% berberine chloride concentration was clinically effective when two drops three times daily for three weeks were applied locally in the eyes by Babbar and others in 1982 to treat trachoma, a blinding disease caused by *Chlamydia trachomatis*.

Giardiasis in children aged five months to fourteen years was relieved by berberine given in oral doses of 10 mg/kg/day for ten days. No unpleasant side effects were noted by Gupte in this 1975 study, but 17% relapsed after one month.

Antisecretory

NONALKALOIDAL EXTRACT

In 1886 Dr. Jeancon applied a colorless, nonalcoholic goldenseal extract with its alkaloids removed to the cervical os and canal. This gradually reduced excessive secretions until they ceased. Improvement in cervical erosion, extreme urethritis, and aphthous ulceration of the mouth and pharynx followed local application. His experiments demonstrated the important effects of components in goldenseal other than the prominent alkaloids berberine and hydrastine.

ALKALOID: BERBERINE

In randomized, controlled clinical trials by Rabbani and others in 1987 using a single dose of 400 mg berberine sulfate, 33 patients with *E. coli* diarrhea who used berberine had a reduced stool volume, and more had their diarrhea stopped within 24 hours than among the 30 controls. The same berberine dose for cholera patients was not as effective when compared to controls. In a placebo-controlled, double-blind, randomized clinical trial by Khin and others in 1985, 100 mg of berberine hydrochloride given four times daily reduced liquid stools by one liter but was inferior to 500 mg four times daily of tetracycline for 185 cholera patients.

Berberine hydrochloride was compared by Lahiri and Dutta in 1967 to chloramphenicol for the treatment of epidemic cholera and severe diarrhea in children and adults. The adult dose was a 50 mg tablet of berberine hydrochloride every eight hours for two days, then one tablet twice daily for three more days. Berberine was superior to chloramphenicol in lowering the mortality rate of vibrio-negative patients in serious condition. It was also better in cases of true cholera one year, but the next the two drugs were equivalent. Berberine reduced volume and duration of diarrhea, period of hydration, intake of intravenous fluid, and convalescence period. It produced no side effects or toxicity.

In 100 cases of diarrhea in children, 50 children were given 25 mg berberine tannate orally four times daily and compared with 50 similar patients receiving sulphonamide, sulphonamide plus streptomycin, chloromycetin plus streptomycin, or the furoxone form of furazolidine. All mild and moderate cases using berberine had recovered within three to five days, respectively, comparable to the positive controls using antibiotics. Of the severe cases two were fatal in the berberine group and three in the group receiving antibiotics. Adverse effects with berberine consisted of vomiting in three children, leading to their withdrawing from this 1970 study by Sharda.

Heart Tonic

Alkaloid: Berberine

In 1988 berberine was studied by Marin-Neto and others in 12 patients with congestive heart failure who were refractory to conventional therapy with digitalis and diuretics. The berberine was administered intravenously at 0.02 and 0.2 mg/kg/min for 30 minutes. The 0.2 mg/kg/min rate caused a significant decrease in systemic and pulmonary vascular resistance, as well as left ventricular and right atrium end-diastolic pressures. Besides decreasing peripheral resistance and blood pressure, it also had a positive inotropic effect by increasing cardiac index, stroke index, and left ventricular ejection fraction. These acute beneficial effects were offset by ventricular tachycardia that developed in 4 patients 1–20 hours after administration ended.

Zeng and Zeng in 1999 looked at effective oral dosing of berberine for 56 patients with severe congestive heart failure. Giving 1.2 grams berberine daily for 2 weeks, in addition to the ACE inhibitors and loop diuretics that each received (as well as digoxin in 51 and nitrates in 46), the authors measured plasma berberine concentrations and compared these with outcomes. A decrease in ventricular premature beats and increase in left ventricular ejection fraction was enjoyed by all of the patients but was significantly better in the 31 with plasma concentrations of berberine higher than 0.11 mg/L 2.4 hours after administration compared with those lower than this. No side effects or arrhythmias were detected.

In 2003 Zeng and others gave 1.2 grams berberine daily in 4 divided doses as tablets to 79 congestive heart failure patients on ACE inhibitors along with diuretics / spironolactone in 77, digoxin in 76, and nitrates in 71. This significantly increased left ventricular ejection fraction and exercise capacity, improved dyspnea-fatigue index, and reduced frequency of ventricular premature complexes compared with 77 patients using only comparable conventional medications. The mortality of the berberine group decreased significantly as well, and there were no apparent side effects.

Safety Concerns

Ellingwood indicated that with extreme irritability of the stomach fluid preparations were preferable, and the use of small doses (1–2 drops in solution) was required. Felter believed that while advantageous in chronic gastritis, acutely inflamed tissues of the GI tract contraindicated goldenseal's internal use. Other cases aggravated by goldenseal included local employment for anal fissures, rectal ulcers and proctitis unless it was administered carefully in small amounts. Acute purulent otitis media was the one exception of its contraindication for acute mucosal inflammation.

When taken for an extended period, toxicity symptoms reported for hydrastis in a book edited by Grunewald and others include digestive disorders, constipation, excitatory states, hallucinations and occasionally delirium. High dosages are claimed to induce vomiting, difficulty breathing, spasms, bradycardia, and central paralysis. However, the form of hydrastis, the duration of its use, the doses, and the species affected in this manner are not specified by this source. Grieve noted that large amounts of the dried root can be very poisonous. Lust warns that eating the fresh plant can produce ulcers and inflammation of mucous membranes locally.

Goldenseal has developed a reputation for masking drug use, particularly opiods. Foster described a study in 1975 that showed goldenseal given with the opiate alkaloid codeine failed to alter the detection of this opiate in a urine drug screen. He also related that in a 1982 study on racehorse drug detection, the inclusion of an efficient hydrolysis step in urinalysis prevented a decrease in measured total morphine excretion 5–6 hours after goldenseal consumption. In testing liver microsomal conversion of morphine, Turova and others in 1964 found berberine failed to change the rate of morphine conversion.

Alkaloid Kinetics and Safety Issues

In infant rabbits berberine sulfate given orally at 500 mg/kg was absorbed as shown by Bhide and others in 1969. It reached maximum levels in the blood after eight hours, and remained after 72 hours. The highest tissue levels were found in the heart, followed by the pancreas and liver. It was excreted through the urine and stools mostly in the first day, but was still being eliminated after 48 hours. When Schein and Hanna in 1960 gave berberine sulfate orally to rats at up to 1 gm/kg, it was very poorly absorbed.

Only extreme doses of the alkaloids are reported by Felter and Ellingwood to have caused convulsions and death in lower animals. Though the alkaloids, particularly hydrastine, were actively poisonous in animals under experimental conditions, hydrastis did not have this effect on humans in ordinary medicinal doses.

In 1962 Turova and others reported that berberine sulfate given orally to cats at 25 mg/kg caused a general depression within one hour, lasting 6–8 hours. At 50 mg/kg it caused salivation and occasional vomiting. When given 100 mg/kg the vomiting lasted 6–8 hours and all animals died within 8–10 days. Higher doses caused serous-hemorrhagic inflammation in the small and large intestines. The lethal dose for half the rats given berberine sulfate was determined by Kowalewski and others to be greater than 1 gm/kg orally, but only 88.5 mg/kg when injected intraperitoneally and 14.5 mg/kg injected intramuscularly. Six weeks of 0.5 gm/kg oral daily doses caused no histopathological changes in the tissues and organs of rats.

Berberine hydrochloride administered intraperitoneally by Shanbhag and others to cats produced sedation, retching, urination and defecation within 3–5 minutes at all dose levels tested: 5, 20, and 40 mg/kg. Intraperitoneal injection of 5 mg/kg resulted in sedation after five minutes in mice under amphetamine stimulation. It increased the sleeping time in mice given the sedative pentobarbitone.

Berberine has been shown by Chan in 1993 to be a potent displacer of bilirubin from albumin in test tubes. Berberine significantly reduced bilirubin serum protein binding when given IP to rats. For this reason berberine-containing herbs should be avoided in pregnant women and jaundiced neonates to avoid increasing the risk of kernicterus. Berberine has also been shown in several studies by Lin and others in 1999 to reduce retention of the chemotherapeutic drug rhodamine 123 by hepatoma cells *in vitro* and retention of taxol by oral, gastric, and colon cancer cell lines due to increased efflux by P-glycoprotein. Therefore, it is best to avoid these combinations.

Late nineteenth century research with frogs reported by the Lloyds showed that 200 mg of hydrastine hydrochlorate stimulated the central nervous system and caused rapid muscular rigidity, convulsions, and death from respiratory tetany, with similar results in rabbits. Hydrastine given by Poe and Johnson in 1954 to 1.5-month-old rats using intraperitoneal (IP) injection caused no deaths at 50 mg/kg. However, it induced convulsions and death in 40–100% of cases dose-dependently in amounts ranging from 100–250 mg/kg. The lethal dose for half receiving this form was 104 mg/kg.

Canadine (tetrahydroberberine) IP injection by Chin and others of 40-65 mg/kg in mice increased sleeping time from hexobarbital and reduced spontaneous activity. It inhibited metrazole convulsions but aggravated strychnine convulsions. The acute IP LD_{50} in mice was 566 mg/kg. In rats they orally administered 150 or 300 mg/kg/day of canadine for 30 days, and little visual visceral change was found, only very slight microscopic swelling in the heart. After oral administration to monkeys of 180 or 206 mg/kg, sedation, tremor, and catatonia occurred within 0.5–1.0 hour and disappeared in 24–48, 12–24, and 5 hours, respectively.

Endangerment Versus Cultivation

The area where goldenseal was abundant and harvested in the 19th century was very limited in scope. The plant grew in large patches initially, but, with clearing of the forest for cultivation, the easily accessible sources were soon decimated. By the late 19th century between 140,000–150,000 pounds were annually supplied, of which 25,000–28,000 pounds were used solely to extract the alkaloids. Remote mountain areas remained where subsistent dwellers continued to supply the demand. According to McGuffin, annual wild harvest of dried goldenseal root has been estimated at between 200,000–400,000 pounds dry weight on four occasions in the 20th century (1908, 1927, 1949 and 1998). On the other hand, Cech reports that commercial planting in Oregon and Washington during this time have been relatively successful.

Concannon and DeMeo describe how over-collection, road intrusion, urbanization, and recreational use of the land, populations of goldenseal have been dramatically reduced. As a consequence, the listing of goldenseal under Appendix II of the Convention in Trade in Endangered Species (CITES) became effective in September, 1997, regulating ethical and sustainable supply in world trade. Exportation of crude goldenseal from the United States or Canada now requires an export permit that is granted only on the basis of legal and non-detrimental harvesting.

Thornton insisted in 1998 that the cultivation of goldenseal is necessary to insure the continuing availability of this valuable plant resource as its market demand grows worldwide. Using High Performance Liquid Chromatography (HPLC) analysis the cultivated goldenseal appears to have, on average, equivalent or higher levels of active constituents, compared to wildcrafted sources. The average time to harvest after transplantation was calculated to be 3.6–3.8 years. McGuffin reported in 1999 that plans to expand cultivated acreage could provide an even greater percentage of the total supply from commercial growing ventures.

Table 4 Goldenseal Root and Derivatives—Summary of Medicinal Uses and Pharmacology

GOLDENSEAL *Hydrastis canadensis* L.	Native American Uses	Physiomedical and Eclectic Medical Uses	Modern Clinical Studies	Laboratory Research Findings
Whole Root Powder	Tonic Chapped lips	Digestive tonic Liver tonic Gall stones Biliary catarrh Uterine bleeding from fibroids or subinvolution		
Water Extracts	Fever Pneumonia Dyspepsia Liver trouble Diarrhea Whooping cough Locally: Ear aches Sore eyes Skin sores	Urinary infections Locally: Skin ulcers Wounds Discharges Eye infections Skin conditions Mouth ulcers		

Continued on next page

Table 4—*Continued*

GOLDENSEAL *Hydrastis canadensis* L.	Native American Uses	Physiomedical and Eclectic Medical Uses	Modern Clinical Studies	Laboratory Research Findings
Hydroalcoholic Extracts		Liver tonic Dyspepsia Constipation Alcoholism Myalgia	Gastric tonic	Anti-adrenergic Anti-serotonergic Genito-urinary, respiratory, and uterine relaxant
Glycerine / Water Extract (Liquid Hydrastis)		Uterine fibroids		Enhanced IgM antibody response
Nonalkaloidal Extract			Antisecretory Anti-ulcer	Astringent
ISOLATED ALKALOIDS				
Berberine		Tonic Dyspepsia Gonorrhea Malaria Locally: conjunctivits	Choleretic Cholagogic Antitrachoma Anti-giardial Antidiarrheal Positive inotropic Vasodilation	Anti-adrenergic Cholinergic Antisecretory Antimicrobial Anti-adherence Pro-macrophage COX-2 inhibition
Hydrastine		Dyspepsia		Anti-adrenergic antagonist Uterine tonic
Canadine and/or Canadaline				Anti-adrenergic Anti-serotonergic Cholinergic Antimicrobial Uterine relaxant

References

BOOKS

Barton, BS. *Collections for an Essay Towards a Materia Medica of the United States*, 1798 and 1804, Bulletin of the Lloyd Library, Cincinnati, OH., No. 1, 1900.

Cook, WH. *The Physio-Medical Dispensatory* (1869), Eclectic Medical Pub., Portland, OR., 1985.

Ellingwood, F. *American Materia Medica, Therapeutics and Pharmacognosy* (1919 edition), Eclectic Medical Pub., Sandy, OR., 1994.

Felter, HW. *The Eclectic Materia Medica, Pharmacology and Therapeutics* (first published 1922), Eclectic Medical Pub., Sandy, OR., 1994.

Felter, HW and Lloyd, JU. *King's American Dispensatory*, 1898 version, Eclectic Medical Pub., Sandy, OR., 1983.

Grieve, M. *A Modern Herbal*, 1931 version, Dover Pub., New York, 1971.

Gruenwald, J et al (eds.). *PDR for Herbal Medicines*, 1st ed., Medical Economics Co., Montvale, N.J., 1998.

Kuts-Cheraux, AW. *Naturae Medicina and Naturopathic Dispensatory*, American Naturopathic Physicians and Surgeons Assoc., Des Moines, Iowa, 1953.

Lloyd, JU and Lloyd, CG. *Hydrastis Canadensis* (1884), Bulletin of the Lloyd Library, Cincinnati, OH., No. 10, 1908.

Lust, J. *The Herb Book*, Bantam Books, New York, 1974.

Moerman, DE. *Medicinal Plants of Native America*, Vol. 1, Univ. of Michigan Museum of Anthropology, Ann Arbor, Mich., 1986.

Powers, JL, (Chair., Comm. On National Formulary). *The National Formulary*, 8th ed., American Pharmaceutical Assoc., Washington, D.C., 1946.

ARTICLES

Abdel-Haq, H et al. Relaxant effects of Hydrastis canadensis L. and its major alkaloids on guinea pig isolated trachea. *Pharmacol. Toxicol.*, 87:218–222, 2000.

Akhter, MH et al. Possible mechanism of antidiarrhoeal effect of berberine. *Indian J. Med. Res.*, 70:233–41, 1979.

Amin, AH et al. Berberine sulfate: antimicrobial activity, bioassay, and mode of action. *Can. J. Microbiol.*, 15:1067–76, 1969.

Babbar, OP et al. Effect of berberine chloride eye drops on clinically positive trachoma patients. *Indian J. Med. Res.*, 76(Suppl.):83–8, 1982.

Baldazzi, C et al. Effects of the major alkaloid of Hydrastis canadensis L., berberine, on rabbit prostate strips. *Phtyother. Res.*, 12:S89–S91, 1998.

Bhide, MB et al. Absorption, distribution and excretion of berberine. *Indian J. Med. Res.*, 57:2128–31, 1969.

Bloyer, WE. Hydrastis canadensis. *Ecl. Med. J.*, 57:679–83, 1897.

Bolle, P et al. Response of rabbit detrusor muscle to total extract and major alkaloids of Hydrastis canadensis. *Phytother. Res.*, 12:S86–S88, 1998.

Cech, R. An ecological imperative – growing a future for native plant medicinals. *Unit. Pl. Sav. Newslett.*, 1(2):1, 4–5, 1997.

Chan, E. Displacement of bilirubin from albumin by berberine. *Biol. Neonate*, 63(4):201-208, 1993.

Chan, MY. The effect of berberine on bilirubin excretion in the rat. *Comp. Med. East West*, 5(2): 161–8, 1977.

Chin, K-C et al. Pharmacologic actions of tetrahydrobererine on the central nervous system. *Sheng Li Hsueh Pao*, 25(3):182–90, 1962 (*Chem. Abs.* 59:13249g).

Cometa, MF et al. Acute effect of alkaloids from Hydrastis canadensis L. on guinea-pig ileum: structure-activity relationships. *Phytother. Res.*, 0:S56–8, 1996.

Cometa, MF et al. Spasmolytic activities of Hydrastis canadensis L. on rat uterus and guinea-pig trachea. *Phytother. Res.*, 12:S83–S85, 1998.

Concannon, JA and DeMeo, TE. Goldenseal: facing a hidden crisis. *Endang. Spec. Pull.*, 22(6):10–2, 1997.

Dutta, NK et al. Berberine in toxin-induced experimental cholera. *Br. J. Pharmac.*, 44:153–9, 1972.

El-Masry, S et al. Colorimetric and spectrophotometric determinations of Hydrastis alkaloids in pharmaceutical preparations. *J. Pharm. Sci.*, 69(5):597–8, 1980.

Fearn, J. Mangifera indica and Hydrastis canadensis. *Ecl. Med. J.*, 70:378, 1910.

Felter, HW. Hydrastis in ice-water dyspepsia. *Ecl. Med. J.*, 56:343–4, 1896.

Felter, HW. Hydrastis and black haw in menorrhagia. *Ecl. Med. J.*, 66:93, 1906.

Foster, S. Goldenseal masking of drug tests. *HerbalGram*, 21:7, 35, 1989.

Fukuda, K et al. Inhibition by berberine of cyclooxygenase-2 transcriptional activity in human colon cancer cells. *J. Ethnopharmacol.*, 66:227–233, 1999.

Gentry, EJ et al. Antitubercular natural products: berberine from the roots of commercial Hydrastis canadensis powder. Isolation of inactive 8-oxotetrahydrothalifendine, canadine, beta-hydrastine, and two new quinic acid esters, hycandinic acid esters-1 and –2. *J. Nat. Prod.*, 61:1187–93, 1998.

Ghosh, AK et al. Effect of berberine chloride on Leishmania donovani. *Indian J. Med. Res.*, 78:407–16, 1983.

Gibbs, OS. On the curious pharmacology of hydrastis. *Fed. Proc.*, 6:332, 1947.

Gillis, E and Langenhan, HA. A phytochemical study of Hydrastis canadensis (goldenseal). *J. Am. Pharm. Assoc.*, 20:210–24, 329-38, 1931.

Govidan, M and Govindan, G. A convenient method for the determination of the quality of goldenseal. *Fitoterapia*, 71:232–5, 2000.

Gupte, S. Use of berberine in treatment of giardiasis. *Am. J. Dis. Child.*, 129:866, 1975.

Haginiwa, J and Harada, M. Pharmacological studies on crude drugs. V. Comparison of the pharmacological actions of berberine type alkaloid-containing plants and their components. *Yakugaku Zasshi*, 82:726–31, 1962. (*Chem. Abs.* 57:9145b).

Howes, PE. Hydrastis canadensis. *Trans. Nat. Ecl. Med. Assoc.,* 32:76–8, 1904.

Imaseki, I et al. Effect of berberine alkaloids on intestine and uterus in mice. *Yakugaku Zasshi,* 81:1281–4, 1961 (*Chem. Abs.* 565:5372c).

Jeancon, JA. Researches on hydrastis. *Ecl. Med. J.,* 46:576–7, 1886.

Johnson, CC et al. Toxicity of alkaloids to certain bacteria II. Berberine, physostigmine, and sanguinarine. *Acta pharmacol. et toxicol.,* 8:71–8, 1952.

Kaneda, Y et al. In vitro effects of berberine sulphate on the growth and structure of Entamoeba histolytica, Giardia lamblia and Trichomonas vaginalis. *Ann Trop. Med. Parasitol.,* 85(4):417–25, 1991.

Khin, MU et al. Clinical trial of berberine in acute watery diarrhoea. *Br. Med. J.,* 291:1601–5, 1985.

Kowalewski, A et al. Toxicity of berberine sulfate. *Acta Pol. Pharm.,* 32(1):113–20, 1975 (*Chem. Abs.* 83:91108u).

Kulz, F. Differences in the pharmacological effects of drugs upon animals and man. *Ecl. Med. J.,* 85(9):429–34, 1925.

Kumazawa, Y et al. Activation of peritoneal macrophages by berberine-type alkaloids in terms of induction of cytostatic activity. *Int. J. Immunopharmac.,* 6(6):587–92, 1984.

Lahiri, SC and Dutta, NK. Berberine and chloramphenicol in the treatment of cholera and severe diarrhoea. *J. Indian Med. Assoc.,* 48(1):1–11, 1967.

Leone, MG et al. HPLC determination of the major alkaloids extracted from Hydrastis canadensis L. *Phytother. Res.,* 10:S45–6, 1996.

Lin, HL et al. Up-regulation of multidrug resistance transporter expression by berberine in human and murine hepatoma cells. *Cancer,* 85:1937–42, 1999.

Lin, Hl et al. Berberine modulates expression of mdr1 gene product and the responses of digestive track cancer cells to Paclitaxel. *Br. J. Canc.,* 81(3):416–22, 1999.

Lloyd, JU. Hydrastis canadensis. *Ecl. Med. J.,* 58:316–20, 1898.

Mahajan, VM et al. Antimycotic activity of berberine sulphate: an alkaloid from an Indian medicinal herb. *Sabouraudia,* 20:79–81, 1982.

Marin-Neto, JA et al. Cardiovascular effects of berberine in patients with severe congestive heart failure. *Clin. Cardiol.,* 253–60, 1988.

McGuffin, M. AHPA goldenseal survey measures increased agricultural production. *HerbalGram,* 46:66–7, 1999.

Merrell, WS. Hydrastis canadensis. *Ecl. Med. J.,* 21:244–5, 1862.

Palmery, M et al. Effects of Hydrastis canadensis L. and the two major alkaloids berberine and hydrastine on rabbit aorta. *Pharmacol. Res.,* 27(Suppl. 1):73–4, 1993.

Palmery, M et al. Further studies of the adrenolytic activity of the major alkaloids from Hydrastis canadensis L. on isolated rabbit aorta. *Phytother. Res.,* 10:A47–9, 1996.

Palmery, M et al. Antiserotoninergic activity of the major alkaloids from Hydrastis canadensis L. on isolated rabbit aorta. *Pharmacol. Res.,* 35(Suppl.):28, 1997.

Poe, CF and Johnson, CC. Toxicity of hydrastine, hydrastinine, and sparteine. *Acta pharmacol et toxicol.,* 10:338–346, 1954.

Rabbani, GH et al. Randomized controlled trial of berberine sulfate therapy for diarrhea due to enterotoxigenic Escherichia coli and Vibrio cholerae. *J. Infect. Dis.,* 155(5):979–84, 1987.

Rehman, Jet al. Increased production of antigen-specific IgG and IgM following in vivo treatment with the medicinal plants Echinacea angustifolia and Hydrastis canadensis. *Immunol. Lett.,* 68: 391–5, 1999.

Sabir, M et al. Experimental study of the antitrachoma action of berberine. *Indian J. Med. Res.,* 64: 1160–7, 1976.

Sabir, M et al. Antagonism of cholera toxin by berberine in the gastrointestinal tract of adult rats. *Indian J. Med. Res.,* 65:305–13, 1977.

Sack, RB and Froehlich, JL. Berberine inhibits intestinal secretory response of Vibrio cholerae and Escherichia coli enterotoxins. *Infect. Immun.,* 35(2):471–5, 1982.

Scazzocchio, F et al. Antimicrobial activity of Hydrastis canadensis extract and its major isolated alkaloids. *Fitoterapia,* 49 Suppl. (5):58–9, 1998.

Scazzocchio, F et al. Antibacterial activity of Hydrastis Canadensis extract and its major isolated alkaloids. *Planta Med.,* 561–4, 2001.

Schein, FR and Hanna, C. The absorption, distribution, and excretion of berberine. *Arch. Intern. Pharmacodynamie,* 124:317–25, 1960 (*Chem. Abs.* 54:14473e).

Scudder, JM. Hydrastis canadensis. *Ecl. Med. J.,* 30:155, 1870.

Scudder, JM. Colorless hydrastis. *Ecl. Med. J.,* 46:347–8, 1886.

Scudder, JM. Fluid hydrastis. *Ecl. Med. J.,* 47:45, 1887.

Shanbhag, SM et al. Pharmacological actions of berberine on the central nervous system *Jap. J. Pharmac.,* 20:482–7, 1970.

Sharda, DC. Berberine in the treatment of diarrhoea of infancy and childhood. *J. Indian Med. Assoc.,* 54(1):22–4, 1970.

Shin, D-H et al. A paradoxical stimulatory effect of berberine on guinea-pig ileum contractility: possible involvement of acetylcholine release from the postganglionic parasympathetic nerve and cholinesterase inhibition. *Life Sci.,* 53:1495–1500, 1993.

Subbaiah, TV and Amin, AH. Effect of berberine sulphate on Entamoeba histolytica. *Nature,* 215: 527–8, 1967.

Sun, D et al. Influence of berberine sulfate on synthesis and expression of pap fimbrial adhesin in uropathogenic Escherichia coli. *Antimicrob. Agents Chemother.,* 32(8):1274-7, 1988.

Sun, D et al. Berberine sulfate blocks adherence of Streptococcus pyogenes to epithelial cells, fibronectin, and hexadecane. *Antimicrob. Agents Chemother.,* 32(9):1370–4, 1988.

Supek, Z. Effect of berberine on the uterus in test animals. *Farmakol. I Toksikol.,* 9(6):12–4, 1946 (*Chem. Abs.* 41:6987g).

Swabb, EA et al. Reversal of cholera toxin-induced secretion in rat ileum by luminal berberine. *Am. J. Physiol.,* 241:G248-52, 1981.

Tai, Y-H et al. Antisecretory effects of berberine in rat ileum. *Am. J. Physiol.,* 241:G253–8, 1981.

Turova, AD et al. Berberine. *Lekarstv. Sredstva iz Rast.,* pp. 303–7, 1962. (*Chem. Abs.* 58:2763b).

Turova, AD et al. Berberine, an effective cholagogue. *Med. Prom. SSSR,* 18(6):59–60, 1964 (*Chem. Abs.* 61:15242f).

Velluda, CC et al. Effect of Berberis vulgaris extract, and of the berberine, berbamine, and oxyacanthine alkaloids on liver and bile function. *Lucrarile prez. Conf. Natl. farm., Buch.,* pp. 351–4, 1958 (*Chem. Abs.* 53:15345a).

Wolf, S and Mack, M. Experimental study of the action of bitters on the stomach of a fistulous human subject. *Drug Standards,* 24(3):98–101, 1956.

Zeng, X and Zeng, X. Relationship between the clinical effects of berberine on severe congestive heart failure and its concentration in plasma studied by HPLC. *Biomed. Chromatogr.,* 13:442–4, 1999.

Zeng, X-H et al. Efficacy and safety of berberine for congestive heart failure secondary to ischemic or idiopathic dilated cardiomyopathy. *Am. J. Cardiol.,* 92:173–6, 2003.

WESTERN ECHINACEA—Infection Fighter of the Great Plains
Echinacea angustifolia DC —roots

Summary

Western echinacea root and its hydro-alcoholic extract were traditionally used both orally and topically. Research results shown with direct application to cells in the laboratory are more likely to be duplicated in local applications. The internal administration of echinacea enhances systemic immune function, and this supports the healing process. The current popularity of echinacea and research focuses on its use for colds and flu. This has reduced appreciation of its usefulness in other infectious conditions. Though beneficial when taken alone, echinacea may also help if used with necessary antimicrobial drugs. The established safety of echinacea products given orally has produced only theoretical contraindications and rare individual sensitivities to restrict oral use.

The variety of active constituents in the whole root and their effects are complementary. The mild local anesthetic effect of the alcohol-soluble isobutylamides gives immediate pain relief, while the anti-inflammatory activity of these components produces an extended reduction in pain and swelling. While the isobutylamides have immune enhancing activity, echinacoside contributes local antibacterial and antiviral effects. The anti-hyaluronidase activity of the polyphenolic caffeic acid derivatives helps keep certain bacteria, tumors, and toxins from penetrating into the tissues. Certain polyphenols have some antiviral effects as well. The polyphenols and pentadecadiene add some antitumor activity. In aqueous solutions the high molecular weight polysaccharides and glycoproteins can add further anti-inflammatory, antitumor, and immune stimulant activitities. Even though echinacea may have no direct anti-venin, cell proliferant, or antibiotic activity, it can still play an important role in treating bites, wounds, and infections by contributing other effects to the healing process.

Original Uses and Identification

The species *Echinacea angustifolia,* Western or narrow-leafed echinacea, was originally used by many tribes throughout its native Great Plains habitat as documented by Moerman. Most of the recorded uses were local applications. The Dakota, Omaha, Pawnee, and Winnebago used Western echinacea for bites from snakes and other venomous pests and as a poultice over enlarged glands. They used the plant topically as a toothache remedy, as the Teton Sioux and Comanche used the root. Great Plains tribes including the Crow, Sioux, Omaha, Pawnee, Ponca, Cheyenne, Kiowa and Comanche chewed the root for painful mouth, tooth, gum and throat conditions and used it internally for bowel pain.

Attempts to classify the echinacea species began with T. Nuttall and A. DeCandolle from 1834 to 1841. At the beginning of the 20th century, identification of the different species was challenging in commercial trade, then considered as belonging to the *Brauneria* genus. *E. angustifolia* and *E. pallida* were the only echinacea species approved for medicinal use. Moser and also Heyl and Staley proposed identifying characteristics to pharmacists for distinguishing these species from *E. purpurea* and adulterants such as *Parthenium integrifolium* that were being supplied by Missouri wildcrafters.

Recent genetic evidence has led to the proposal that *E. angustifolia* be renamed in conformity with the conclusion made in 1955 by the botanist Arthur Conquist as *Echinacea pallida* (Nutt) Nutt. var. *angustifolia* (DC.) Cronq. Though *E. angustifolia* and *E. pallida* (pale echinacea) share many of the same traditional uses and some overlay in their geographic distribution along the eastern edge of the Great Plains, their roots have distinctively different chemical profiles as demonstrated by Bauer and Remiger in 1989. Western echinacea root and its extracts contain alkamides called isobutylamides that produce a characteristic numbness and tingling sensation on the tongue, whereas pale echinacea lacks these compounds and their sensory effects. Instead, pale echinacea root and its extracts contain 2-ketoalkenes and 2-alkynes, often described as polyacetylenes, with similar immune enhancing effects as the alkamides in Western echinacea.

Acceptance by Doctors

In 1885 the eminent pharmacist John Uri Lloyd first introduced commercial Western echinacea extracts to medicine. Initially, Echinacea was known as a medicine of Eclectic doctors, since its most prominent practitioners such as John King and Finley Ellingwood were some of its most ardent advocates. However, its popularity soon moved beyond the realm of "irregular" medical practice. In a survey by Lloyd Brothers Pharmacists published in 1912 to which over 10,000 physicians of all types responded, echinacea was listed by 5,065 physicians and ranked eleventh among all botanical drugs in importance.

The first significant clinical research done with *Echinacea angustifolia* was from 1913–1916 by the Eclectic physician von Unruh. He used a Lloyd Bros. medication called Subculoyd Echinacea (1.0 ml) and Inula Compound (1.33 ml) in the treatment of tuberculosis patients, injected either intramuscularly or intravenously. In 150 patients he claimed to have 100% recovery in incipient pulmonary cases, 50% arrested in moderately advanced cases, but no success in cases far advanced. In his microscopic research of conducting over 500 differential and cell counts in over four years, he found injected echinacea increased the phagocytic power of leucocytes, improved both high and low white blood cell counts, and normalized the percentage of mature neutrophilic white blood cells.

Thereafter, Western echinacea was included in the *National Formulary* as an official drug from 1916 to 1950. Even though Unruh's research conflicted with findings in 1921 animal experiments by Couch and Giltner, by 1924 it was noted that the sales of their echinacea extract were seven times greater than those of any other product made by the Lloyd Brothers.

Medicinal Preparations

Root Powder

The *National Formulary* (NF) 4th edition established the root powder as an official drug in 1916. In the 8th edition in 1946 the dried rhizome and roots were included there for the last time. In the *NF8* as in previous editions, *Echinacea pallida* was listed along with *E. angustifolia*. The average dose of the dried rhizome and roots was given as one gram.

Decoction

Lust notes that the root should not be used once it has lost its odor. Naturopaths sometimes used this form, simmering 4 grams dried root in 4 ounces of water and consuming 1–2 ounces 3 times daily according to Kuts-Cheraux.

Tincture

The tincture has typically been made with the fresh root, going back to the Eclectics but also emphasized by Grieve. Its dose ranged from 0.5–1.0 teaspoon (2–4 ml) every 2–4 hours as indicated by the Eclectics or 1–2 ml every 1–3 hours according to Lust. The strength and alcohol content vary depending on the manufacturer.

SPECIFIC MEDICINE

Lloyd determined the best solvent to extract the root was four parts alcohol to one part water. His extract was known as Specific Echinacea, also called Specific Strength Medicine Echinacea. It was the same drug strength as a fluid extract (1:1) but was improved due to removal of inert material by Lloyd's special process. The final product contained 65% alcohol.

Internally, the recommended dose of Specific Echinacea was 5–60 drops in a little water every 1–4 hours. For infected wounds or venomous bites and stings, where its beneficial effects were often instant and marked, 15–60 drops were given internally in a little water every 15–30 minutes. A bandage over the affected area was kept saturated first at full strength, then later mixed with three parts water.

FLUID EXTRACT

The *NF* 4th edition made the fluid extract an official medicine in 1916. The solvent consisted of four parts alcohol to one part water with a final content of 65% alcohol. The average dose was one milliliter, equivalent to 15 minims. The Eclectic Felter indicated the fluid extract dosage range was 5–30 minims, while the naturopathic physician Kuts-Cheraux gave from 10–60 minims. The *NF8* dropped the fluid extract of *E. angustifolia* in 1946.

Early Anglo Uses

TINCTURE

The introduction of *Echinacea angustifolia* to Anglo medicine was in 1887 by a German, Dr. H.C.F. Meyer from Pawnee City, Nebraska, in an article co-authored by Dr. John King in the *Eclectic Medical Journal*. Meyer had used the root for sixteen years as an alterative and antiseptic. He used its tincture internally and externally for boils, carbuncles, ulcers of the throat and extremities, hemorrhoids, and wasp and bee stings. Meyer claimed that in 613 cases of rattlesnake poisoning in humans and animals, recoveries occurred from between two to twelve hours.

Doctors used echinacea tincture for almost every type of infection. Dr. Charles Billingslea of South Fork, Ark., found prior to 1910 that it aided in recovery of three cases of puerperal sepsis, three cases of appendicitis, eighteen cases of typhoid fever, and two cases of uremia. When echinacea was given from beginning to end, and other treatments were also prescribed as indicated, these cases ended as cures. The tincture was given every two hours in doses of 10–15 drops for septic fever, 5–10 drops for typhoid fever, 10 drops in appendicitis, and 15–20 drops in uremia.

Dr. C.H. Rigg administered tincture of fresh echinacea root to treat fever that arose after labor due to the sepsis. The naturopathic doctor A. Shramm noted the fresh root tincture of Western echinacea was beneficial in diphtheria and fevers. For septicemia following childbirth he recommended one half to one teaspoon every two to four hours.

SPECIFIC MEDICINE

Following its medical introduction, Western echinacea was used internally to treat serious infections that are now the province of antibiotics. A case in point occurred in 1896 when severe boils in a 40-year-old man developed into carbuncles that appeared 3–4 at a time. Dr. E.R. Waterhouse treated them with a 1:7 dilution of Specific Echinacea in water given in teaspoonful doses every three hours. The carbuncles dried up gradually and completely disappeared.

Dr. Henry Reny of Biddeford, Maine, used Specific Echincacea in water and glycerine in doses of 5 drops every 1–3 hours to help resolve seven cases of appendicitis. Specific Echinacea was used in seven serious septicemia cases following births or abortions along with other treatments common between 1894–1896. Five cases resulted in rapid, complete recovery, one recovery was slow, and one patient died.

Together with a large number of physicians, Dr. Finley Ellingwood advocated its employment for typhoid fever. By 1913 after 5–15 years of experience using Western echinacea for this condition from beginning to end, it followed only a mild course of fever throughout the entire period. Ellingwood and later the naturopathic doctor M. Holmes both noted that other normally resistant and challenging infections including diphtheria, scarlet fever, and measles were also effectively treated with this remedy.

In anaphylaxis resulted from the diphtheria antitoxin, Ellingwood found echinacea to be a direct antidote. He believed that Western echinacea worked like a tonic due to its blood purifying effects, antagonizing streptococci and other microbes, while contributing strongly to resistance of disease by increasing leucocytosis without any side effects. Cases of infected wounds, snakebites, and boils were reported by Dr. W.N. Holmes in 1917 to be cured with Specific Echinacea used internally and externally.

By 1933 Specific Echinacea was still described in Eclectic medical literature as the remedy of choice for acute septic infection and was also endorsed as a local application to recent trauma or infected areas. In 1934 using healthy students at the Eclectic Medical College in Cincinatti, Ram studied the effects of echinacea by taking for four days Specific Echinacea in water in doses equivalent to 2–15 grains of the dried root. An increase in the total white blood cell count was evident which reached a peak in two thirds after 24 hours and in the other third after 48 hours. For all subjects the leukocyte increase from 24–48 hours was accounted for mostly by neutrophils after 24 hours and by lymphocytes after 48 hours.

FLUID EXTRACT

Dr. W.L. Lewis of Canton, Penn., reported in 1907 that teaspoonful doses of echinacea fluid extract every four hours and a 25% solution applied locally reversed the course of what otherwise was proving to be a fatal course of external anthrax.

Ellingwood recommended it topically in an ointment along with its internal use for all sorts of ulcerations of the skin. The fluid extract was also used in naturopathy to treat boils and carbuncles. Dr. Schramm of Los Angeles indicated his usual dose was 2 ml 3–6 times daily. It could be combined with simple syrup for flavor and used in conjunction with local treatment.

Topical Medical Uses

While Western echinacea preparations have become widely used internal remedies for colds and flu throughout Europe and America in recent years, their local applications and other uses have not been emphasized, at least in America. In studying the development of its traditional use in clinical practice, it becomes obvious that Western echinacea was commonly applied both locally and internally for many conditions, especially all types of infections. Early reports published for the medical profession demonstrate the great potential of this botanical remedy.

It is interesting to note that when Western echinacea was first introduced to clinical medicine in the late 19th century, scant mention was made of its use for simple upper respiratory infections. When it was recommended for colds, it was used as a local application. In 1906 Dr. A.F. Stephens tried a colorless echinacea preparation, with just enough alcohol to preserve it, as a nasal douche repeatedly for 3–4 hours on the first day of a bad cold that disappeared by the next morning. He used this successfully with patients, unequalled by any other remedy for cleansing the nasal cavities in chronic rhinitis, due to its anesthetic and seemingly antiseptic qualities. In 1918 Dr. W.W. Houser of Lincoln, Neb., upon contracting a cold with nasal burning and a copious, clear, watery discharge, applied echinacea fluid extract on a cotton swab to the inner lining of his nose 4–5 times with intervals of one hour. The next morning found him free from any cold symptoms.

For various local maladies such as gangrene, deep suppurating wounds, fistulas, varicose ulcers, epithelioma, abscess ulcers, and all forms of skin disease, Dr. G. Rounsville of Mottoon, Ill., in 1919 applied echinacea ointment containing two drams of tincture in each ounce prior to bandaging. In deep wounds or fistulas, the ointment was heated to a consistency of cream and injected when cool, then applying a compress and bandage.

Western echinacea was popular for its local effects on boils. Its early anesthetic use locally for the pain of cancer and inflammatory conditions is also noteworthy. Dr. W. Holmes from Nashville, Tenn., used Specific Echinacea over carcinomas to help prevent extension into new tissue, relieve the pain, and eliminate the odor. Naturopathic doctor Milton Holmes recommended Specific Echinacea as a local application for snakebites, cuts, wounds, and insect and bee stings while giving 20 drops internally every 3–4 hours as well.

Water Soluble Versus Alcohol Soluble Components

Much of the research on echinacea's constituents has focused on the water-soluble high molecular weight (large) polysaccharides. In its original uses by native American Indians, echinacea root was chewed, applied as a poultice, or extracted and consumed as a tea. In these forms the large polysaccharides exert their influence. Arabinogalactans and other polysaccharides along with glycoproteins contribute to some extent to the anti-inflammatory, antiviral, and immune modulating activities of Western echinacea.

Fructans, also known as fructofuranosides, are water-soluble fructose polymers. Giger and others found in 1989 that these polysaccharides are about ten times higher in Western echinacea roots than in the above-ground plant. Some smaller fructans are present in alcoholic tinctures made from the fresh herb.

The Eclectics used a high alcohol extract of *E. angustifolia* root. Since a 50% or more alcohol concentration precipitates high molecular weight polysaccharide components, such precipitates are removed by filtration in the process of producing commercial botanical extracts. Therefore, most polysaccharide activity does not apply to high alcohol extracts.

Alcohol soluble components that contribute greatly to echinacea's anti-inflammatory and immune effects are a group of alkamides characterized as isobutylamides. In 2001 Perry and others showed that echinacoside was the main phenolic compound with small amounts of cynarin, cichoric acid, and chlorogenic acid also present. Cheminat and others found that these provide important antiviral activity, while Facino and others showed their connective tissue protective effects. Cynarin is the characteristic phenolic for this *Echinacea* species. The compound 1,8–pentadecadiene has demonstrated some anti-cancer properties.

Laboratory Research—Root Extracts, Fractions and Isolates

Immune Enhancement

TINCTURE

A study in 1988 by Bauer and others of the effects of the 90% ethanolic extracts of *E. angustifolia* roots showed that it improved phagocytic activity in mice when given orally. This effect correlated strongly with the isobutylamide fraction. The polar fraction containing polyphenols had a lesser effect.

SPECIFIC MEDICINE

The combined effects of all the components help explain the local and internal effects of echinacea roots against infections. In 1999 Rehman and others used a 1:1 strength Specific Echinacea extract in the drinking water of mice for six weeks. When challenged with an antigen, the mice drinking echinacea had significantly higher levels of antigen-specific IgG from day 7 to day 27 and a somewhat higher level of IgM than those mice not drinking the extract in their water.

POLYSACCHARIDES

A study by Wagner and others in 1985 of large polysaccharides of various types from the water extract of *E. angustifolia* root showed significant immunostimulant activities. These root polysaccharides caused a greater increase in phagocytosis (consumption of particles by white blood cells as a means of removing foreign substances) than those from other parts of the plant.

A mixture of polysaccharides and glycoproteins obtained in 1993 by Bodinet and others as filtrates from a 30% ethanolic extract of *E. angustifolia* roots produced a number of results in isolated cells of the immune system. These included an increase in the production of important cytokines like interleukins and interferons, increased growth of mouse spleen cells, and increased antibody production.

Anti-inflammatory

POLYSACCHARIDES

In studies from 1985 to 1988 Tragni, Tubaro and others applied a fraction from a water extract of *E. angustifolia* roots topically to inflamed skin in mice. This fraction inhibited swelling in proportion to the dose used. This anti-inflammatory activity was shown to be due to large polysaccharides in this aqueous fraction.

ALKAMIDES

In 1989 Wagner and others found Western echinacea isobutylamides inhibit 5-lipoxygenase activity, thereby partially accounting for the anti-inflammatory effect. In 1994 Muller-Jakic found the hexane extract of *E. angustifolia* roots to act as a dual inhibitor of both 5-lipoxygenase and cyclooxygenase. The isolated isobutylamides were less potent than the echinacea root extract, indicating other active compounds were also present. This isobutylamide activity helps to account for reductions in redness, pain, and swelling by *E. angustifolia*. (Isobutylamides are not found in *E. pallida* roots which therefore lack the tongue-tingling effect.)

Antiviral and Antibacterial

POLYSACCHARIDES

A mixture of polysaccharides and glycoproteins had an antiviral effect against herpes simplex virus.

PHENOLICS

Cheminat and others showed that echinacoside from this polar fraction has antiviral and cell growth inhibitor activity. In 1950 the *E. angustifolia* compound echinacoside had been isolated by Stoll and others who showed it was mildly active against *Staphylococcal* and *Streptococcal* bacteria.

Antihyaluronidase

PHENOLICS

Hyaluronidase breaks down hyaluronic acid, the binding substance between cells. A significant effect of *E. angustifolia* alcoholic root extracts is due to its phenolic derivatives that inhibit hyaluronidase. This was shown by Facino and others in 1993 using fractions of the root made with ethylacetate, butylacetate and chloroform. Cichoric acid and caftaric acid had the greatest anti-hyaluronidase activity, while chlorogenic acid demonstrated a lesser effect.

According to Mekkes and Nahuys in 2001, hyaluronic acid helps speed wound healing. The importance of echinacea phenolics blocking hyaluronidase goes beyond wound healing. Hyaluronidase is found in snake and spider venom, in malignant tissues, and in some pathogenic bacteria secretions promotes their penetration into tissue. Bacteria that secrete hyaluronidase include *Streptococcus pyogenes* (responsible for lymph infections associated with red streaks, cellulitis, and sometimes gangrene), *Staphylococcus aureus* (causative agent in boils, carbuncles, and occasionally cellulitis), and *Clostridia perfringens* (associated with anaerobic cellulitis and gas gangrene following wound infection).

Anesthetic

ALKAMIDES

In 1954 the component causing the numbing effect on the tongue caused by echinacea was identified by Jacobson as an isobutylamide. The numbness following the initial tingling produces a mild anesthetic effect after local application. Its above-ground parts contain similar compounds but in lesser amounts than the roots. In 1989 Bauer and Remiger have shown *E. angustifolia* roots contain different types of alkamides including over a dozen isobutylamide constituents.

Antitumor

OIL

In the roots Voaden and Jacobsen also found 1,8-pentadecadiene, inhibitory to carcinosarcoma and lymphocytic leukemia in rodents.

Modern Clinical Studies with Root Products for Colds and Flu

MIXED POWDER

Ordinary drying of echinacea root appears to not be an adequate means of supplying an effective herb product. Barrett and other in 2002 provided 492 mg of dried Western echinacea root combined with 496 mg of equal parts dried *Echinacea purpurea* root and above-ground herb which was taken as 4 capsules 6 times the first day of early cold symptoms. Then the same single dose of this combination was used 3 times daily thereafter for up to 10 days. There was no significant difference among the 148 college students using this product and dosing schedule compared to those taking a 1.3 gram doses of alfalfa on the same schedule.

HYDROALCOHOLIC EXTRACTS

As reported in a review by H. Wagner in 1997, most of the recent clinical studies on Western echinacea use low strength alcoholic root extracts and have looked at their effects on colds and flu. In one clinical study using a homeopathic liquid Echinacea preparation to prevent infections, one 12 ml dose daily of a liquid extract with 1.5 gm of *E. angustifolia*, 0.35 gm *Eupatorium perfoliatum*, 0.24 gm *Baptisia tinctoria*, and 0.0024 gm homeopathic Arnica was taken by 303 patients for 8 weeks who were compared to 306 subjects given placebo. Significantly fewer using the *E. angustifolia* product fell ill; 14.8% fewer initial infections and 27.3% fewer recurrent infections occurred. Treating colds and influenza with this preparation in two placebo-controlled, double-blind randomized studies with 100 subjects each showed that in the echinacea group most of the 15 symptoms measured in one study and 3 of 7 in the other were significantly better than placebo.

In a placebo-controlled, double-blind, randomized study with 302 healthy volunteers in 1998, Melchart and others used a 1:11 strength liquid extract of *E. angustifolia* roots made with 30% ethanol. This was given in 50-drop doses twice daily five days per week for twelve weeks to study its value to prevent upper respiratory tract infections. At this dosage only slight improvements were noted. About 37% of the placebo group developed an infection, compared to 32% of the *E. angustifolia* group, a difference lacking statistical significance.

Potential Contraindications and Drug Interactions

In reviewing clinical trials and considering the extensive popular use of *Echinacea* spp. with so few reported side effects, it was concluded by Barrett and others in 1999 that the estimated risk of adverse effects from oral consumption is quite small. According to Gallo and others in 2000, those using *Echinacea* spp. products during pregnancy did not show an increased fetal risk. The German Commission E monograph gives no contraindications for external use but describes the internal use as contraindicated "in principle" for systemic diseases such as multiple sclerosis, collagenosis, leukosis, autoimmune disorders, AIDS and HIV infection, and tuberculosis. The Commission E states that injection of echincacea is contraindicated in pregnancy and in allergic tendencies, especially allergies to members of the Asteraceae family. One case using a combination of 96% whole plant Western echinacea (*E. angustifolia*) extract and 4% purple coneflower (*E. purpurea*) root extract was associated with anaphylaxis by Mullins in 1998.

According to the respected herbalist Kerry Bone's assessment, the oral contraindications are disputable for complex high alcohol extracts used in living subjects. Based on Eclectic empirical experience, the use for tubercular conditions seems safe. Though potential allergic sensitivity suggests echinacea may be a risk to some asthmatics, it appears to many herbal prescribers to be beneficial in conditions such as asthma that can be exacerbated by infections. The current belief that echinacea extracts act primarily as a stimulus to phagocytosis supports the argument that its use in autoimmune conditions is safe. However, new evidence by Rehman and other in 1999 that *E. angustifolia* high alcohol extract significantly increases antigen-specific IgG antibody production in rats suggests that the effects may not be limited to non-specific immune enhancement.

Speculative reports suggesting that *E. angustifolia* root extracts may lead to increased blood levels of some drugs is based on a study by Budzinski and others in 2000. They monitored the effect of a commercial extract in test tubes and found this preparation was fourth out of 19 extracts studied in its ability to inhibit the metabolize isozyme CYP 3A4. However, not only are the results of this study preliminary and questionable based on the simple test tube procedure used, but St. John's wort extract was ranked as the second greatest inhibitor. It is known from human studies that St. John's wort has the opposite effect; it induces, rather than inhibits, CYP 3A4.

Cultivation and Wildcrafting

Cultivation of Echinacea angustifolia, E. pallida and E. purpurea has increased rapidly due to the demand and monetary value. According to Dana Hurlburt of the Kansas Biological Survery, wild E. angustifolia remains abundant in central Kansas with a stable harvest over a 100–year history, in spite of recent booms in digging prior to 1999. Fire suppression, grazing, exotic species and herbicide use have probably contributed more to local population declines than has over-harvesting. This contrasts with North Dakota and Montana where three years of over-harvesting on reservations is suspected to have depleted local Western echinacea populations. North Dakota and Montana have recently passed legislation to prevent plant poaching on private lands, with restitution and penalties up to $10,000 or fines on a per diem basis, respectively.

Table 5   Western Echinacea Root and Derivatives—
            Summary of Medicinal Uses and Pharmacology

WESTERN ECHINACEA *Echinacea angustifolia* DC	Native American Uses	Early Medical Uses (Locally and internally)	Early Medical Uses (Internal only)	Modern Clinical Studies	Laboratory Research Findings
Whole Root	Locally: Enlarged glands Snakebites Toothaches Sore gums, mouth, throat Internally: Bowel pain				
Tincture (Hydroalcoholic)		Boils Carbuncle Epithelioma Fistulas Gangrene Hemorrhoids Snakebites Stings Skin ulcers Wounds	Appendicitis Diphtheria Puerperal fever Septicemia Typhoid fever Uremia	Colds Flu	Increases phagocytosis
Specific Medicine (Hydroalcoholic)		Carbuncles Snakebites Stings Wounds	Appendicitis Diphtheria Measles Scarlet fever Septicemia Typhoid fever		Increases neutrophils, lymphocytes, IgG antibodies
Fluid Extract (Hydroalcoholic)		Anthrax Boils Carbuncles Skin ulcers		Colds	

Table 5—*Continued*

WESTERN ECHINACEA *Echinacea angustifolia* DC	Native American Uses	Early Medical Uses (Locally and internally)	Early Medical Uses (Internal only)	Modern Clinical Studies	Laboratory Research Findings

FRACTIONS AND ISOLATED CONSTITUENTS

Polysaccharides and/or Glycoproteins					Antiviral Anti-inflammatory Increases phagocytosis, cytokines, spleen cells, antibodies
Alkamides					Anti-inflammatory Increases phagocytosis
Phenolic Derivatives					Antiviral Antibacterial Inhibits hyaluronidase

References

BOOKS

Anon. *Dose Book,* Lloyd Brothers, Pharmacists Inc., Cincinnati, Ohio, 1932.

Boyd, RF, and Hoerl, BG. *Basic Medical Microbiology,* Little, Brown and Co., Boston, Mass., 1977.

Brinker, F. *Herb Contraindications and Drug Interactions*, 3rd ed., Eclectic Med. Pub., Sandy, OR., 2001.

Comm. On National Formulary. *The National Formulary,* 4th ed., American Pharmaceutical Assoc., Washington, D.C., 1916.

Ellingwood, F. *American Materia Medica, Therapeutics and Pharmacognosy* (1919), Eclectic Medical Pub., Sandy, OR., 1994.

Felter, HW. *The Eclectic Materia Medica, Pharmacology and Therapeutics* (1922), Eclectic Medical Pub., Sandy, OR., 1994.

Felter, HW, Lloyd JU. *King's American Dispensatory* (1898), Eclectic Medical Pub., Sandy, OR., 1992.

Grieve, M. *A Modern Herbal*, 1931 version, Dover Pub., New York, 1971.

Hobbs, C. *Echinacea Monograph* from *Eclectic Dispensatory of Botanical Therapeutics* (Alstat E, comp.), vol. 1, Eclectic Medical Pub., Portland, OR., 1989.

Kuts-Cheraux, AW. *Naturae Medicina and Naturopathic Dispensatory*, American Naturopathic Physicians and Surgeons Assoc., Des Moines, Iowa, 1953.

Lloyd, JU. *A Treatise on Echinacea*, Lloyd Brothers, Cincinnati, Ohio, 1917.

Lloyd, JU. *Echinacea,* Lloyd Brothers, Cincinnati, Ohio, 1923.

Lust, J. *The Herb Book*, Bantam Books, New York, 1974.

Moerman, DE. *Medicinal Plants of Native America,* vol 1, Univ. Mich. Mus. of Anthrop., Ann Arbor, 1986.

Powers JL (Chair.). *The National Formulary*, 8th ed., Am. Pharm. Assoc., Washington, D.C., 1946.

ARTICLES

Barrett, B et al. Echinacea for upper respiratory infection. *J. Fam. Pract.*, 48(8):628–35, 1999.

Barrett, B et al. Treatment of the common cold with unrefined Echinacea. *Ann. Intern. Med.*, 137:939–46, 2002.

Bauer, R et al. Immunological in vivo and in vitro examinations of Echinacea extracts. *Arzneim.-Forsch.*, 38:276–81, 1988. [in German]

Bauer, R et al. Alkamides from the roots of Echinacea angustifolia. *Phytochem.*, 28:505–8, 1989.

Bauer, R and Remiger, P. TLC and HPLC analysis of alkamides in Echinacea drugs. *Planta Med.*, 55:367–71, 1989.

Billingslea, CL. The influence of Echinacea. *Ellingwood's Ther.*, 4:222, 1910.

Blankmeyer, HH. Echinacea as a local anesthetic. *Ellingwood's Ther.*, 3:468, 1909.

Bodinet, C et al. Host-resistance increasing activity of root extracts from Echinacea species. *Planta Med.*, 59(Suppl.):A672–3, 1993.

Bone, K. Echinacea: when should it be used? *Eur. J. Herb. Med.*, 3(3):13–17, 1997/98.

Budzinski, JW et al. An in vitro evaluation of human cytochrome P450 3A4 inhibition by selected commercial herbal extracts and tinctures. *Phytomed.*, 7(4):273–282, 2000.

Cheminat, A et al. Caffeoyl conjugates from Echinacea species: structures and biological activity. *Phytochem.*, 27:2787–94, 1988.

Couch, JF, Giltner T. An experimental study of Echinacea therapy. *Am. J. Pharm.*, 93:227–8, 1921.

Daniel, TJ. Echinacea in snake bites. *Ecl. Med. J.*, 70:348, 1910.

Ellingwood, F. Echinacea in typhoid and infection. *Ellingwood's Ther.*, 7:414–5, 1913.

Ellingwood, F. Tonic effect of Echinacea. *Ellingwood's Ther.*, 10:190, 1916.

Ellingwood, F. Echinacea. *Ellingwood's Ther.*, 12:216, 1918.

Facino, RM et al. Direct charaterization of caffeoyl esters with antihyaluronidase activity in crude extracts from Echinacea angustifolia roots by fast atom bombardment tandem mass spectrometry. *Farmaco*, 48:1447–61, 1993. (*Chem. Abs.* 120:294112w).

Gallo, M et al. Pregnancy outcome following gestational exposure to Echinacea. *Arch. Intern. Med.,* 160:3141–3, 2000.

Giger, E et al. Fructans in Echinacea and in its phytotherapeutic preparations. *Planta Med.,* 55:638-9, 1989.

Heyl, FW and Staley JF. Analysis of two Echinacea roots. *Am. J. Pharm.,* 86:450–5, 1914.

Holmes, ME. Echinacea augustiflora [sic] *Naturopath Her. Health,* 41:17, 1936.

Holmes, WN. Physiologic and specific actions. *Ellingwood's Ther.,* 11:77–9, 1917.

Houser, WW. Echinacea in acute choryza [sic]. *Ellingwood's Ther.,* 12:19, 1918.

Hurlburt, D. Endangered Echinacea—what threat, which species, and where? *United Plant Savers Newsletter,* pp. 4 and 6, Summer, 1999.

Jacobson, M. Occurrence of a pungent insecticidal principle in American coneflower roots. *Science,* 120:1028–9, 1954.

Johnston, BA and Malone, D. States pass legislation curtailing harvest of wild Echinacea. *HerbalGram,* 46:67, 1999.

Kindscher, K. Ethnobotany of purple coneflower (Echinacea angustifolia, Asteraceae) and other Echinacea species. *Econ. Bot.,* 43(4):498–507, 1989.

Lewis, WL. Anthrax and its treatment. *Ellingwood's Ther.,* 1(2):1907.

Li, TSC. Echinacea: cultivation and medicinal value. *HortTechnology,* 8(2):122–9, 1998.

Lloyd, JU. Vegetable drugs employed by American physicians. *J. Am. Pharm. Assoc.,* 1:1228–41, 1912.

Mekkes, JR and Nahuys, M. Induction of granulation tissue formation in chronic wounds by hyaluronic acid. *Wounds,* 13(4):159–64, 2001.

Melchart, D et al. Echinacea root extracts for the prevention of upper respiratory tract infections. *Arch. Fam. Med.,* 7:541–5, 1998.

Meyer, HCF, King J. Echinacea angustifolia. *Ecl. Med. J.,* 47:209–10, 1887.

Moser, J Jr. Echinacea and a spurious root that appeared in the fall of 1909. *Am. J. Pharm.,* 82:224-6, 1910.

Muller-Jakic, B et al. In vitro inhibition of cyclooxygenase and 5-lipoxygenase by alkamides from Echinacea and Achillea species. *Planta Med.,* 60:37–40, 1994.

Mullins, RJ. Echinacea-associated anaphylaxis. *Med. J. Austral.,* 168:170–1, 1998.

Perry, NB et al. Echinacea Standardization: analytical methods for phenolic compounds and typical levels in medicinal species. *J. Agric. Food Chem.,* 49:1702–6, 2001.

Ram, NH. Echinacea—its effect on the normal individual—with special reference to changes produced in the blood picture. *Ecl. Med. J.,* 95:34–6, 1935.

Rehman, J et al. Increased production of antigen-specific immunoglobulins G and M following in vivo treatment with the medicinal plants Echinacea angustifolia and Hydrastis canadensis. *Immunol. Lett.,* 68:391–5, 1999.

Rigg, CH. Echinacea. *Ecl. Med. J.,* 56:166, 1896.

Rounsville, GLB. Echinacea. *Ellingwood's Ther.,* 13:169–70, 1919.

Schramm, A. Echinacea. *J. Naturopath. Med.,* p. 15, Feb., 1957.

Shalaby, AS et al. Response of Echinacea to some agricultural practices. *J. Herbs, Spices Med. Plants,* 4(4):59–67, 1997.

Stephens, AF. Acute rhinitis—Echinacea. *Ecl. Med. J.,* 66:115, 1906.

Stoll, A et al. Isolierung und konstitution des echinacosids, eines glykosids aus den wurzeln von Echinacea angustifolia D.C.. *Helv. Chim. Acta,* 33:1877–93, 1950. [in German]

Tragni, E et al. Evidence from two classic irritation tests for an anti-inflammatory action of a natural extract, echinacina B. *Fd. Chem. Toxic.,* 23:317–9, 1985.

Tragni, E et al. Anti-inflammatory activity of Echinacea angustifolia fractions separated on the basis of molecular weight. *Pharm. Res. Comm.,* 20(S. 5):87–90, 1988.

Tubaro, A et al. Anti-inflammatory activity of a polysaccharidic fraction of Echinacea angustifolia. *J. Pharm. Pharmacol.,* 39:567–9, 1987.

Unruh, Vv. Echinacea angustifolia and Inula helenium in the treatment of tuberculosis. *Nat. Ecl. Med. Assoc. Quart.,* 7:63–70, 1915.

Unruh, Vv. Observations on the laboratory reactions in test made of Echinacea and Inula upon tubercle bacilli and other germs. *Ellingwood's Ther.,* 12:126–30, 1918.

Voaden, DJ and Jacobson, M. Tumor inhibitors. 3. Identification and synthesis of an oncolytic hydrocarbon from American Coneflower roots. *J. Med. Chem.,* 15:619–23, 1972.

Wagner, H. Herbal immunostimulants for the prophylaxis and therapy of colds and influenza. *Eur. J. Herb . Med.,* 3:22–30, 1997.

Wagner, H et al. Immunostimulating polysaccharides (heteroglycans) of higher plants. *Arzneim.-Forsch.,* 35:1069–75, 1985. [in German]

Wagner, H et al. In vitro inhibition of arachidonate metablism by some alkamides and prenylated phenols. *Planta Med.,* 55:566–7, 1989.

Waterhouse, ER. Specific Echinacea. *Ecl. Med. J.,* 56:524–5, 1896.

Watkins, L & Niederkorn JS. Echinacea. *Ecl. Med. J.,* 93:293, 1933.

Zeumer, EP. Echinacea locally. *Ecl. Med. J.,* 84:23–4, 1924.

CRANBERRY—A Food That Became a Medicine

Vaccinium macrocarpon Aiton—fruit

Summary

As a northern native American food, the cranberry, *Vaccinium macrocarpon*, has become part of the cultural heritage celebrating the bounty of the New World at Thanksgiving. A number of Vaccinium species provide berries for food with particular health value throughout North America and Europe, including bilberries, blueberries, and lingonberries. They are especially high in antioxidant flavonoids and anthocyanins. The leaves of many Arctostaphylos species in the same heath family as Vaccinium have been used primarily as remedies for urinary tract infections. While phytochemical components are in many aspects similar between these two genera, there are notable differences. The arbutin in the leaves of V. vitis-idaea (lingonberry) in Canada and lack of arbutin in the leaves and ursolic acid in the berries of the Mexican A. pungens seem to cross over the generic distinctions. Cranberry fruit resembles the fruit of this southern Arctostaphylos species in its common use for urinary tract conditions.

Early studies associated cranberry's organic acid content with lowering urinary pH. Its established use as a food was expanded when the commercial production of its juice increased in the 20th century, and it became popular as a sweetened diluted beverage, or cocktail. Since anthocyanins gave cranberries and their juice the characteristic ruby red color, the commercial extraction was concerned with a standard content of these components for appearance sake. Eventually, cranberry juice products developed a regional and then national reputation for ameliorating chronic recurrent urinary tract infections. Human studies first focused on cranberry juice acidifying the urine to reduce ammonia odor and prevent urinary crystals and stone formation. The pure juice proved more effective than the diluted cocktail for increasing urine acidity.

Though the acidic components characterize the cranberry flavor and are carefully assayed to assure appropriate content in the juice, those present are inadequate for producing antibacterial effects. The triterpenic ursolic acid in the whole berries contributes antibacterial activity. Inhibition of adhesion by bacteria to the urinary mucous membrane by the juice was discovered to be a major contributing factor for preventing and treating these infections. Other compounds present in the juice are responsible for this effect. The most important of these was determined to be the proanthocyanidins (tannins), concentrated in the skin and seeds of cranberries. Proanthocyanidins, rather than the red anthocyanin pigments, have much to do with helping reduce the incidence and severity of Eschericia coli infections of the urinary tract. Similar to ursolic acid that is left behind in the pomice after the juice is expressed, these compounds are only partially extracted in the juice. The antioxidant effects of the anthocyanin and flavonol components also have implications for cardiovascular health, but little of the flavonols are retained in the commercial juice cocktail.

Names and Traditional Uses

The genus name for cultivated cranberry has an uncertain origin. It may be derived from the Latin words *vacca* for cow or *bacca* for berry. The species name *macrocarpon* is derived from Greek and refers to its large (*makro*) fruit (*karpos*). Its former scientific name was *Oxycoccus macrocarpus*, referring to a large acidic berry.

The red juicy berry of this 1–3 feet tall plant are very tart. The wild species known as small cranberry is 12–20 inches tall and is designated as *Vaccinium oxycoccos* (formerly *Oxycoccus microcarpus*), since its red berries are small and very sour. Both creeping plants have evergreen leaves, grow in bogs, and sport small pink flowers with recurved petals from June to August. The stamens' appearance is believed to account for its earlier name of craneberry, since they look like crane bills. The berries at the end of thin stalks produce a characteristic nodding motion.

Angier notes that cranberry is considered the most important berry of the North, from Alaska to Newfoundland. *V. macrocarpon* grows in acidic soil in bogs and swamps and along wet shores. It is native from Newfoundland west to Minnesota and south as far as North Carolina. Cranberry is cultivated in Canada, Wisconsin, New England, and the Pacific Northwest, and it has been introduced into Europe.

Best known as an accompanying side dish served with turkey on Thanksgiving, cranberries have become part of this traditional American feast. Angier reports that the Pilgrims shipped ten barrels of this easy-to-keep fruit to England for King Charles II. Native Americans of the Great Lakes region and Northeast often used cranberries to flavor a staple preparation called pemmican, made by pounding dried venison or buffalo meat and mixing this with berries and hot fat.

Besides using the fruit for food, the *American Herbal Pharmacopoeia* reports that the Montagnais used a decoction of the branches for pleurisy. Angier also declares that a tea made from the leaves of cranberry species was considered a spring tonic by native Americans and pioneers. This tea was thought to be diuretic and was used for many kidney disorders and to prevent kidney stones and gravel in the bladder.

History of the Fruit As a Remedy

Angier notes the cranberry fruit was believed to remove blood toxins and to help control liver ailments. An old recipe for convalescents and invalids involved simmering crushed cranberries in water with a little oatmeal, sugar, sherry, and lemon peel for 30 minutes, straining, and serving chilled as a beverage. The *American Herbal Pharmacopoeia* describes early reports by Sterns in 1801 and Rafinesque in 1830 regarding cranberry as an antiscorbutic food, its use for fevers, and its laxative effect when taken in large amounts. Rafinesque also mentioned a diuretic activity. The *AHP* also noted the *material medica* written Eclectic Henry Hollembaek in 1865 confirmed these uses and added antiseptic and mild astringent to the list of cranberry's effects. He also described using the berries as a poultice for local inflammations and gangrene.

The Eclectics did not widely utilize the fruit of this plant. Felter and Lloyd noted, however, that it was frequently used as a home remedy for inflammatory swellings, particularly erysipelas. Cranberry poultice was also applied for tonsillitis, scarletinal sore throat, enlarged cervical glands, and poor-healing skin ulcers. A split cranberry was applied with paste to boils on the tip of the nose by several noted physicians of the late 19th century. In 1974 the naturopath John Lust still recommended a poultice of fresh cranberries as part of the means for treating erysipelas.

It was reported by Bodel and others in 1959 that cranberry juice had been used widely as a folk remedy around Cape Cod in Massachusetts for the treatment of urinary tract infections. In 1963 Dr. Sternlieb indicated that from his experience cranberry juice is a simple and effective method for preventing and treating kidney infections and stones, though he noted potential problems for some with products that contain high amounts of calories and carbohydrates. The popularity of cranberry for urinary tract problems led to clinical trials that grew in number over the next several decades, so that by 1999 a monograph for cranberry liquid preparation was included in the 19th edition of the *National Formulary*. This preparation was described in the *NF* as a bright red juice derived from the fruits of *Vaccinium macrocarpon* or *V. oxycoccos* and containing no added substances.

Vaccinium Species Fruit Content and Activities

A number of species in the genus *Vaccinium* have fruit that has been utilized as food. This includes the blueberry which has several species and many cultivars. Like the red cranberry, there are two major American blueberry species: the highbush (*Vaccinium corymbosum*) and the lowbush (*V. angustifolium*). The berries of both were first used by native Americans of the upper Midwest, Northeast, and Atlantic coast as a food, and now they are grown commercially along with rabbiteye blueberry (*V. ashei*). The European species sometimes referred to as blueberry, but more commonly known as bilberry (*V. myrtillus*), has been used for medicinal purposes since the time of St. Hildegard of Bingen in the 12th century. Much therapeutic research has been carried out on bilberry extracts, mostly utilizing an extract standardized to 36% anthocyanin (anthocyanoside) content, equivalent to 24% anthocyanidins after the sugar moieties are removed. The 15 main bilberry anthocyanins include the six found in cranberries. Bilberry anthocyanins are prone to oxidation and enzymatic degradation when the fruits are dried or in aqueous solution. A good quality standardized bilberry product is made as a dry extract from the fresh fruit.

In 1998 Prior and others showed by analysis of the fresh berries of these species that the various commercial cultivars of highbush blueberry had on average higher content of anthocyanins but lower yield of phenolics than lowbush, and rabbiteye blueberries had the highest phenolics, while the oxygen radical absorbance capacity was equivalent for all three. By comparison, bilberry had over twice the anthocyanins, over one and a half times the phenolics, and by far the greatest antioxidant activity compared to the American blueberry species. In general the authors found these species to be one of the richest antioxidant sources of all the fresh fruits and vegetables studied.

As a measure of anticancer activity in test tubes, extract fractions of *Vaccinium* species were compared by Bomser and others in 1996 to determine their ability to induce the phase II detoxification enzyme quinone reductase. Crude extracts, anthocyanin and proanthocyanidin fractions were not active. The ethyl acetate extract potencies decreased from the blue bilberry to the red lingonberry (*Vaccinium vitis-idaea*) to cranberry to lowbush blueberry. The hexane/chloroform subfraction of the ethyl acetate extract of bilberry had the greatest potency, while crude flavonoid subfractions had little. However, the other three species showed the greatest potency inducing the enzyme ornithine decarboxylase that blocks a tumor promoter. The crude extracts of these decreased in potency from cranberry to lowbush blueberry to lingonberry, while bilberry was much weaker. For this effect the greatest activity was found in the proanthocyanidin fractions, while the anthocyanidin fractions or ethyl acetate extracts were inactive or weak.

Cranberry is best known for preventing urinary tract infections in association with reducing bacterial adhesion to the mucous membrane of the urinary tract. In a study by Ofek and others in 1991 of seven juices (cranberry, blueberry, grapefruit, orange, pineapple, guava, and mango) and their effect on adherence of a strain of *E. coli* that causes infections of the kidney, only cranberry juice and blueberry juice contained the high-molecular-weight inhibitor of the MR adhesin on the hair-like protrusion of the bacteria. Cranberry juice inhibited the adhesion of all thirty *E. coli* isolates from the urinary tract, but only four of twenty of the bacterial isolates from the bowel. The proanthocyanidin extract of cranberry juice and other *Vaccinium* species including blueberries prevent this common urinary bacterial pathogen from adhering to the mucosa. This was determined by Howell and others in 1998 in their comparative study of these condensed tannins in *Vaccinium* juices versus other fruit and vegetable derivatives. In 1996 Zopf and Roth indicated that such specific adhesin-binding anti-infective agents provide a potentially revolutionary adjunctive approach to treating infections.

Heath Family Herbs/Phytochemicals for the Urinary Tract

As mentioned, a tea made with cranberry leaves was used by pioneers for kidney and bladder disorders. Bilberry (V. myrtillus) leaves were also used in Europe for mucosal inflammation and atony of the bladder. Bilberry leaves were analyzed in 1954 by Ramstad and found to contain malic acid, citric acid, ursolic acid, and oleanolic acid, hydroquinone but not arbutin, and condensed tannins. Likewise, the leaves of the northern American and Canadian lingonberry, Vaccinium vitis-idaea, have been used similarly. Vaccinium is a genus in the heath family, Ericaceae. The heath family includes another genera, Arctostaphylos, with species whose leaves have been traditionally used for urinary tract infections. Best known of this group in Europe and America is the leaves of uva ursi or bearberry, Arctostaphylos uva-ursi. The extracts of leaves from uva ursi and lingonberry were both shown by Holopainen and others in 1988 to actively inhibit the urinary bacterial pathogens Escherichia coli and Proteus vulgaris.

Arbutin, and lesser amounts of the antibacterial aglycone hydroquinone which it releases were both found in these species by Sticher and others in 1979. While uva ursi leaves yield up to 18.6% arbutin, in 1983 Fromard determined that *V. vitis-idaea* contains about 10.4%. Besides these phenolic compounds, in 1965 Britton and Haslam described how lingonberry yields cinnamic acid esters, whereas uva ursi leaves contained the phenolics gallic acid, ellagic acid, and their tannins. Both species are known to yield quercetin and other flavonoids. Uva ursi leaves also yield the triterpenes ursolic acid and oleanolic acid as documented by Morimoto and others in 1983. In 1966 Constantine and others demonstrated that the individual components of several *Arctostaphylos* species did not account for the antimicrobial spectrum demonstrated with complex extracts of their leaves.

Apparently, the leaves of several species of *Vaccinium* and *Arctostaphylos* are effective urinary tract antiseptics due to several types of phenolics (i.e., arbutin/ hydroquinone, flavonols, cinnamic acids, anthocyanins, and/or tannins) but also due to triterpenoids (e.g., ursolic acid). However, the gallotannins and ellagitannins of *Arctostaphylos* species are distinct from the condensed catechin tannins of *Vaccinium* species. While the leaves are appreciated as antiseptics, the fruit are not often considered as such. Yet, both cranberry and a similar *Arctostaphylos* species have this capacity.

The fruit called pinguica from the *Arctostaphylos pungens* bush in the southwestern United States and northern Mexico are used to treat urinary tract infections. According to Bye in 1986, a tea of the leaves or fruit is used for kidney or other urinary ailments. That same year Winkelman indicated that the dried fruit of pinguica are also used alone for kidney problems such as nephritis, prostate problems, and urinary tract infections. The fruit are red to reddish brown berries resembling little apples, giving the plant its Spanish name, manzanita. However, in 1983 Dominguez and others had shown that the leaves and fruit of *A. pungens* do not contain arbutin as found in the other *Arctostaphylos* species, but they do contain ursolic acid and tannins. The ursolic acid in the fruit seems to contribute to its usefulness in managing the infections. This compound is held in common with cranberry fruit, but it is not effectively extracted in the juice.

Components—Fruit Versus Juice

The nutritive content of cranberries as reported by Kuzminski in 1996 is somewhat limited.The raw fruit contains considerable carbohydrates and fiber as expected, along with appreciable potassium and vitamin C, but significant quantities of other essential vitamins and minerals are lacking. However, other important components are active and characteristic. Anthocyanin and organic acid profiles can be used to assure preparation authenticity. The first red anthocyanin was identified in 1931 by Grove and Robinson as a 3-glucoside of peonidin. Two other glycosides of peonidin and three with cyanidin compose the anthocyanins. Cranberry content of quinic acid of 0.5–0.8%, along with much smaller amounts of benzoic acid, is converted and excreted as hippuric acid, as described by Fellers CR and others in 1933. In 1989 Hughes and Lawson measured citric acid content as equivalent to quinic acid in the whole fresh frozen berries, while malic acid yield was slightly lower.

As early as 1934, Markley and Sando found that the cranberry pomace or fruit pulp remaining after extracting the juice from the fruit contained free ursolic acid and an unidentified resin acid. In 1953 Wu and Parks isolated both triterpenoids ursolic acid and oleanolic acid from the berries. The flavonol aglycones quercetin and myrecetin along with several of their glycosides were later identified in cranberries. According to the 2003 USDA database for flavonoid content, cranberry and its juice have some of the highest contents of these flavonols of the 225 foods and beverages studied. The anti-adherence proanthocyanidins (procyanidins or condensed tannins) in the fruit are oligomers of epicatechin. These components are concentrated in the seeds and the skins of the fruit.

Single strength cranberry juice has from 2.2–3.3% organic acids. As reported by Kuzminski in 1996, cranberry juice contains about 2.8% glucose and 0.8% fructose, an unusual ratio (about 3.5) for a fruit juice. In addition, the proportions of quinic acid (1.1%), citric acid (1.1%), and malic acid (0.8%) are important for the flavor. The anthocyanins vary from 0.02–0.05% and are made up of the six glycosides of the anthocyanidins cyanidin and peonidin. The juice also contain proanthocyanidins.

According to Kuziminski, half of the carbohydrates and almost all of the fiber and vitamin C are lost in the juice, but the potassium content is somewhat elevated as compared to the whole fruit. The 2003 USDA database for flavonoid content indicates that little of the quercetin and myricetin found in raw cranberries and raw cranberry juice is retained in the bottled cranberry juice cocktail.

Product Forms and Doses

Whole Berries

In addition to their fiber content, Hughes and Lawson confirmed that whole cranberries contain about one third of the carbohydrates and calories and 50% more total organic acids (citric acid, malic acid, quinic acid) than an equivalent amount of the juice cocktail with its added sugar. About 3 ounces of the frozen berries provide an equivalent amount of juice (2 ounces) as 6 fluid ounce of the juice cocktail.

JUICE

Bodel and others in 1959 indicated that one liter of juice can be obtained from pressing 1,500 grams of cranberries. Sweetened undiluted juice is known in the industry as "Cran." It is produced by first freezing the berries, and then thawing them prior to pressing. This causes cellular rupture that results in much greater juice and anthocyanin yield. In various studies, 5–6.5 ounces lowered urine pH, 11 ounces further acidified the urine and decrease alkaline pH crystals, 16 ounces acidified the urine, reduced urine odor, and effectively treated urinary tract infections (UTIs), 25 ounces reduced bacterial biofilm and adhesion, and 32 ounces diminished ionized calcium excretion.

JUICE COCKTAIL

Early cranberry juice cocktail (from at least 1959–1968) was 33% juice in 1967. Now, it contains 25% of native cranberry juice along with flavor and nutrient additives: 5% fructose, 7% glucose, 0.32 mg/ml vitamin C. The pH of this juice cocktail is 2.5–3.0. Staples and Francis confirmed in 1968 that the color of the cocktail is due to the anthocyanin pigments, and juice color varies following the mixing of different proportions of the four different colors of cranberries (white, pink, red, and dark red). When the juice is pressed from frozen-thawed cranberries, about 40% of the red anthocyanin pigment remains in the press cake, called pomace.

According to Chiriboga and Francis in 1970, multiple extractions with acidic methanol remove over 90% of this pigment from the pomace; these red anthocyanins are subsequently concentrated. These authors described in 1973 how the reclaimed freeze-dried pigment concentrate consists of 17% anthocyanins, 18% flavonols, and 36% tannins. This powdered extract can be added as a colorant to the juice for production of standard-colored cranberry cocktail. The flavonols help the cocktail to retain the pigment in solution longer, and the flavonols were more stable than the anthocyanins.

Doses in various positive open-label clinical studies ranged from 4–32 ounces daily. Doses ranging from 4–6 ounces prevented UTIs, while 300 ml (10 oz.) daily was the effective dose for treating UTIs. A single dose of 15 ounces reduced *E. coli* adherence to cells in the urinary tract. Daily use of 32 ounces reduced infective urinary stones and slightly lowered urine pH, but one study showed this acidifying effect with as little as 12 ounces while another was negative when using 10 ounces.

POWDERED CONCENTRATE

Characterization of these products and their dosage is extremely inadequate in most clinical studies. Hughes and Lawson determined that hard gelatin encapsulated cranberry powder produced by rapid drying contained about one fourth the carbohydrates/calories and 5% as much benzoic acid as an equivalent amount (6 ounces) of the cocktail. The total organic acids in the hard capsule cranberry powder were 50% greater than in the juice cocktail, and the powder also provided some fiber content (about half that of the fresh berries). Twelve hard gelatin capsules (6.9 grams) of this cranberry powder were equivalent to 6 fluid ounce (180 ml) of the juice cocktail. Doses of powdered juice concentrate range from 7.5 grams (plus 1.7 grams lingonberry juice powder) to 9.6 grams daily to prevent UTIs.

A powdered cranberry extract was given for anti-adherence in a partially effective dose of 1.2 grams daily with 90 mg additional vitamin C. This product was likewise partially effective in preventing UTIs, but the dose of the 400 mg capsules was unspecified.

Laboratory Pharmacological Research

Antibacterial

URSOLIC ACID

Following its identification in cranberries again by the Russians Murav'ev and others in 1972, ursolic acid was shown to have antibacterial activity in test tubes in 1976 by Kowalewski and others. They found it effective against Gram-positive *Staphylococcus* and Gram-negative bacteria as well as yeast. In 1986 the Russians Zaletova and others again showed it inhibits Gram-positive *S. aureus* and Gram-negative bacteria but not some yeast such as *Candida albicans* and *Microsporium lenosum*.

Inhibiting Bacterial Adherence

FRESH JUICE AND CONCENTRATE

Sobota in 1984 showed in test tubes that cranberry fresh juice, cocktail, and concentrate all significantly reduced adherence of *Escherichia coli* to cells from the lining of the urinary tract at dilutions of 1:100 or less. The fresh juice was more potent than the concentrate at all concentrations and more effective than the cocktail at 4 of the 6 concentrations tested.

JUICE COCKTAIL

The cocktail inhibited adherence by 75% or more for 60% of the 77 different clinical isolates of *E. coli*, as shown by Sobota in 1984. While the fructose concentrations from 0.02–0.20 gm/ml sometimes inhibited bacterial adherence, 0.15 gm/ml added to 33% juice did not have an additive effect. Vitamin C had no anti-adherence effect from 0.1–10 mg/ml. Urine from mice given cranberry cocktail for 14 days in place of water inhibited *E. coli* adherence by 80%.

PROANTHOCYANIDINS AND FRUCTOSE

Zafriri and others found in 1989 that fructose is responsible for inhibiting adherence due to type 1 *E. coli* fimbriae (MS adhesin), whether it is from cranberry, orange, or pineapple juice. Ofek and others discovered that a high-molecular-weight, nondialysable polymer from *V. macrocarpon* inhibits the MR adhesion associated with pyelonephritogenic strains of *E. coli*. This polymer acts on *E. coli* type P fimbriae that bind by lectins with specificity to uroepithelial cells. In 1998 Howell and others determined that the proanthocyanidin extract contained this polymer that was not available in orange, pineapple, or non-*Vaccinium* juices.

This nondialyzable material derived from cranberry juice concentrate was also tested by Weiss and others in 1998 with bacteria responsible for causing dental plaque. Interspecies adhesion or coaggregation that contributes greatly to plaque stability was reversed in 58% of 84 coaggregating bacterial pairs. It was especially effective against pairs where one or both members were Gram-negative anaerobic bacteria involved in periodontal disease. The effective concentration range of the active component was 0.6–2.5 mg/ml.

In a study by Burger and others in 2000, a high molecular weight nondialyzable component of cranberry juice was also tested to determine its effect on the adherence of the pathogenic *Helicobacter pylori* bacteria to human gastric mucus and red blood cells in test tubes. Three strains of *H. pylori* tested utilize a sialic acid-specific adhesin that was inhibited by the cranberry constituent.

In several studies in 2000 Foo and others described the active proanthocyanidin oligomers as having mainly 4 or 5 epicatechins with at least one A-type linkage and procyanidin A2 as the common terminal unit, but some contained 3, 6, or 7 epicatechins and/or had a terminal unit with a single epicatechin. The epicatechin monomer and procyanidin B2 dimer were inactive as antiadherence agents, whereas the epicatechin dimer procyanidin A2 was weakly active.

Antioxidant

JUICE

In 1998 Wilson and others used a juice made from pressing cranberries that had been frozen, pasteurized, and filtered to study its anti-oxidant protective effects for serum lipoproteins. This extract consisted of 5.6% soluble solids of mostly sugars and contained 1.58 mg polyphenols per liter; it was bright red and had a pH of

2.5. Diluting this juice to 0.05% produced significant reduction in test tubes of low density lipoprotein (LDL) relative electrophoretic mobility independent of pH, a sign of reduced oxidation of the LDL. Similarly, thiobarbituric acid reactive substance formation from LDL by cupric sulfate was reduced at a juice dilution of 0.1%, another indication of diminished LDL oxidation. This suggests a potential application for prevention of cardiovascular disease.

URSOLIC ACID

Acute liver damage from carbon tetrachloride in mice was reduced by subcutaneous injection of 10 mg/kg ursolic acid, according to Ma and others in 1986.

Anti-inflammatory

URSOLIC AND OLEANOLIC ACIDS

In 1980 Iwu and Ohiri associated oleanolic acid and ursolic acid with anti-arthritic effects of a methanol extract from a different botanical. Ringbom and others found in 1998 that these triterpenoids produced significant direct cyclooxygenase-2 (COX-2) inhibition in test tubes. The concentrations of ursolic acid and oleanolic acid required to inhibit COX-2 by 50% were less than those needed for COX-1 by factors of 0.6 and 0.8, respectively. Their effect on COX-2 prostaglandin biosynthesis was exposure time-dependent, whereas their COX-1 inhibition was not.

Antiviral

JUICE

Commercial cranberry drink has also been found to inactivate poliovirus type 1 in a preliminary study by Konowalchuk and Speirs in 1978.

URSOLIC AND OLEANOLIC ACIDS

These triterpenoids demonstrated equivalent anti-HIV activity in test tube studies by Kashiwada and others in 1998, but ursolic acid had a low therapeutic index bases on its slight toxicity. Their derivatives were found to be more effective by Kashiwada and others in 1998 and 2000.

Human Pharmacological Studies

Increasing Urine Acidity

BERRY SAUCE

The observation of this effect by Blatherwick and Long in 1923 in one subject fed 305 grams of cranberry sauce was associated with increased secretion of organic acids, particularly hippuric acid. They also believed that the hippuric acid excretion found after eating 300-450 grams of prunes was a derivative of the quinic acid. In 1933 Fellers and others found consumption of whole or strained cranberry sauce by six subjects did not significantly lower urinary pH. Likewise, urinary volume was not directly affected. However, after establishing baseline levels on a standard diet, increasing consumption from 22 grams to 32.7 grams to 54 grams (fresh weight) daily for several days cause progressively greater, though slight, increases in hippuric acid secretion. Giving 100 grams or more of the sauce in 24 hours increased the content of acids in the urine up to 15%. Over five days of adding more cranberries to the basal diet, going from 100 to 150 to 200 to 250 to 300 grams daily, excretion of hippuric acid rose steadily each day. Hippuric acids returned to normal several days after a single ingestion of 250 grams.

JUICE

In 1964 Kraemer described how 16 ounces of cranberry juice reduced pH in 5 of 6 normal subjects after a single consumption. This amount also reduced the pH to 6.0 or less in 5 of 6 subjects with chronic urinary tract disorders. DuGan and Cardaciotto found no significant objective change in pH measurements when using from 3–6 ounces per day with 220 patients in 1966.

Compared to baseline, a prescribed regime of cranberry juice and/or ascorbic acid given in 1975 by Nickey to ten volunteers found that the average pH was reduced equivalently with either cranberry juice or vitamin C. However, the greatest and most consistent reduction to a urinary pH of 5.0–5.5 or lower was achieved with a combination of the two. Amounts used were not indicated, as the volunteers followed their usual 3-meal daily diets with no snacks over the 15-day duration. The pH was measured daily in a consistent manner.

In 1979 Kinney and Blount studied four groups of ten each using either 150, 180, 210, or 240 ml of juice with each meal. The juice was actually a sweetened 80% juice preparation. The pH was first measured for six days on a controlled diet and then for six days using the same menu plus juice, with each subject serving as their own control. The differences in urinary pH were significant for each group between the baseline control and cranberry use. The reductions were equivalent for the 180–240 ml groups (from about 5.95 to 5.43) that were greater than the 150 ml group (from 5.85 to 5.49).

In 2002 Kebler and others tested 12 healthy men in trial periods of five days in which they compared the effects on 24-hour urine samples of intake of 330 ml of either mineral water (control) or cranberry juice. Creatinine was assayed to assure compliance with standard dietary intake. Cranberry juice acidified the urine in comparison to the control.

JUICE COCKTAIL

A 1959 study by Bodel and others showed consumption of 1200–1500 ml (40–50 oz.) of cranberry juice cocktail (33% juice) in one day caused only a slight decrease in pH in the three subject tested and led to excretion of 3–4 grams of hippuric acid. Surprisingly, 4000 ml of the cocktail caused a slight pH increase in one subject. High hippuric acid concentrations in the urine were not consistently achieved because of the increased volume of urine from the large quantity of diluted juice. Concentrating the hippuric acid is needed to achieve a low pH of at least 5 to produce a bacteriostatic effect for common urinary tract pathogens. Thus, reduction of excessive fluid intake is necessary while using cranberry juice with its accompanying active components, if this antibacterial acidifying effect was to be attained. A slightly greater decrease in pH occurred when 600 ml of the sweetened juice was consumed undiluted.

Reduction of urinary pH was again shown to be minor in study with four people by Kahn and others in 1967. Using 1500–4000 ml (50–133 ounces) of cranberry cocktail containing 33% juice produced transient lowering of the urinary pH in three subjects and a sustained effect in one subject. In 1968 at the end of a 9-year study by Zinsser and others, it was reported that one quart of cranberry cocktail per day used by 53 patients was able to maintain a urinary pH of 6 or lower.

A double-blind, randomized trial by Avorn and others in 1994 using 300 ml (10 ounces) daily of standard commercial cranberry juice cocktail for 6 months with 153 women found no significant difference in the acidification of the urine when compared to placebo. Then, in 1997 Jackson and Hicks studied 21 elderly men in a nursing home who had a positive history of UTIs or were catheterized. They served as there own controls in a double crossover study. After four weeks with no cranberry product, they each received 118.3 ml of juice cocktail three times daily with meals (355 ml or 12 ounces daily) for four weeks, followed by another four weeks without the cocktail. The pH of the first morning urine was measured daily over these twelve weeks and was found to be significantly lower during the period when the juice cocktail was consumed. In 2002 Howell and Foxman tested the properties of urine following consumption of 240 ml (8 ounces) of the commercial juice cocktail. Urine pH was not affected.

JUICE CONCENTRATE

A liquid cranberry juice concentrate was given by Schlager and others in 1999 in 2-ounce containers that were comparable to 300 ml cranberry juice cocktail. The pH of the urine was not significantly different with the juice concentrate than with the placebo.

Urinary Crystal Formation

JUICE

A study by Kahn and others in 1967 found four of six people consuming 2 pints of the juice daily for one month showed elevated total calcium excretion and two of six had elevated oxalate, but in five ingesting up to 5 pints of undiluted juice the percentage of ionized urinary calcium did not increase significantly. In 1973 Light and others studied the effects of giving cranberry juice on the presence of ionized calcium in the urine. Normal individuals had about 32% of urinary calcium in ionized form, and 2–5 pints of the juice given to 5 of these did not change the amount or percentage. However, in 10 patients with kidney stones, 55% of their urinary calcium was ionized. In these kidney stone patients given 2 pints of cranberry juice weekly for one month, the amount of ionized calcium was reduced by half. This significant reduction was considered valuable for preventing stone formation.

The juice was believed to benefit some urinary tract calculi due to lowering urine pH. In 2002 Kebler and others tested 12 healthy men with 4 trials of five days each following 4-day adaptation periods. Creatinine was assayed to assure compliance with standard dietary intake. The four trials compared the effects on 24-hour urine samples of intake of 330 ml (11 ounces) of either mineral water (control), blackcurrant, plum, or cranberry juice. Blackcurrant juice caused significant alkalinity of the urine and increased citric acid and oxalic acid excretion, but did not affect the relative supersaturation of urinary crystal sources. Plum juice had no significant effect on the parameters measured. Cranberry juice acidified the urine, increased oxalic acid secretion, increased the relative supersaturation of uric acid, but decreased the relative supersaturation of struvite and brushite. The juices did not change excretion of calcium, magnesium, and uric acid. The authors suggested that blackcurrant juice was preferable for prevention of uric acid stones due to its alkalinity, whereas cranberry juice acidity made it useful for prevention of apatite, brushite, and struvite stones. They also noted these conclusions should be tested in stone-forming patients, rather than healthy subjects.

JUICE COCKTAIL

A study by Kahn and others in 1967 with four people used 1500–4000 ml (3-8 pints) of cranberry cocktail containing 33% juice. Urinary calcium excretion increased in two.

Inhibiting Bacterial Adherence

JUICE

In 2001 Reid and others looks at the effect that cranberry juice had on bacterial biofilm on urinary tract mucosal cells in spinal cord injured patients. In this type of patient population, UTIs are common and sometimes fatal. Fifteen of these subjects consumed a 250 ml glass of water three times daily for one week, followed by three 250-ml glasses (25 ounces) of cranberry juice daily for an additional week. The cranberry juice reduced the biofilm load and diminished adhesion of both Gram-negative and Gram-positive bacteria to the cells, while water had neither effect.

JUICE COCKTAIL

As shown by Sobota in 1984, a total of 15 out of 22 human subjects drinking 15 oz of cranberry cocktail had significant inhibition of *E. coli* adherence by urine collected 1-3 hours after consumption. This urine was tested with bacteria adhering to cells in test tubes. A study in 1988 by Schmidt and Sobota examined cranberry juice cocktail's ability to inhibit adherence of urinary isolates of the Gram-negative bacteria *E. coli, Proteus,* and *Klebsiella* to uroepithelial cells as a potential benefit independent of urine acidification and bacterial inhibition. Adherence was reduced by urine collected from humans 2 hours after drinking 12 ounces of cranberry juice cocktail. When pre-incubated with the bacteria, urine was effective against all strains. However, 1 of 2 strains of *E. coli* and *Proteus* but both strains of *Pseudomonas* showed reduced adherence after urinary epithelial cells were exposure to urine collected following cranberry cocktail consumption. However, residual bacteria always remained on the cells, even when they were directly exposed to the cocktail.

In 2002 Howell and Foxman decided to test the anti-adhesion properties of urine following cranberry juice cocktail consumption against antibiotic-resistant isolates of *E. coli.* Following consumption of 240 ml (8 ounces) of the commercial juice cocktail, urine was collected over a 12-hour period, and isolates were exposed to the urine for 20 minutes. Adhesion was prevented in 31 of 39 total isolates (80%) including 19 of 24 that were antibiotic-resistant. The anti-adhesion activity was present in the urine within 2 hours and lasted for up to 10 hours after consuming the cranberry cocktail.

CRANBERRY EXTRACT

In 1999 Habash and others studied the urine of ten healthy males in four separate trials for 2.5 days each in separate weeks over a 4-week period. The trials include a control, 500 ml water 3 times daily, 400 mg cranberry extract 3 times daily, and 500 mg vitamin C twice daily. Urine was collected on the third day after the last dose for each, chemically assessed, and then exposed to silicone rubber along with various urinary pathogens to determine adherence. Only the vitamin C led to consistently acidic urine. Increased water led to lower urine protein content. The urine from vitamin C and cranberry extract supplementation reduced the deposition and adherence of *E. coli* and *Enterococcus faecalis,* but not *Staphylococcus epidermidis, Psuedomonas aeruginosa,* or *Candida albicans.* The urine following increased water vastly increased deposition and adherence of *E. coli* and *E. faecalis.*

Altering Blood Lipids

JUICE

Vinson and Holland reported at the American Chemical Society national meeting in New Orleans in March, 2003, that two servings daily of cranberry juice with either artificial sweetener or sugar in 19 adults with high cholesterol both increased serum HDL cholesterol and lowered LDL cholersterol, but had no effect on total cholesterol. One serving daily for one month had no effect of these lipid levels, but three servings per day of the sugar-sweetened juice were associated with increased triglyceride levels.

Preventive and Therapeutic Clinical Trials

Reducing Ammoniacal Odor

JUICE

Several studies note the important effect of cranberry juice in subjectively reducing the ammoniacal urinary odors frequently encountered in geriatric patients, particularly in nursing homes. In 1964 Kraemer described how 16 ounces of cranberry juice in 5 of 6 subjects with chronic urinary tract disorders caused a noticeable reduction in turbidity and ammoniacal odor. Tested in a nursing home and in a hospital incontinent ward the cranberry juice used in 5-day periods noticeably reduced the odor of ammonia, according to assessments by supervisory personnel.

In 1966 DuGan and Cardaciotto found that using only 3-6 ounces of the juice per day produced no significant objective change in chemical measurements including ammonia with 110 male and 110 female patients. However, even this small amount reduced the odor from the wards that housed these patients. Also, patients who had complained of burning sensations on urination were no longer subject to this discomfort called dysuria.

Reducing Stone-associated Infections

JUICE COCKTAIL

As reported in 1968 on a 9-year study by Zinsser and others, one quart of cranberry cocktail (1 part juice to 2 parts water) per day had been used with 53 patients to lower and prevent recurrences of infective stones. Of these patients 8% worsened, 32% of the cases were arrested, and 60% improved. During this process the intervals of recurrence were prolonged from 21 to 44 months. Cranberry juice cocktail was superior to other acidifying agents (ammonium chloride, methenamine mandelate with or without sulfamethizole, and potassium acid phosphate) in this regard when used for up to ten years. Larger quantities of undiluted juice were more effective in preventing UTI.

Preventing Urinary Tract Infections

JUICE COCKTAIL

A dose of 4–6 ounces (120–180 ml) of cranberry juice cocktail almost daily appears to help prevent urinary tract infections (UTI) in high-risk populations of long-term care facilities as shown by Gibson and others in 1991. Of 28 nursing home patients, 19 avoided Gram-negative bacilli urinary infections during the seven weeks they consumed the juice cocktail.

POWDERED JUICE CONCENTRATES

Twelve 800 mg capsules daily of a powdered juice concentrate given to 21 subjects by Kilbourn in 1986 prevented infections in all except one, but when given to 6 patients with pre-existing UTI, none were cured. This evidence suggests that cranberry juice alone may be more effective as a preventive measure than as a treatment.

In a 2001 open, randomized controlled trial with a 12-month follow up, Kontiokari and others gave 50 ml daily of a combination juice concentrate to 50 women for six months. The preparation consisted of 7.5 grams of cranberry juice concentrate and 1.7 grams of lingonberry juice concentrate added to 50 ml of water with no sugars. They were advised to add this to an additional 200 ml of unsweetened water to make it more palatable. Another 50 received a lactobacillus drink for five days each week for one year, and another group of 50 had no intervention. All 150 women had a history of UTI caused by *E. coli*. The first recurrence occurred before 6 months with 16% of the women using juice, 39% of the lactobacillus group, and 36% of the control group. After 12 months 24% of the juice group, 43% of the lactobacillus group, and 38% of the control group had experienced reoccurrence of the UTI. So even though those using the juice concentrate had stopped after six months, the recurrence rate did not approach the levels of the other two groups over the next six months.

In 2001 Stothers and Stothers compared the use of concentrated cranberry tablets with cranberry juice and placebo for 150 women with recurrent URIs in a randomized and blinded clinical trial. Both the tablets and the juice were effective in significantly reducing the annual frequency of URIs and antibiotic consumption. For prevention the cranberry tablets proved to be twice as cost effective as the juice.

LIQUID CONCENTRATE

Surprisingly, the efficacy of a liquid concentrate was not the same as powdered forms. A liquid cranberry juice concentrate was given by Schlager and others in 1999 to 15 children with neurogenic bladder given intermittent catheterization in a double-blind, placebo-controlled crossover study. They received the concentrate or placebo (liquefied artificial cranberry-flavored gelatin) for 3 months each. The juice concentrate was dispensed in 2-ounce containers that were comparable to 300 ml cranberry juice cocktail. The frequency of bacteria in the urine and number of infections were not significantly different with the liquid juice concentrate, compared to the placebo.

CRANBERRY EXTRACT

In 1997 Walker and others used 400 mg capsules of concentrated cranberry extract solids to treat 10 women with a history of recurrent UTIs. After antibiotic treatment of a UTI each woman was randomly and blindly assigned to either the placebo or cranberry extract group. After 3 months they switched groups. The cranberry extract significantly reduced the incidence of infection. Over the 6 months of the study 21 UTIs occurred: 6 in the cranberry group and 15 in the placebo group.

Treating Urinary Tract Infections

JUICE

A clinical study by Papas PN and others in 1966 of 60 adults diagnosed with acute infection of the urinary tract utilized 16 oz of cranberry juice per day for 3 weeks. This completely relieved symptoms in 32 (53%) and led to moderate improvement in 12 others (20%). Of these 44, 17 (39%) were infection-free at a six-week follow-up. All tolerated the regimen exceptionally well.

JUICE COCKTAIL

A placebo-controlled, double-blind, randomized trial by Avorn and others in 1994 using 300 ml daily of standard commercial cranberry juice cocktail for 6 months was undertaken with 153 elderly women. A baseline urine sample and 6 monthly clean-voided specimens were collected and tested for pyuria and bacteriuria. Those completing the study included 60 in the cranberry group and 61 in the placebo group with similar medical histories. Bacteria in the urine along with white blood cells was found in 28.1% of the urine samples for the placebo group compared to 15.0% for the cranberry group. Significant differences between the groups using these parameters were noted after the first month.

Potential Adverse Effects

No adverse side effects have been found with prolonged use. On the contrary, both DuGan and Cardaciotto along with Papas and others reported the beneficial side effect of burning sensations during urination disappearing in those who had this complaint. One report in 2001 by Davies and others described immune thrombocytopenic purpura in a 68-year-old man who had used cranberry juice for 10 days. This resulted in his hospitalization for oral and urinary bleeding and extensive

278 Complex Herbs—Complete Medicines

discoloration on his shins. Tests indicated that the cranberry juice induced IgM and IgG anti-platelet antibodies in this patient's serum. This was considered good evidence for an immune mechanism for the low platelet count. A cranberry juice constituent was believed to act as a hapten.

Possibly the greatest concern about potential harm from regular consumption of cranberries and/or the juice is due to residues and their combinations from pesticides that are used in non-organic commercial cultivation. Safety information provided in 2000 by the pesticide chart produced for Oregon and Washington growers by the Cranberry Institute in Massachusetts indicates recommended rates of application, timing intervals in regard to both pre-harvest and field re-entry, and maximum number of applications, along with advisory notes. Of the 20 insecticides listed as used for cranberry producing beds, 7 are considered relatively safe, but 2 are extremely toxic to people, 5 are moderately toxic to people, 4 are extremely toxic to birds, 1 is moderately toxic to birds, 8 are extremely toxic to bees, 4 are moderately toxic to bees, 3 are extremely toxic to fish, and 5 are moderately toxic to fish. Five of these insecticides are toxic to humans, birds, bees and fish, while two others are extremely toxic to humans, bees and fish. Of the 9 herbicides listed for producing beds 7 are considered relatively safe, but 1 is moderately toxic to humans and 1 is moderately toxic to fish. Of the 15 fungicides listed 2 are relatively safe, but 4 are extremely toxic to fish, and 9 are relatively toxic to fish. These relative toxicities are determined based on single pesticide exposures, not on the combinations of several that might be used together. The greatest risk appears to be for the wildlife and humans who living near the cranberry bogs. Consumption of commercial cranberry products has not been shown to increase health risks.

Table 6 Cranberry Fruit and Derivatives—Summary of Medicinal Uses and Pharmacology

CRANBERRY *Vaccinium macrocarpon* Aiton	Traditional Uses	Modern Clinical Studies	Laboratory Research Findings

Whole Fruit	Nutritive
	Liver problems
	Detoxification Con-
	valescence
	Diuretic
	Antiseptic
	Locally:
	  Inflammation
	  Gangrene
	  Erysipelas
	  Sore throat
	  Skin ulcers
	  Boils
			Contains vitamin C, fiber, flavonols, potassium, & carbohydrates
			Increases total urinary acids

Fruit Juice	Nutritive Urinary tract infections (UTIs) Kidney stones	Reduces urine odor Reduces dysuria Reduces infective stones Relieves UTIs	Contains flavanols, potassium, & carbohydrates Inhibits bacteria adhesion Increases urine acidity Reduces urinary struvite, brushite, & ionized calcium Improves cholesterol profile Inactivates polio virus
Juice Cocktail	Nutritive	Reduces infective stones Prevents UTIs Relieves UTIs	Contains potassium & carbohydrates Inhibits bacteria adhesion Increases total urinary acids

Continued on next page

Table 6 *Continued*

CRANBERRY *Vaccinium macrocarpon* Aiton	Traditional Uses	Modern Clinical Studies	Laboratory Research Findings
Powdered Juice Concentrate		Prevents UTIs	
Solid Extract		Prevents UTIs	Inhibits bacteria adhesion
FRACTIONS OR ISOLATED CONSTITUENTS			
Proanthocyanidins (Procyanidins)			Enhances ornithine decarboxylase Inhibits bacterial adhesion
Ursolic Acid			Antibacterial Anti-HIV Anti-inflammatory Reduces liver toxicity

References

BOOKS

Angier, B. *Field Guide to Medicinal Wild Plants*. Stackpole Books, Harrisburg, Penn., 1978.

Felter, HW and Lloyd, JU. *King's American Dispensatory*, 1898 version, Eclectic Medical Pub., Portland, OR., 1983.

Lust, J. *The Herb Book*, Bantam Books, New York, 1974.

Upton, R (ed.). *Cranberry*, American Herbal Pharmacopoeia, Santa Cruz, Cal., 2002.

USP Revision Comm. *The National Formulary*, 19th ed., U. S. Pharmaopeial Convention, Inc., Rockville, MD, 2000.

ARTICLES

Avorn, J et al. Reduction of Bacteriuria and Pyuria After Ingestion of Cranberry Juice. *JAMA*, 271:751–4, 1994.

Blatherwick, NR and Long, ML. The increased acidity produced by eating prunes and cranberries. *J.Biol. Chem.*, 57:815–8, 1923.

Bodel, PT et al. Cranberry juice and the antibacterial action of hippuric acid. *J. Lab. Clin. Med.,* 54:881–8, 1959.

Bomser, J et al. In vitro anticancer activity of fruit extracts from Vaccinium species. *Planta Med.,* 62:212–6, 1996.

Britton, G and Haslam E. Gallotannins. Part XII. Phenolic constitutents of Arctostaphylos uva-ursi L. Spreng. *J. Chem. Soc.,* pp. 7312–9, 1965.

Burger, O et al. A high molecular mass constituent of cranberry juice inhibits Heliobacter pylori adhesion to human gastric mucus. *FEMS Immunol. Med. Microbiol.,*29:295–301, 2000.

Bye, RA Jr. Medicinal plants of the Sierra Madre: Comparative study of Tarahumara and Mexican market plants. *Econ. Bot.,* 40(1):103–24, 1986.

Chiriboga, C and Francis, FJ. An anthocyanin recovery system from cranberry pomace. *Amer. Soc. Hort. Sci.,* 95(2):233–6, 1970.

Chiriboga, CD and Grancis, FJ. Ion exchange purified anthocyanin pigments as a colorant for cranberry juice cocktail. *J. Food Sci.,* 8:464–7, 1973.

Constantine, GH Jr et al. Phytochemical investigation of Arctostaphylos columbiana Piper and Arctostaphylos patula Greene (Ericaceae). *J. Pharm. Sci.,* 55(12):1378–82, 1966.

Davies, JK. A juicy problem. *Lancet,* 358:2126, 2001.

Dominguez, XA et al. Mexican medicinal plants. Part XLVII. Terpenoids of fruits and leaves of "pinguica", Arctostaphylos pungens H.B.K. *Rev. Latinoam. Quim.,* 14(1):37–9, 1983.

DuGan, CR and Cardaciotto, PS. Reduction of ammoniacal urinary odors by the sustained feeding of cranberry juice. *J. Psychiat. Nurs.,* 34:467–70, 1966.

Fellers, CR et al. Effect of cranberries on urinary acidity and blood alkali reserve. *J. Nutrit.,* 6:455–63, 1933.

Foo, LY et al. A-type proanthocyanidin trimers from cranberry that inhibit adherence of uropathogenic P-fimbriated Escherichia coli. *J. Nat. Prod.,* 63:1225–8, 2000.

Foo, LY et al. The structure of cranberry proanthocyanidins which inhibit adherence of uropathogenic P-fimbriated Escherichia coli in vitro. *Phytochem.,* 54:73–81, 2000.

Fromard, F. Arbutin and methylarbutin in Arctostaphylos uva-ursi and some other Ericaceae. Qualitative and quantitative analyses in chromatography. *C.R. Congr. Natl. Solc. Savantes, Sect. Sci.,* 108(3):251–67, 1983. (*Chem. Abs.* 102:163768v).

Gibson, L et al. Effectiveness of cranberry juice in preventing urinary tract infections in long-term care facility patients. *J. Naturop. Med.,* 2:45–7, 1991.

Grove, KE, and Robinson, R. An anthocyanin of Oxycoccus macrocarpus Pers. *Biochem. J.,* 25:1706–11, 1931.

Habash, MB et al. The effect of water, ascorbic acid, and cranberry derived supplementation on human urine and uropathogen adhesion to silicone rubber. *Can. J. Microbiol.,*45:691–4, 1999.

Hakkinen, S and Auriola, S. High-performance liquid chromatography with electrospray ionization mass spectrometry and diode array ultraviolet detection in the identification of flavonol aglycones and glycosides in berries. *J. Chromatog.,*829:91–100, 1998.

Holopainen, M et al. Antimicrobial activity of some Finnish ericaceous plants. *Acta Pharm. Fenn.,* 97(4):197–202, 1988. (*Chem. Abs.* 111:36508w).

Howell, AB and Foxman, B. Cranberry juice and adhesion of antibiotic-resistant uropathogens. *JAMA,* 287(23):3082–3, 2002.

Howell, AB and Vorsa, N. Inhibition of the adherence of P-fimbriated Escherichia coli to uroepithelial-cell surfaces by proanthocyanidin extracts from cranberries. *NEJM,* 339:1085–1086, 1998.

Hughes BG and Lawson, LD. Nutritional content of cranberry products. *Am. J. Hosp. Pharm.,* 46:1129, 1989.

Iwa, MM and Ohiri, FC. Anti-arthritic triterpenoids of Lonchocarpus cyanescens: benth. *Can. J. Pharm. Sci.,* 15(2):39–42, 1980. (*Chem. Abs.* 93:197689f).

Jackson, B and Hicks, LE. Effect of cranberry juice on urinary pH in older adults. *Home Healthcare Nurse,* 15(3):199–202, 1997.

Kahn, HD et al. Effect of cranberry juice on urine. *J. Am. Diet. Assoc.,* 51:251, 1967.

Kashiwada, Y et al. Anti-AIDS Agents. 30. Anti-HIV activity of oleanolic aid, pomolic acid, and structurally related triterpenoids. *J. Nat. Prod.,* 61:1090–5, 1998.

Kashiwada, Y et al. Anti-AIDS Agents. 38. Anti-HIV activity of 3-O-acyl ursolic acid derivatives. *J. Nat. Prod.,* 63:1619–22, 2000.

KeBler, T et al. Effect of blackcurrant-, cranberry- and plum juice consumption on risk factors associated with kidney stone formation. *Eur. J. Clin. Nutrit.,* 36:1020–3, 2002.

Kilbourn, JP. Cranberry juice appears to prevent urinary tract infections. *CCML Newslett.,* January, 1986.

Kinney, AB and Blount, M. Effect of cranberry juice on urinary pH. *Nursing Res.,* 28(5):287-9. 1979.

Konowalchuk, J and Speirs, JI. Antiviral effect of commercial juices and beverages. *Appl. Envir. Microb.,* 35:1219–20, 1978

Kontiokari, T et al. Randomised trial of cranberry-lingonberry juice and Lactobacillus GG drink for the prevention of urinary tract infections in women. *Br. Med. J.,* 322:1571–5, 2001.

Kowalewski, Z et al. Antibiotic action of beta-ursolic acid. *Arch. Immunol. Ther. Exp.,* 24:115–9, 1976. (*Chem. Abs.* 84:160059p)

Kraemer, RJ. Cranberry juice and the reduction of ammoniacal odor of urine. *Southwest. Med.,* 45:211–2, 1964.

Kuzminski, LN. Cranberry juice and urinary tract infections: Is there a beneficial relationship? *Nutr. Rev.,* 54(11):A87–S90, 1996.

Light, I et al. Urinary ionized calcium in urolithiasis—Effect of cranberry juice. *Urology,* 1(1):67–70, 1973.

Ma, X et al. Preventive and therapeutic effects of ursolic acid (UA) on acute liver injury in rats. *Yaoxue Xuebao,* 21(5):332–5, 1986. (*Chem. Abs.* 105:72646z).

Markley, KS and Sando, CE. Petroleum ether- and ether-soluble constituents of cranberry pomace. *J. Biol. Chem.,* 105:643–53, 1934.

Morimoto, K et al. Triterpenoid constituents of the leaves of Arctostaphylos uva-ursi. [Japanese] *Mukogawa Joshi Daigaku Kiyo, Yakugaku Hen,* 31:41–4, 1983 (*Chem. Abs.* 101:107343v).

Murav'ev, IA et al. Spectrometric determination of ursolic acid. *Khim. Prir. Soedin.,* (6):738–40, 1972. (*Chem. Abs.* 78:84570g).

Nickey, KE. Urinary pH: Effect of prescribed regimes of cranberry juice and ascorbic acid. *Arch. Phys. Med. Rehabil.,* 56:556, 1975.

Ofek, I. et al. Anti-Escherichia coli adhesin activity of cranberry and blueberry juices. *New Engl. J. Med.,* 324:1599, 1991.

Papas, PN et al. Cranberry juice in the treatment of urinary tract infections. *Southwest. Med.,* 47:17–20, 1966.

Prior, RL et al. Antioxidant capacity as influenced by total phenolic and anthocyanin content, maturity, and variety of Vaccinium species. *J. Agric. Food Chem.,* 46:2686–93, 1998.

Puski, G and Francis, FJ. Flavonol glycosides in cranberries. *J. Food Sci.,* 32:527–30, 1967.

Ramstad, E. Chemical investigation of Vaccinium myrtillus L. *J. Am. Pharm. Assoc.,* 43:236–40, 1954.

Reid, G et al. Cranberry juice consumption may reduce biofilms on uroepithelial cells: pilot study in spinal cord injured patients. *Spinal Cord,* 39:26–30, 2001.

Ringbom, T et al. Ursolic acid from Plantago major, a selective inhibitor of cyclooxygenase-2 catalyzed prostaglandin biosynthesis. *J. Nat. Prod.,* 61:1212–5, 1998.

Schlager, TA et al. Effect of cranberry juice on bacteriuria in children with neurogenic bladder receving intermittent catheterization. *J. Pediatr.,* 135:698–702, 1999.

Schmidt, DR and Sobota, E. An examination of the anti-adherence activity of cranberry juice on urinary and nonurinary bacterial isolates. *Microbios,* 55:173, 1988.

Sobota, AE. Inhibition of bacterial adherence by cranberry juice: potential use for the treatment of urinary tract infections. *J. Urol.,* 131:1013, 1984.

Staples, LC and Francis, FJ. Colorimetry of cranberry cocktail by wide range spectrophotometry. *Food Technol.,* 22:77–80, 1968.

Sternlieb, P. Cranberry juice in renal disease. *New Eng. J. Med.,* 268:57, 1963.

Sticher, O et al. High-performance liquid chromatographic separation and quantitative determination of arbutin, methylarbutin, hydroquinone and hydroquinone-monomethylether in Arctostaphylos, Bergenia, Calluna and Vaccinium species. *Planta Med.,* 35:253–61, 1979.

Stothers, K and Stothers, L. A cost effectiveness analysis of naturopathic cranberry products used as prophylaxis against urinary tract infection in women. *J. Urol.,* 165(5 Suppl.):10, 2001.

Vinson, J and Holland, G. Cranberries: excellent source of polyphenol antioxidants: single dose and supplementation studies with cranberry juice relevant to heart disease. Batz F (ed.), *Natural Medicine News,* March 28, 2003.

Walker, EB et al. Cranberry concentrate: UTI prophylaxis. *J. Fam. Pract.,* 45(2):167–8, 1997.

Weiss, EI et al. Inhibiting interspecies coaggregation of plaque bacteria with a cranberry juice constituent. *J. Am. Dent. Assoc.,* 129:1719–23, 1998.

Wilson, T et al. Cranberry extract inhibits low density lipoprotein oxidation. *Life Sci.,* 62(24): 381–6, 1998.

Winkelman, M. Frequently used medicinal plants in Baja California. *J. Ethnopharmacol.,* 18:109–31, 1986.

Wu, BYT and Parks, LM. Oleanolic acid from cranberries. *J. Am. Pharm. Assoc.,* 42:602–3, 1953.

Zafriri, D et al. Inhibitory activity of cranberry juice on adherence of type 1 and type P fimbriated *Escherichia coli* to eucaryotic cells. *Antimicrob Agents Chemother,* 33:92–8, 1989.

Zaletova, NI et al. Preparation of some derivatives of ursolic acid and their antimicrobial activity. *Khim.-Farm. Zh.,* 20:568–71, 1986 (*Chem. Abs.* 106:18867e).

Zinsser, HH et al. Management of infected stones with acidifying agents. *N.Y. St.ate J. Med.,* 68:3001–10, 1968.

Zopf, D and Roth, S. Oligosaccharide anti-infective agents. *Lancet,* 347:1017–1021, 1996.

CHARTS

Anonymous. 2000 Northwest United States Cranberry Pesticide Chart. Cranberry Institue, Wareham, Mass., February, 2000.

Anonymous. USDA database for the flavonoid content of selected foods. www.nal.usda.gov/fnic/foodcomp March, 2003.

5
AMERICAN HERBS ACCLAIMED
ACROSS THE ATLANTIC

The survey by the Lloyd Brothers of American doctors to assess the frequency of use of hundreds of botanical remedies [*JAPA*, 1912, pp.1235–1241] indicated that, like goldenseal (#2) and echinacea (#11), saw palmetto (#25) and black cohosh (#30) were rated among the most popular. One of the interesting phenomena of botanical medicine is how herbs come into and fall out of fashion over time. Some herbs become wildly popular during one era but may fall from view in the next, only to re-emerge with even greater demand at some point later down the line. Others maintain a low profile for years, and then are thrust into the spotlight through new investigation and successful product promotion. Black cohosh and saw palmetto along with purple coneflower echinacea are prime examples of these occurrences with American botanical medicines that have once again become popular largely through European clinical application and research.

While introduction of American herbal remedies to Europe typically occurred in the late 19th century via Physiomedicalists in Great Britain and homeopaths on the continent, the 20th century has seen a strong reversal of this process. Often, European utilization has involved an emphasis on a particular therapeutic application. The cross pollination of American botanical agents with European medical science has resulted in a distinctly narrow approach to their use when compared to the traditional American applications. The three herbs discussed here characterize the short and well-documented history of recent widespread popularity resulting from scientific scrutiny.

Black cohosh is one of the foremost traditional American remedies whose popularity grew from an appreciation of its uses by indigenous Americans. While known now as a remedy that influences female function, its early applications were generalized more for spastic and inflammatory conditions. Larger doses of the root attended these problems. This is one case where the most recognized modern form of product is actually quite dilute and is used in small doses compared to earlier extracts of the root.

Purple coneflower (*Echinacea purpurea*) is an illustration of an American plant similar to the traditional medicinal species (*E. angustifolia*) that underwent a separate and unique development. This has led to current misunderstanding and controversy over traditional views versus modern clinical studies. The comparison of these two echinacea species illustrates how modern marketplace generalities blur differences between empirical uses and active phytochemical content based on a failure to properly distinguish species, part, and preparation.

Saw palmetto is unusual in that its primary use by native Americans, like cranberry, appears to have been as a food. Observations of animals led to its therapeutic consumption to enhance nourishment of fatty tissue. The effects on both male and female organs led to recognition of its hormonal activity for which is now mainly known. An effect of its lipid fraction involves its inhibition of smooth muscle spasms that contribute to urinary problems. At the same time the whole berry contains water-soluble compounds that influence the immune system.

While the uses of each of these herbs have changed over time, the current perception of the usefulness is perceived as particular conditions that have been specifically researched. Their broader use has yet to be examined scientifically. Current perceptions of their limitations are a result of therapeutic type casting. More earnest examination of their potential should involve investigations of their empirical uses.

BLACK COHOSH—
Remedy for Muscle Pain and Women's Concerns

Cimicifuga [*Actaea*] *racemosa* L.—roots and rhizome

Summary

Native Americans and the pioneers used fresh or dried black cohosh root or relied on a water extract for treating rheumatism, chorea, and menstrual problems. Eclectics and others developed alcoholic extracts in the form of tinctures or fluid extracts, or even concentrated solid extracts insoluble in water made from these alcoholic extracts, for treating these same conditions. Active cinnamic acid derivatives are water soluble, while its triterpenic compounds extract with alcohol. Currently, standardized liquid and solid hydro-alcoholic extracts are being clinically researched for menopause. Tolerance is good at doses effective for menopausal symptoms, but large doses can produce adverse effects.

Names

Linnaeus classified this plant as *Actaea racemosa*. *Actaea* is from the Greek word for elder which has similar leaves; *racemosa* refers to its flowers that are in racemes. Frederick Pursh later placed this species in the Linnaean genus *Cimicifuga* (bugbane) as *C. serpentaria* (snake-like). Thomas Nuttal is credited with combining these names as *Cimicifuga racemosa*, the scientific synonym that has long been utilized until a recent return to the Linnaean name.

Benjamin Barton in 1801 referred to it as squaw root, noting that Indians valued this remedy highly for the diseases of women. In 1812 Peter Smith used the terms squaw root, rattleweed, and black snakeroot, the latter the most popular early common name. According to the Lloyds, C. S. Rafinesque in 1808 proposed its placement in a new genus *Macrotrys*. The popular American botancy author, Amos Eaton, misspelled this name as "Macrotys," which consequently became the most common name used by Eclectics from 1840–1940. Now, the root is most commonly known by the Indian-derived name of black cohosh. The rhizome, or enlarged underground stem, was long referred to as a root in the medical literature as is still done in modern times (and will sometimes be done here also for brevity's sake). The actual roots appear as rootlets attached to the rhizome, and they are used together.

The Chinese have a traditional remedy called sheng-ma that is the rhizome of *Actaea* [syn. *Cimicifuga*] *foetida* or similar species such as *A. dahurica* and *A. heracleifolia*. The Japanese refer to the Chinese crude drug as "shoma," the rhizome of *Cimicifuga simplex* or other species of the genus. The Chinese species have traditional medical applications primarily as an antipyretic and analgesic. Some authors such as McKenna and others in 2001 describe these Chinese species as black cohosh and discuss them interchangeably with the American species, even though their clinical equivalence has not been established. Nonetheless, the high demand of American black cohosh has led to substitution of these spurious Chinese species in its place.

Early Uses of the Root and Tea

Cimicifuga racemosa is abundant mostly on hillsides in woodlands east of the Mississippi River, except in New England and the deep South. Early medical uses were learned from the Indians. It was native Americans who first used the root chiefly for rheumatism, to initiate menstrual periods, and to aid in giving birth. Moerman describes its uses by various tribes. The Micmac and Penobscot used the root for kidney trouble. The Cherokees made an infusion of the root to stimulate menstruation, for fatigue, coughs, colds, and consumption, and as an anodyne for rheumatic pains. The Iroquois also used an infusion of the root, which was taken for rheumatism and to promote milk flow in nursing women.

In 1785 the German author, Johann Schoepf, writing in Latin, was the first to publish information on uses of the root as a diuretic and for pain. In 1801 Benjamin Barton described the root as astringent, the decoction being used as a gargle for sore throat. The "Indian doctor" Peter Smith in 1812 noted the root was famous for curing chronic rheumatism with moderate use. As implied by one of its names, the root was applied to snakebites as a poultice while also taken internally in small amounts. In 1818 William Hand recommended the fresh root be made into a strong infusion for chronic rheumatism, flatulent colic, and conditions.of hysteria.

The Lloyds describe how early uses emphasized the powdered root and its tea. Bigelow fully noted its uses for rheumatism, dropsy, and other conditions in 1820. Dr. T.S. Garden described *Actaea racemosa* uses in 1823 and thirty years later was still giving it for pulmonary tuberculosis. Dr. N. Chapman noted its reputation as an expectorant for treating consumption, asthma, and other pulmonary diseases in 1825. In 1828 Rafinesque described use of the root as a poultice by Indians for snakebites. He later indicated the root decoction was used as an auxiliary in acute and chronic rheumatism and as valuable for dropsy, hysteria, and locally as a gargle.

According to the Lloyds, the root was included as either *Actaea* or *Cimicifuga* in the two separate revisions of the *United States Pharmacopeia* in 1830. (It remained in the *USP* until the eleventh revision in 1930.) Dr. Young brought attention to black cohosh for chorea in 1831. As *Cimicifuga* it was included in the first edition of the *Dispensatory of the United States of America* in 1833. Dr. Wooster Beach, the father of Eclecticism, included it in his *American Practice of Medicine* in 1833. In 1832 Horton Howard cites case studies of the efficacy of the decoction in smallpox. By 1842 Dr. Hildreth confirmed black cohosh for the treatment of TB., asthma, and chorea. In 1848 Dr. N.S. Davis declared it to be a pure sedative. In 1856 Dr. G.B. Wood considered it a standard remedy for chorea, as did J.D. O'Connor in 1858 when he also advocated it for rheumatic and neuralgic pains.

Hydroalcoholic Extracts and Solid Extracts—Professional Acceptance

Some frontier practitioners found obtaining and transporting the dried root convenient. Many medical doctors, including Eclectics, came to prefer alcoholic extracts over water extracts. Dr. Thomas Morrow, first Dean of the Eclectic Medical Institute from 1842–1850, that he was called "Old Macrotys." Subsequently, black cohosh became a favorite remedy of Dr. John King. He established the root tincture and the solid resinoid extract in the Eclectic profession by his writings in the 1840s and in the *Eclectic Dispensatory of the United States of America,* published with Dr. Robert Newton in 1852. Extracts of the root later became official in the USP into the twentieth century, including the 1:1 fluid extract (beginning in 1860) and a 1:5 strength tincture (beginning in 1880). Black cohosh dried rhizome and roots and its fluid extract were both official in the *National Formulary* from the fifth edition in 1926 through the eighth in 1946.

Root and Rhizome Preparations and Doses

ROOT POWDER

Lust recommended that the root be collected in the fall after the fruit has disappeared and the leaves have died. The naturopathic dose range of the dried root (rhizome and its rootlets) was from 65 mg to 1.3 grams, with an average dose 1.0 gram as indicated by the 1946 edition of the *NF*.

WATER EXTRACT

Two teaspoons of dried roots/rhizome is simmered in one pint of water as directed by Lust. From 2–3 tablespoonful are taken cold, up to six time daily. Boiling water partially extracted its active principles; alcohol did so more completely.

TINCTURE

The official tincture in the 1942 *NF* was a 1:5 extract using 82% alcohol; the average dose was 4 ml. This far exceeded the naturopathic dose recommended by Kuts-Cheraux in 1953 of 0.07–1.33 ml, who described black cohosh as one of naturopathy's most useful botanicals.

ECLECTIC HYDROALCOHOLIC EXTRACTS

John M. Scudder insisted that the fresh roots/rhizome be used to make the tincture, and Grieve later noted the fresh root dug in October is used for tinctures. The tincture was given in doses of about one teaspoonful or 4 ml. The Lloyd Brothers Pharmacists produced their popular 1:1 strength Specific Medicine extract using 77% alcohol to extract the roots and rhizome. Though technically the same strength as the fluid extract, this preparation was the produced by a distinct but undefined special process. Their recommended dose was up to 0.65 ml, but Dr. H.W. Felter described a dosage range up to double their suggested maximum dose.

FLUID EXTRACT

The official 1:1 strength *NF* extract of the roots/rhizome with an alcohol content between 71% to 78% was given in doses from 0.07 ml to 2.0 ml with an average dose of 1.0 ml. Again the naturopathic dose given by Kuts-Cheraux was lower, from 0.3–1.0 ml.

RESINOID

Dr. King had believed a high concentration of alcohol (90%) was important for making the most effective extract called a saturated tincture. Such extracts were only of value when made from recently dried roots/rhizome. In 1835 by adding the alcoholic extract to cold water King discovered a resinous precipitate from the root that was insoluble in water. This resinoid product, under the name cimicifugin or macrotin, came into general use about 1850. The resinoid was taken as a dry, insoluble powder in doses of 11–33 mg. The resinoid did not exert the complete effect of the tincture and was considered by some to be ineffective.

SOLID EXTRACT

A popular solid extract of the roots/rhizome made by using 40% isopropanol and water is standardized to 1 mg triterpenes calculated as 27-deoxyacteine per 20 mg tablet.

Rheumatic and Nervous Conditions—Traditional Forms Used

ROOT POWDER

Black cohosh root was known to be most effective in chronic muscle pain that seemed to arise from a contracted state of the muscle fibers. This was typically associated with stiffness. Typically low back pain of this type would respond well, as would painful stiffness in the loins and thighs. It was also effective for soreness of muscular tissues that felt as if bruised.

WATER EXTRACT

Grieve and Lust noted that the infusion and decoction have been used to treat rheumatism. Lust also indicated these forms were used for chronic bronchitis and were noteworthy for their emetic effect.

ECLECTIC HYDROALCOHOLIC EXTRACTS

The best extract of the rhizome was believed by most to be made with water and alcohol rather than a simple water decoction. For rheumatic and neuralgic conditions Dr. John King believed the fluid extract and the decoction were both less effective than the tincture. He used the alcoholic extract for fifty years to treat chorea, preferring this form to others including his own resinoid extract.

Beside acting as an antispasmodic, the saturated tincture of the root was indicated for the pain of neuralgia and inflammation. For successful use in persistent neuralgia, especially where there is spinal irritation, Scudder believed the tincture had to be given until it produced cerebral symptoms consisting of weight and fullness with a dull headache.

The consensus among the Eclectic doctors like Felter was that the Specific Medicine alcoholic extract was extremely effective for muscular pains of a rheumatoid character: heavy, tensive, aching, dull, sore, and stiff. Felter states that the rheumatic indications for black cohosh Specific Medicine also applied to salicylates, and the two could be used together.

FLUID EXTRACT

According to the Lloyds, of five cases of chorea that had undergone other treatments, four responded positively to the fluid extract of black cohosh. However, in only one of ten cases of epilepsy treated with black cohosh did any improvement take place.

RESINOID

Dr. Price reported cases in 1910 of chorea that began in a child and low back pain in an adult that resolved in thirty and three days, respectively, when 11 mg were taken every two hours. In 1861 Parrish reported a case of insomnia lasting several months following the death of a close friend. This condition had been resistant to conventional treatments but was cured by black cohosh resin in 16 mg doses 3–4 times daily, though it produced occasional headaches.

Women's Reproductive Conditions—Traditional Uses

ROOT POWDER

Dr. John King believed the powdered root overcame uterine inertia to help accelerate labor, though he admitted that it occasionally failed in this action. Commonly, the root was used for dull aching pains of the uterus and ovaries, being considered one of the best remedies for the latter, and was even used for pains in the breast.

ECLECTIC HYDROALCOHOLIC EXTRACTS

Uterine pains that were rheumatoid in character, that is, heavy, tensive, aching, dull, sore, and stiff were indications for black cohosh during the menstrual period. It was also used for uterine congestion with radiating pains. Besides dysmenorrhea, black cohosh hydro-alcoholic extract was highly regarded for the treatment of a variety of female reproductive disorders. This included amenorrhea, especially in young teenagers.

Eclectic physicians of the late 19th and early 20th centuries had differing opinions about its uterine stimulant effects during pregnancy. Dr. John King described the tincture as ecbolic, inducing abortion when used every three hours, while Dr. Moxley claimed an abortifacient potential when the root was administered as a decoction in doses that produced headaches. Dr. A.J. Howe and Dr. Haifley declared that in their experience it was not abortive.

Black cohosh tincture made from the fresh root was considered a useful influence before, during and after labor. Black cohosh tincture was commonly and effectively given as a preparation for birth in the last four weeks before the expected date of delivery. The dose was sometimes as low as 1–2 drops every 2–4 hours or 5–6 drops every 3–4 hours and continued until a month after delivery. This seemed to improve labor outcome compared to previous deliveries in women who had given birth multiple times, but applied especially to women with previous difficult labors and a lax uterus with the fetus hanging low. Its preparatory use for weeks prior to labor diminished postpartum hemorrhage according to Dr. Leister.

In 100 cases of labor Dr. J.S. Niederkorn reported in 1910 that to increase the frequency and force of expulsive contractions in labor within 60-90 minutes, 5–10 drops should be given every 15–20 minutes. Black cohosh not only seemed to ease labor, but also to speed the delivery of the placenta and to prevent postpartum complications including hemorrhage. It was administered for both false and ineffective labor, as well as for after pains.

According to Drs. Scudder, King and Whitney, following delivery it could be employed as a uterine tonic to treat subinvolution. Subsequently, it was used to correct malposition after manually restoring the uterus to its proper place.

Among its many uses as reported in 1923 by Dr. Bowles, when the time of reproductive potential was past, it was used to treat the hot flashes and other problems of menopause. As indicated by Webster and many doctors black cohosh was often combined with other herbal remedies.

FLUID EXTRACT

In observations from 160 labors reported by Dr. J.S. Knox in 1885, the fluid extract, given in doses of 1.0 ml with 3.0 ml compound syrup of sarsaparilla every night for four weeks prior to confinement, helped to mildly sedate the women, reduced discomfort in the first stage, increased the rhythm of the second stage, relaxed the soft tissue, and reduced lacerations.

RESINOID

According to Dr. Price, the resinoid was considered especially effective for dysmenorrhea and associated symptoms such as ovarian neuralgia as well as for treating the hot flashes and insomnia occurring at menopause. Its originator, Dr. King, used this form extensively for women's problems.

Active Compounds Isolated from the Roots and Rhizome

Of probable significance in the anti-inflammatory activity of black cohosh root is the salicylic acid content. This component helps explain black cohosh benefits in myalgias and neuralgias. However, an even greater impact may derive from the rhizome's cinnamic acid phenolic derivatives like caffeic acid and isoferulic acid or when formed as esters of piscidic acid and fukiic acid (cimicifugic acids A, B, and F), especially fukinolic acid. These water-soluble compounds all dissolve well in a 50% solution of water and ethanol.

Of the phytoestrogenic isoflavones biochanin, but not genistein, has been reported in the hydroalcoholic extracts, according to Liske in 1998. He noted that formononetin, a phytoestrogenic isoflavone component once described as a component, is not found in ethanolic or isopropyl alcohol extracts. Kennelly and others in 2002 indicated formononetin is not apparent in black cohosh, since analysis of methanolic extracts from roots and rhizomes from 13 locations in the eastern USA failed to detect this isoflavone or its glucoside.

A number of triterpenoids of the resin that extract well in alcohols (ethanol or methanol) were discovered or confirmed in 2000 by several groups of researchers: Bedir and Khan, He and others, and Shao and others. Along with previously known triterpene glycosides including cimicifugoside, actein, 27-deoxyactein, and cimiraceroside A, of which 27-deoxyactein has the greatest relative yield, 9 more of these compounds were identified including cimiracemosides A-H. Cimicifugoside M was declared by He and others to serve as a specific indicator for identification of *Cimicifuga racemosa*, whereas the chromone cimifugin not found in black cohosh is specific to the Chinese species *C. foetida*. They analyzed over 30 commercial black cohosh products and found extracts of *C. racemosa*, *C. foetida*, and a combination of the two.

Laboratory Research—Extracts and Compounds from the Roots/Rhizome

Hormonal Effects

METHANOLIC / ETHANOLIC / ISOPROPANOLIC HYDROALCOHOLICEXTRACTS

The effect of black cohosh on female reproductive conditions was initially described as hormonal influence. Jarry and others showed that in rats with ovaries removed a methanol extract of the rhizomes reduced the serum concentration of pituitary luteinizing hormone (LH). This extract contained three substances that bind to estrogen receptors. One of these phytoestrogens was believed to be formononetin that, however, did not lower serum LH. A methanolic extract was dried and extracted with chloroform in 1991 by Duker and others to concentrate the hormonal activity. The extract contained phytoestrogens with an acute but no chronic LH effect along with nonphytoestrogens that reduced LH with chronic use.

In a 1960 study by Siess and Seybold an ethanolic extract of *C. racemosa* used chronically in rats provided no evidence of direct or indirect influence on genital growth or function. Einer-Jensen and others in 1996 showed no estrogenic effects in mice or rats given the ethanolic extract. No formononetin was found in 1997 by Struck and others in ethanolic extracts of the rhizomes. In 1999 Kruse and others showed fukinolic acid from a 50% ethanolic extract of the rhizomes does have mild estrogenic activity in cell cultures. Still, a study by Zava and others of estrogen receptor-binding with a 1:5 strength 50% ethanolic extract found little activity.

To evaluate the potential hormonal effects from using different doses of a common isopropanolic extract of the roots, in 2002 Freudenstein and others used three different doses (0.714 mg/kg, 7.14 mg/kg, 71.4 mg/kg) to compare with a vehicle control and an active estrogenic control (mestranol) in rats with estrogen-dependent mammary gland tumors. Unlike mestranol, after six weeks none of the extract doses had stimulated tumor growth. Rather, for rats receiving the extract, the number and size of the tumors were no different than for rats given the inactive vehicle. In addition, uterine weight and endometrial growth were unaffected, and prolactin, follicle stimulating hormone, and LH levels were unchanged.

Again in 2002, Bodinet and Freudenstein found that the isopropanolic extract was non-estrogenic and significantly inhibited human breast cancer cell (MCF–7) proliferation in test tubes due to an estrogen-antagonistic effect. This extract even enhanced the anti-proliferation effect of the drug tamoxifen against these cells in test tubes.

According to a report by Bone in 2001, based on studies of rats described at the 3rd International Congress on Phytomedicine in Munich, October 11–13, 2000, black cohosh contains selective estrogen receptor modulators (SERM). The SERM compounds primarily interact with the estrogen beta-receptors and affect bone, liver, brain, and arteries, but the components did not interact with estrogen alpha-receptors of the uterus. In 2002 Zierau and others tested the isopropanolic extract on estrogen receptor-positive MCF-7 cell proliferation and demonstrated that it was not only non-estrogenic but anti-estrogenic when given with estradiol, similar to tamoxifen. When tested for estrogen-dependent gene transcription in two types of estrogen alpha-receptor cells, this extract was again shown to be both non-estrogenic and anti-estrogenic. However, the ethanolic extract activity differed in terms of active extract concentration. Also, in one of the alpha-receptor cell assays the ethanolic black cohosh extract, though non-estrogenic, was not anti-estrogenic. These results not only confirmed the lack of alpha-receptor stimulation by black cohosh isopropanolic and ethanolic extracts, but also showed differences in their activities based on dosage and anti-estrogenic effects.

Muscle Relaxant

FLUID EXTRACT

In 1932 Macht and Cook showed that following the marked primary contraction of uteri from animals, the fluid extract of black cohosh produced a rapid relaxation and depression of this isolated organ. It also produced a mild central depression in rats.

RESINOID

The resinoid produced no effect on either the isolated intestinal or uterine muscles of animals according to Macht and Cook.

Vasodilator

TRITERPENES

Acteina, a resinous component of the root extracted with chloroform in 1962 by Genazzani and Sorrentino, was hypotensive in rabbits and cats but not in dogs or humans, though it acted as a peripheral vasodilator in the latter two. This demonstrates that biological effects cannot be directly extrapolated between species. Eclectics asserted that the effects of black cohosh as studied in animals gave no hint of its relationship to practical therapy and clinical worth.

Anti-inflammatory

PHENOLIC DERIVATIVES

Caffeic acid, isoferulic acid, and esters formed with these and fukiic and piscidic acids (fukinolic acid and cimicifugic acids A, B and F), extracted using a 50% ethanolic solution, were shown by Loser and others in 2000 to inhibit elastase. Elastase is released by neutrophilic white blood cells at the beginning of inflammation, contributing to the destruction of connective tissues in rheumatic disorders.

Menopause—Modern Clinical Studies

STANDARDIZED LIQUID HYDROALCOHOLIC EXTRACT

A large open study reported in 1982 by Stolze, concerning 629 female patients seeing 131 different doctors, found that use of 40 drops twice daily for 6–8 weeks of a 60% ethanolic black cohosh extract standardized to contain 1 mg per of triterpenes per 20 drops reduced or eliminated a number of menopausal symptoms. Conditions such as hot flashes, headache, tinnitus, vertigo, heart palpitation, sleep disturbances, irritability, depression, and profuse perspiration were eliminated in 42%–55% of the women, depending on the symptom. At least some improvements in these symptoms were found in 82%–93%. It took up to four weeks to notice some benefits and from six to eight weeks for complete recovery from certain conditions, depending on the patient. Only 7% of the women reported experiencing mild stomach trouble, and this was only temporary.

A comparative study in 1985 by Warnecke using 40 drops twice daily of the standardized black cohosh liquid extract, conjugated estrogens (0.625 mg daily), or diazepam (2 mg daily) each in twenty different menopausal patients for twelve weeks looked at the impact of menopausal symptoms. The black cohosh extract was superior to diazepam and estrogen in relieving the depressive symptoms. Black cohosh also was better at reducing the constellation of other symptoms associated with menopause when these symptoms were considered together as a whole.

Both Liske and Foster report on several other open, noncontrolled studies with a total of 88 patients using the same hydroalcoholic extract and dose. Patients began to have beneficial effects after 4 weeks that became clinically relevant after 12 weeks. The extract was well tolerated, with only 4 patient complaints of mild GI problems at the beginning. The scientific research lends support to traditional Eclectic use of black cohosh hydroalcoholic extracts for menopause.

STANDARDIZED SOLID EXTRACT

A dried hydro-ethanolic extract of black cohosh rhizome standardized to 2 mg triterpenes was shown by Duker and others in 1991 to reduce LH secretion in menopausal women (mean age of 52 years) after eight weeks. However, according to Foster in 1999, other more extensive studies with this extract contradict these findings, and no LH inhibition is evident with this form.

A solid extract described by Liske in 1998 is made from a 40% isopropanolic and 60% aqueous extract, each tablet standardized to 2 mg triterpenes. This was more effective after three months in treating menopause symptoms than conjugated estrogens (0.625 mg daily) in one study when 2 tablets were taken twice daily. In another study after six months of using the same black cohosh product and dose, 56% of women no longer required hormone injections (4 mg estradiol valerate and 200 mg prasterone-nantate) to treat menopausal symptoms. Following hysterectomy, no significant difference in symptoms was discovered between those using the same black cohosh extract and dose versus those taking estriol (1 mg), conjugated estrogens (1.25 mg) or a hormone combination (2 mg estradiol and 1 mg norethisterone acetate) daily. This black cohosh extract, however, does not contain phytoestrogenic isoflavones nor have estrogenic effects. On the contrary it appears to block estrogen receptors, making it suitable to use in breast cancer patients with or without tamoxifen.

Table 7   Black Cohosh Roots and Derivatives—
Summary of Medicinal Uses and Pharmacology

BLACK COHOSH *Actaea racemosa* L.	Native American Uses	Folk Remedy Uses	Early Medical Uses	Modern Clinical Studies	Laboratory Research Findings
Whole Rhizome/ Roots	Rheumatism Menses Labor Kidneys	Snake bites	Rheumatism Tuberculosis Asthma Edema Chorea Neuralgia Labor		
Water Extract	Rheumatism Menses Labor Nursing Coughs Fatigue	Rheumatism Sore throat Hysteria Colic Chronic bronchitis Emetic	Rheumatism Sore throat Asthma Edema Chorea Neuralgia Smallpox		
Eclectic Tinctures and Specific Medicine (Hydro- alcoholic)			Rheumatism Neuralgia Inflammation Chorea Dysmenorrhea Amenorrhea Labor Pre-labor and post-labor Menopause		
Fluid Extract (Hydro- alcoholic)			Chorea Pre-labor		Uterine relaxant Depressant
Standard- ized Liquid Extract (Hydro- alcoholic)				Menopause	

Continued on next page

Table 7   *Continued*

BLACK COHOSH *Actaea racemosa* L.	Native American Uses	Folk Remedy Uses	Early Medical Uses	Modern Clinical Studies	Laboratory Research Findings
Standardized Solid Extract (Hydro-isopropenolic)				Menopause	Anti-estrogenic
Resin			Rheumatism Dysmenorrhea Menopause Neuralgia Chorea		Lowers LH Estrogenic

ISOLATED CONSTITUENTS

Triterpenes					Vasodilation
Cinnamic Acid Derivatives					Estrogenic Anti-inflammatory
Isoflavones				Estrogenic	Estrogenic
Salicylates			Rheumatism Neuraliga	Rheumatism Neuralgia	Anti-inflammatory

A much-publicized study by Jacobson and others in 2001 investigated the effect of a black cohosh product versus placebo on hot flashes in 85 breast cancer survivors of which 59 used tamoxifen. The greatest problem with this study was its failure to characterize the product beyond describing its dose as one tablet twice daily for 60 days. Though described simply as black cohosh, it is more likely that a tablet would be a solid extract. The results failed to demonstrate efficacy for hot flashes, but sweating was improved significantly for those using the black cohosh product as compared to the placebo group.

In 2002 the 40% isopropanolic extract of the root was given by Liske and others to perimenopausal and postmenopausal women in one of two daily doses (representing 39 mg or 127.3 mg of the dried root) to determine relative efficacy and assess estrogenic activity. Both doses were well tolerated. The reduction of menopausal symptoms based on responder rating was 70% and 72%, respectively. The lack of changes in vaginal cells also indicated a nonestrogenic effect. Likewise, no significant changes in serum hormone levels relevant to sexual function were noted.

Adverse Effects Based on Doses

The Eclectics such as Felter and the Lloyds indicated that full doses of the roots, tincture, fluid extract, or the resinoid can produce a severe, frontal headache with a full or bursting sensation which passes after administration of the medicine is stopped. Toxic doses cause nausea, vomiting, vertigo, impaired vision, and reduced circulation. In Stolze's 1982 study about 7% of those using 40 drops twice daily of the standardized hydro-alcoholic extract experience brief stomach and intestinal complaints.

The Lloyd's reported a personal investigation by Dr. E.E. Sattler at Miami Medical College of Cincinnati. He took 0.67–1.33 ml of black cohosh fluid extract internally that produced no sensible effects. However, 4.0 ml of this medicine after twenty minutes produced both an upset stomach and dizziness with a sense of fullness in the head and temples. Ten minutes later another 4.0 ml was consumed. In another fifteen minutes nausea and vertigo were strongly manifested, accompanied by an intense headache that lasted eight hours. Slight diarrhea and drowsiness followed. A pulse of 80 when the first dose was taken diminished in thirty minutes after the second dose to 62 beats per minute. However, the pulse became more forceful. This experiment was repeated several times with similar results.

Several patients of this doctor experienced like symptoms after taking 20–50 drops of the fluid extract. Small doses gradually increased or frequently repeated were found to give the best results with the least adverse effects. The side effects were much stronger when black cohosh fluid extract was taken on an empty stomach.

One case of jaundice due to liver failure that required liver transplantation after using a black cohosh product for one week was reported in 2002 by Whiting and others. Due to the sudden unprecedented serious impact on the liver of this 47-year-old menopausal women and the failure to positively identify the contents of the product, it is highly unlikely that black cohosh was responsible for this adverse outcome.

References

BOOKS

Anon, *Dose Book,* Lloyd Brothers Pharmacists, Inc., Cincinnati, Ohio, 1932.

Boyle, W. *Herb Doctors,* Buckeye Naturopathic Press, East Palestine, Ohio, 1988.

Boyle, W. *Official Herbs,* Buckeye Naturopathic Press, East Palestine, Ohio, 1991.

Council on Pharmacy and Chemistry of A.M.A. *Epitome of the Pharmacopeia and National Formulary,* American Medical Assoc., Chicago, Ill., 1944.

Felter, HW. *The Eclectic Materia Medica, Pharmacology and Therapeutics,* 1922 ed., Ecletic Medical Publications, Sandy, OR., 1994.

Grieve, M. *A Modern Herbal,* 1931 version, Dover Pub., New York, 1971.

Kuts-Cheraux, AW. *Naturae Medicina and Naturopathic Dispensatory,* American Naturopathic Physicians and Surgeons Assoc., Des Moines, Iowa, 1953.

Lloyd, JU and Lloyd, CG. "Cimicifuga racemosa" in *Drugs and Medicines of North America,* vol. 1, pt. 2, pp. 244–291, (1884-85 ed.), Lloyd Library Bull. No. 30, Cincinnati, OH., 1931.

Lust, J. *The Herb Book,* Bantam Books, New York, 1974.

Moerman, DE. *Native American Ethnobotany,* Timbers Press, Portland, OR., 1998.

Powers, JL (Chair, Comm. on N.F.). *The National Formulary,* 8th ed., American Pharmaceutical Assoc., Washington, D.C., 1946.

Revolutionary Health Comm. of Hunan Province. *A Barefoot Doctor's Manual,* rev. and enlarged ed., Cloudburst Press, Seattle, 1977.

Smith, P. *The Indian Doctor's Dispensatory,* Lloyd Library Bull. No. 2, Cincinnati, OH., 1901.

ARTICLES

Bedir, E and Khan, IA. Cimiracemoside A: a new cycloanostanol xyloside from the rhizome of Cimicifuga racemosa. *Chem. Pharm. Bull.,* 48(3):425–427, 2000.

Bodinet, C and Freudenstein, J. Influence of Cimicifuga racemosa on the proliferation of estrogen receptor-positive human breast cancer cells. *Breast Canc. Res. Treat.,* 76:1–10, 2002.

Bone, K. Debate over black cohosh. *Br. J. Phytother.,* 5(4):215–7, 2001.

Bowles, T. Some uses for macrotys. *Ecl. Med. J.,* 83:429–31, 1923.

Duker, E et al. Effects of extracts from Cimicifuga racemosa on gonadotropin release in menopausal women and ovariectomized rats. *Planta Med.,* 57:420–4, 1991.

Einer-Jensen, N et al. Cimicifiga and Melbrosia lack estrogenic effects in mice and rats. *Maturitas,* 25(2):149–53, 1996.

Foster, S. Black cohosh: Cimicifuga racemosa – a literature review. *HerbalGram,* 45:35–50, 1999.

Freudenstein, J et al. Lack of promotion of estrogen-dependent mammary gland tumors in vivo by an isopropanolic Cimicifuga racemosa extract. *Cancer Res.,* 62:3448–52, 2002.

Genazzani, E and Sorrentino, L. Vascular action of acteina: active constituent of Actaea racemosa L. *Nature,* 194:544–5, 1962.

Haifley, WH. Cimicifuga racemosa. *Ecl. Med. J.,* 70:119–20, 1910.

Howe, AJ. Cimicifuga and abortion. *Ecl. Med. J.,* 45:501–2, 1885.

Jacobson, JS et al. Randomized trial of black cohosh for the treatment of hot flashes among women with a history of breast cancer. *J. Clin. Oncol.,* 19(10):2739–45, 2001.

Jarry, H and Harnischfeger, G. Studies on the endocrine effects of constituents from Cimicifuga racemosa. 1. Influence on the serum concentration of pituitary hormones in ovariectomized rats. *Planta Med.*, (1):46–9, 1985 [in German] (*Chem. Abs.* 102:215969h).

Jarry, H et al. Studies on the endocrine effects of the contents of Cimicifuga racemosa. 2. In vitro binding of compounds to estrogen receptors. *Planta Med.*, (4):316–9, 1985 [in German] (C.A. 103:200749h).

He, K et al. Direct analysis and identification of triterpene glycosides by LC/MS in black cohosh, Cimicifuga racemosa, and in several commercially available black cohosh products. *Planta Med.*, 66:635–40, 2000.

Kennelly, EJ et al. Analysis of thirteen populations of black cohosh for formononetin. *Phytomed.*, 9(5):461–7, 2002.

Knox, JS. The influence of Cimicifuga racemosa upon parturition. *Ecl. Med. J.*, 45:267, 1885.

Kruse, SO et al. Fukiic and piscidic acid esters from the rhizome of Cimicifuga racemosa and the in vitro estrogenic activity of fukinolic acid. *Planta Med.*, 65:763–4, 1999.

Leister, WL. Macrotys in latter weeks of gestation. *Ecl. Med. J.*, 68:13940, 1908.

Linde, H. Die inhaltsstoffe von Cimicifuga racemosa. *Arch. Pharm.*, 301:335–41, 1968 [in German]

Liske, E. Therapeutic efficacy and safety of Cimicifuga racemosa for gynecologic disorders. *Adv. Nat. Ther.*, 15(1):45–53, 1998.

Liske, E et al. Physiological investigation of a unique extract of black cohosh (Cimicifugae racemosae rhizoma): a 6-month clinical study demonstrates no systemic estrogenic effect. *J. Wom. Health Gender-Based Med.*, 11(2):163–74, 2002.

Loser, B et al. Inhibition of neutrophil elastase activity by cinnamic acid derivatives from Cimicifuga racemosa. *Planta Med.*, 66:751–3, 2000.

Macht, KI and Cook, HM. A pharmacological note on cimicifuga. *J. Am.Pharm. Assoc.*, 21:324–30, 1932.

McKenna, DJ et al. Black cohosh: efficacy, safety, and use in clinical and preclinical applications. *Alternat. Ther.*, 7(3):93–100, 2001.

Mundy, WN. Macrotys. *Ecl. Med. J.*, 83:468–70, 1923.

Niederkorn, JS. Macrotys and caulophyllin. *Ecl. Med. J.*, 70:63–6, 1910.

Parrish, E. Therapeutical and pharmaceutical notes on cimicifuga. *Ecl. Med. J.*, 20:197–200, 1861.

Piancatelli, G. New triterpenes from Actaea racemosa. *Gazz. Chim. Ital.*, 101(2):139–48, 1971 [in Italian].

Price, MG. Macrotin. *Ecl. Med. J.*, 70:486–7, 1910.

Radics, L et al. Carbon-13 spectra of some polycyclic triterpenoids. *Tetrahed. Lett.*, 48:4287–90, 1975.

Schindler, H. Die inhaltsstoffe von heilpflanzen und prufungsmethoden fur pflanzliche tinkturen. *Arzneim.-Forsch.*, 2:547–9, 1952 [in German].

Scudder, JM. Tincture of macrotys in neuralgia. *Ecl. Med. J.*, 24:236–7, 1864.

Scudder, JM. Macrotys in pregnancy and parturition. *Ecl. Med. J.*, 35:477–8, 1875.

Siess, M an Seybold, G. Studies on the effects of Pulsatilla pratensis, Cimicifuga racemosa and

Aristolochia clematitis on the estrus in infantile and castrated white mice. [German] *Arzneim.-Forsch.*, 514–20, 1960.

Shao, Y et al. Triterpene glycosides from Cimicifuga racemosa. *J. Nat. Prod.*, 63:905–10, 2000.

Stolze, H. An alternative to treat menopausal complaints. *Gyne* , 3:14–6, 1982 [in German].

Struck, D et al. Flavones in Extracts of Cimicifuga racemosa. *Planta Med.*, 63:289, 1997.

Warnecke, G. Beeinflussung klimakterischer beschwerden durch ein phytotherapeutikum. *Med. Welt.*, 36:871–4, 1985 [in German].

Webster, HT. Cimicifuga racemosa. *Ecl. Med. J.*, 61:195–8, 1901.

Whiting, PW et al. Black cohosh and other herbal remedies associated with acute hepatitis. *Med. J. Austral.*, 177:432–5, 2002.

Whitney, WH. Cimicifuga (Macrotys) racemosa. *Ecl. Med. J.*, 48:162–4, 1888.

Zava, DT et al. Estrogen and progestin bioactivity of foods, herbs, and spices. *Proc. Soc. Exp. Biol. Med.*, 217:369–78, 1998.

Zierau, O et al. Antiestrogenic activites of Cimicifuga racemosa extracts. *J. Ster. Biochem. Mol. Biol.*, 80:125–130, 2002.

PURPLE CONEFLOWER ECHINACEA—
American Herb, German Serendipity

Echinacea purpurea (L.) Moench. —herb or roots

Summary

As a fairly recent innovation, purple coneflower herb juice has relatively few applications. The oral use of the juice products enhances systemic immune function and thereby supports the healing process. The external application of these echinacea juice products has been shown to be useful for wounds and other local conditions. The plant juice contains more of the water-soluble compounds like polysaccharides and less alcohol-soluble isobutylamides. Like the alcohol-preserved plant juice, internal use of purple coneflower whole fresh plant and root alcoholic extracts has mostly been used for viral upper respiratory conditions.

Studies on the internal use of both *E. purpurea* plant juice and its alcoholic root extracts indicate that these both enhance immune function and resistance to infectious microorganisms. An advantage in treatment can be obtained by their complementary use together with antimicrobial herbs or medications. Purple coneflower products have only theoretical contraindication warnings aside from isolated individual sensitivities among those with atopic conditions such as asthma or eczema.

The various active constituents provide complementary effects when it comes to therapeutic activity. The anti-inflammatory isobutylamides produce an extended reduction in pain and swelling. Enhanced phagocytosis, consumption of debris by white blood cells, is the major immune activity of the isobutylamides. The anti-hyaluronidase activity of cichoric acid and other polyphenolic caffeic acid derivatives and possibly some smaller alcohol-soluble polysaccharides helps keep certain bacteria, tumors, and toxins from penetrating into the tissues. Water-soluble root compounds including large polysaccharides and cichoric acid have some antiviral effects as well. The large polysaccharides and glycoproteins add further anti-inflammatory, antitumor, antihyaluronidase, and immune stimulant activities to the complex of active components in the root.

Limited Root Applications by Native and Anglo Americans

According to both Moerman and Hobbs, in its original uses by native American Indians, *Echinacea purpurea*, or purple coneflower, root was chewed, applied as a poultice, or extracted and consumed as a tea. The Delaware tribe to the east and the Choctaw to the south both used E. purpurea root because it grew closest to their homelands. The Delaware prepared the root as a tea for gonorrhea, and the Choctaw chewed the root for coughs and dyspepsia.

Echinacea purpurea was introduced to medicine by John King in his *American Eclectic Dispensatory* (1852) as *Rudbeckia purpurea*, a folk remedy at times confused with Western small-leaved echinacea, E. angustifolia. The root was considered a useful treatment for syphilis. Fifty years later E. purpurea was still sometimes supplied in place of the preferred E. angustifolia. Echinacea in commercial trade consisted of the three species, E. purpurea, E. angustifolia, and E. pallida (pale echinacea). Moser and Heyl note identifying characteristics that distinguish these from adulterants, such as the spurious *Parthenium integrifolium*, which were supplied from as early as 1909 by Missouri wildcrafters.

German Development and Cultivation

Unlike its wild Western cousin, *Echinacea angustifolia*, E. purpurea is readily cultivated in flower gardens. It is commonly known as purple coneflower for its large attractive flowerheads with dark purple ray flowers (petals). When Dr. Gerhard Madaus traveled to America to obtain echinacea seeds, he had hoped to grow the preferred medicinal species E. angustifolia. However, the seeds that he had obtained were those of E. purpurea, so he began to cultivate this species in Germany in 1939 for medicinal use.

The roots of purple coneflower are small but the above ground plant is large compared to wild Western echinacea. Consequently, Madaus extracted the juice from the above-ground part of the *E. purpurea* plant and preserved it with 22% alcohol. This juice product is distinctive from high-alcohol root extracts, due in part to its content of large polysaccharides. Since purple coneflower juice had not previously been used clinically, he began experimenting serendipitously with this form. Since that time, much European research on echinacea has utilized this purple coneflower juice or similar preparations. Besides oral and topical use, the plant juice has also been administered by injection in Germany.

The German Commission E monographs published in 1989 identified several approved internal uses for *Echinacea purpurea* herb expressed juice. The indications noted were those conditions for which purple coneflower is most well known. These uses as supportive therapy for colds and chronic infections of the respiratory tract are now quite common. Another approved use was for chronic infections of the lower urinary tract.

Growing popularity of purple coneflower in Europe, both for its juice and the homeopathic tincture of the whole fresh plant, followed the German research into it medical effectiveness. Substitution of its root alcoholic extract for that of *E. angustifolia* subsequently occurred. The commercial demand led to indiscriminate harvesting in America. In 1987 Missouri had already made it illegal to harvest *E. purpurea* along highways on, state parkland, state forest lands, and wildlife areas. A call for increased cultivation of this species resulted. Li as well as Shalaby and others documented recently that *E. purpurea* is relatively easy to grow in comparison with the two other medicinal species. Kindscher reports that yields for cultivated, 3-year-old roots of *E. purpurea* grown in Washington state were 1200 pounds per acre.

Preparations

PLANT JUICE

The liquid form of the juice of the above-ground flowering plant requires addition of alcohol for a 22% ethanol content to preserve the juice and prevent fermentation. The dose for this form is 2-3 ml three times daily. The juice is sometimes dehydrated and provided in capsule or tablet form.

JUICE OINTMENT

External semisolid preparations should contain at least 15% pressed juice.

FRESH WHOLE PLANT HYDROALCOHOLIC EXTRACT

A homeopathic extract of the aerial plant and roots is made with the whole fresh plant using 30% ethanol. This tincture is given internally in doses of 10-30 drops (average about 1 ml) in water from 2-5 times daily. It is also applied undiluted to wounds or burns. A dose from 7–48 mg of a solid extract in tablet form has also been shown to be effective for reducing cold symptoms.

Root Powder

At least 333 mg of the dried powdered root should be used 1–3 times daily. Grieve emphasizes that it is the fresh root that should be used.

Root Tincture

A 1:5 strength 55% ethanol extract is effective at 180 drops (about 4.5 ml). Doses vary with strength of the extract. The cichoric acid content declined significantly in this form after seven months at room temperature or higher.

Solid Extracts

These are provided in tablet form by removing the solvent content, whether water/alcohol, hexane, or other. The isobutylamide marker content of the root declined significantly in this form after seven months at room temperature or higher.

Components of Aerial Plant and Roots

While the components are similar in the above ground portion of purple coneflower and its roots, their concentration and proportions vary. Much of the study of purple coneflower above ground plant constituents and their activity has focused on large polysaccharide water-soluble components. Wagner and others in 1985 studied the large polysaccharides from the leaves and roots and found the polysaccharides differed between the plant parts. Classen and Blaschek indicated in 2000 that arabinogalactan proteins are important immunomodulating components in the pressed juice from the aerial plant.

Giger and others in 1989 reported that fructans found in *E. purpurea* have about ten times higher yield in the roots than in above ground parts of purple coneflower. Fructans with a low degree of polymerization are present in fresh plant tinctures. Bodinet and others extracted polysaccharides and glycoproteins from the roots of *E. purpurea* in 1993 using a hydro-alcoholic solvent that contained only 30% ethanol.

Al-Hassan and others showed in 2000 that several alkamides are in the pressed juice of the fresh flowering aerial plant. In 1997 Perry and others found the alkamide (isobutylamide) level of the rhizome of *E. purpurea* is over twice that of the flower, four times that of the stem, and twenty-eight times that of the leaf. Stuart and Wills in 2000 had similar results—70% total alkamides in the root, 20% in the flower, 10% in the stem, and 1% in the leaf. While air-drying works well for the leaf, Kim and others proved in 2000 that freeze-drying the root was the most effective means of preserving its alkamides, when compared with air drying and vacuum microwave drying.

According to Letchamo and others in 1999, the isobutylamides of the flower heads are highest when mature. The lipophilic components of the plant and roots like isobutylamdes and phenolics are found in high alcohol-content extracts. Livesey and others indicated in 1999 that these alkamides are stable in 55% alcohol extracts even at high temperature (40 degrees Celsius) but decline in the powdered extract even at room temperature with very little remaining after 7 months. Perry and others likewise showed in 2000 that the total alkamides in *E. purpurea* chopped dry roots declined greatly at room temperature, from 5.05 to 3.28 to 1.55 to 0.66 mg/gm dry weight over consecutive 16 week intervals. Alkamide levels in whole dried roots went from 5.23 mg/gm to 4.45 mg/gm dry weight after 16 weeks. In 1999 Arnason indicated that potential means of enhancing stability and shelf-life through the manufacturing process included freeze-drying, removing enzymes from plant material, increasing alcohol content of extracts, removing oxygen from products or adding antioxidants.

The purple coneflower phenolic acid compounds, cichoric acid and caftaric acid, are caffeic acid conjugates with tartaric acid that have been identified by Cheminat and others in *E. purpurea* roots. Perry and others in 2001 found that these compounds diminished from summer to autumn in the roots (from 2.7% to 2.0%) and especially in the tops (from 2.8% to 0.7%). Letchamo and others in 1999 showed that the cichoric acid content in the flower heads declines during their development. At maturity Stuart and Wills found in 2000 that the flower and leaf each yielded about 35% of the total cichoric acid, while the root had 20% and the stem contained 10%. Increasing the drying temperature from 35 to 45 degrees C increased the level of cichoric acid in the roots, according to Li and Wardle in 2001. Kim and others found this caffeic acid derivative readily degrades in flowers with high moisture, and freeze-drying was shown to be the best method of reducing moisture and retaining phenolic content when compared to vacuum microwave drying and air drying at various temperature.

In 1999 both Bauer and Kreuter indicated that the activity of the enzyme polyphenol oxidases rapidly breaks down cichoric acid in the cold-pressed fresh juice, as did Nusslein and others in 2000 when they showed it could be preserved in aqueous extracts by adding 50 mM ascorbic acid or 40% ethanol. Only if the juice is heated to destroy the enzyme will cichoric acid be consistently retained. Bauer showed that heat-stabilized juice products had on average a much lower isobutylamide marker content. Kreuter pointed out that clinical research had employed the cold-pressed and unheated *E. purpurea* plant juice, so only juice with little or no cichoric acid has been proven clinically effective. Also in 1999 Livesey and others indicated that cichoric acid diminished in tinctures with 55% alcohol at room temperature after 7 months but was stable in powder during this time even at higher temperatures.

Al-Hassan and others showed in 2000 that the ethyl acetate fraction of the fresh pressed juice of the aerial parts contained as main substances p-coumaric acid and newly discovered compounds vomofoliol-9-ferulate and hydroxy(carboxyethenoyl)-benzoic acid.

Laboratory Research—Plant and Roots, Extracts, Components

Immune Enhancement

POWDERED ROOT OR HERB

A comparison of macrophage stimulation by Rininger and others in 2000 indicated that the root or herb powder effectively stimulated monocyte viablility and tumor necrosis factor production when compared with active and inactive controls, whereas fresh juice and extracts standardized to 4% phenolic compounds did not.

PLANT JUICE

In 1986 Munder gave 10 mg of freeze-dried juice orally to mice for ten days and enhanced spleen cell production. When these spleen cells were mixed with macrophages and tumor cells, the macrophage destruction of the tumor cells increased ten-fold. In 1992 the freeze-dried juice was shown by Stotzem and others to increase phagocytosis by white blood cells. Burger and others showed in 1997 that the alcohol-preserved juice increased cytokine production of cultured macrophages.

ROOT TINCTURE

A 50% alcohol concentration or greater precipitates large polysaccharide components, and such precipitates are removed by filtration and missing in most commercial purple coneflower root extracts. In 1985 Vomel showed that the root extract influenced the phagocytosis dependent mechanism in Kupffer cells from rat liver. In 1988 a 90% ethanolic extract of *E. purpurea* roots used by Bauer and others improved consumption of foreign particles (phagocytosis) in mice when given orally.

ROOT SOLID EXTRACT

In 1999 Sun and other provided an uncharacterized powdered extract of purple coneflower root to mice in doses of 0.45 mg per day mixed with standard chow. After one and two weeks both natural killer cells and monocytes had progressively increased in number in the bone marrow and spleen compared to mice that received no extract.

ALKAMIDES

Phagocytosis of foreign particles in mice correlated strongly with the lipophilic isobutylamides in *E. purpurea* given orally by Bauer and others in 1988; they showed in 1989 that isobutylamides dissolve well in alcohol and are the main alkamides in the roots of *Echinacea purpurea*.

POLYSACCHARIDES

Large white blood cells called macrophages were activated by purified polysaccharide from *E. purpurea* plant water extract studied by Stimpel and others in 1984. A study by Wagner and others in 1985 of different large polysaccharides from the water extract of either the leaves or the roots from *E. purpurea* showed improved phagocytosis from these constituents.

Different polysaccharides have been active in test tube studies. A polysaccharide fraction from the plant with glucuronoarabinoxylan also increased phagocytosis studies by Proksch and Wagner in 1987. According to Parnham, important components in the juice are large arabinogalactan polysaccharides with high molecular weight. Cell cultures of *E. purpurea* yield active arabinogalactans on which many studies have been done, but these cell culture polysaccharides are not identical to those in the plant itself. Giger and others in 1989 reported that oligomeric fructans are also present in fresh plant tinctures.

Polymeric compounds including polysaccharides and glycoproteins from 30% ethanolic extracts of the roots of *E. purpurea* were tested by Bodinet and others in 1993. The polymers produced an increase in the production of the cytokines such as interleukin-1 and -6, tumor necrosis factor-alpha, and alpha- and beta-interferon. They also increased growth of mice spleen cells, increased antibody production, and had antiviral activity against herpes simplex virus. Wacker and Hilbig had shown in 1978 that water extracts of *E. purpurea* roots, as well as the juice from the fresh plant, caused mammalian cells *in vitro* to have 50-80% greater resistance to influenza, herpes, and vesicular stomatitis viruses.

GLYCOPROTEIN

An isolate from pressed juice of the aerial parts of *E. purpurea* designated arabinogalactan-protein type II was shown by Alban and others in 2002 to be a complement activator by both classical and alternative pathways in test tubes. This activity was due largely to the arabinose side chains that form the 3-dimensional structure. This effect may contribute to the immunostimulating effects of the juice.

Anti-inflammatory

STANDARDIZED EXTRACT

In 2000 Rininger and others also found an extract standardized to 4% phenolic compounds was anti-inflammatory. Other standardized extracts including a pressed juice powder demonstrated radical scavenging activity, though it was not as great as isolated caffeic acid or chlorogenic acid.

ALKAMIDES

In the year 1989 Wagner and others found that isobutylamides from the root extracts inhibit 5-lipoxygenase activity, thereby partially explaining the anti-inflammatory effect of purple coneflower in reducing redness, pain, and swelling. Clifford and others in 2002 found that at 100 mcg/ml several alkamides from the roots inhibited in test tubes the enzymes cyclooxygenase I by 36–60% and cyclooxygenase II by 15–46%.

Antihyaluronidase

PLANT JUICE

The juice of purple coneflower exhibited activity in the lab that recommends its local use. In the early 1950s Busing found that *E. purpurea* juice inhibits hyaluronidase secreted by group A streptococci. This activity appeared to be due to large, linear, colloidal polysaccharides, possibly fructans.

PHENOLICS

According to Mekkes and Nahuys in 2001, hyaluronic acid helps speed wound healing. Hyaluronidase catalyzes the breakdown of hyaluronic acid, an intercellular cement substance. Possibly the most significant effect in local application of alcoholic root extract is the hyaluronidase inhibiting activity of its caffeic acid derivatives. Of these polyphenolic echinacea compounds, cichoric acid and caftaric acid have the greatest antihyaluronidase activity, and Cheminat and others found these in *E. purpurea* roots. Hyaluronidase is found in snake and spider venom, in malignant tissues, and in various pathogenic bacteria secretions enhances tissue penetration.

Antimicrobial

PHENOLICS

Cheminat and others showed the same year that cichoric acid from this extract has antiviral and cell growth inhibitor activity.

LIPOPHILIC ROOT EXTRACT

Binns and others showed that a root hexane extract produces phototoxic effects on yeast.

Wound Healing

PLANT JUICE

The juice of purple coneflower exhibited activity in the lab that recommends its local use. In 1956 Tunnerhoff and Schwabe found purple coneflower juice enhanced connective tissue formation in fibrin grafts for wound healing. The plant juice was also shown by Vogel and others in 1968 to reduce exudation associated with the first stage of inflammation. Kinkel and others in 1984 showed the juice in an ointment accelerated the healing rate of surgically-induced skin lesions in guinea pigs after the third, sixth, and ninth days. In 1987 tests done by Meissner on healing skin flaps in animal, the juice of the plant significantly decreased the rate of necrosis.

Immune Enhancement for Internal Use in Colds and Flu

WHOLE PLANT POWDER

Barrett and other in 2002 provided 496 mg of equal parts dried *Echinacea purpurea* root and above-ground herb combined with 492 mg of dried *E. angustifolia* root which was taken as 4 capsules 6 times the first day of early cold symptoms. Then the same single dose of this combination was used 3 times daily thereafter for up to 10 days. There was no detectable benefit among the 148 college students using this product and dosing schedule, compared to 1.3 gram per dose of alfalfa used as a "placebo," as the colds lasted an average of about 6 days with both herbs. In this study ordinary encapsulated dried echinacea plant and root appeared inadequate as an internal treatment, given the debatable assumption that large doses of the nutrient and tonic herb alfalfa did not have a significant beneficial effect.

WATER EXTRACT OF WHOLE PLANT

A study with 95 subjects in 2000 by the Lindenmuths used a proprietary blend of *Echinacea purpurea* and *E. angustifolia* leaves, flowers, and stems along with a water soluble 6:1 dry extract of purple coneflower root and flavoring agents lemongrass and spearmint leaves to treat cold and flu symptoms. An infusion with 8 ounces of boiling water poured over one teabag with this blend was steeped for 10–15 minutes, and 5–6 cups drank the first day. Dosage was reduced daily to one cup by the fifth day. This was compaired to a control tea with peppermint, fennel, ginger, rose hips, papaya leaf, alfalfa, and cinnamon. There was a significant advantage using the echinacea tea for relieving the symptoms, the number of days before the symptoms changed, and how long the symptoms lasted.

SOLID EXTRACT OF FRESH PLANT

Tablets made from a (30% alcoholic) extract of the fresh whole plant consisting of 95% above-ground plant and 5% root were tested by Brinkeborn and others in 1999 in two dosage levels for their overall effect on 12 symptoms of the common cold. The tablets contained either 6.78 mg or 48.27 mg of the extract and were compared with 29.6 mg of an undefined extract of the root only and a placebo in 246 total patients. The fresh whole plant extract was the most effective, with the higher dose resulting in only a slightly greater improvement.

PLANT JUICE

A study by Hoheisel and others in 1997 showed therapeutic benefits for colds when the alcohol-preserved juice product was given in doses of 20 drops every two hours the first day of the cold and then three times daily for up to ten days total. The severity and duration of colds in the echinacea group were significantly less. No significant adverse effect concerns were raised.

In 1992 Schoneberger used 4 ml twice daily of the juice with 54 patients for 8 weeks in a double-blind study to compare its effects to an equal number of patients using placebo in reducing the frequency of colds. With the juice 35% remained healthy compared with 26% of placebo users. For those who did become ill the length of time between infections was 40 days when using the juice versus 25 days for placebo. Juice users also had less severe infections 79% of the time.

Berg and others showed in 1998 that athletes in exhaustive competition (triathlon) given 8 ml of the juice product for 28 days prior had interleukin-related changes and less (no) respiratory infections compared to those receiving magnesium or placebo. To study prevention of respiratory infections 4 ml of the juice product was given orally to subjects twice daily for eight weeks in 1999 by Grimm and Muller. It seemed to reduce infections by decreasing the incidence, duration, and severity of colds but not significantly. Tolerability and adverse effects were similar in placebo and treatment groups of both studies.

Hydroalcoholic Extracts of Root

A clinical study in 1992 by Braunig and others with 180 patients used a 1:5 strength 55% ethanol extract of the roots of *E. purpurea* to treat influenza-like infections. The purple coneflower groups showed different results according to dosage. A dose of 90 drops was no better than placebo, but 180 drops resulted in a significant improvement of flu symptoms including nasal inflammation, frontal sensitivity, and coated tongue after 3–4 and 8-10 days.

In a well-controlled study 1998 study by Melchart and others with 302 healthy volunteers, a 1:11 strength 30% ethanolic extract of the roots of *E. purpurea* was given in doses of 50 drops (about 1 ml of this solution) twice daily five days per week for twelve weeks to study their preventive value for upper respiratory tract infections. A total of 37% of the placebo group had at least one infection, compared to 29% of the *E. purpurea* group. Purple coneflower extract does not seem to work as well in preventing as in treating colds and flus.

In studying the effect on phagocytosis after 5 days, Melchart and others in 1995 used a liquid ethanolic extract of *E. purpurea* roots given as 30 drops orally three times daily for five days, representing one gram per day of the roots. They found this liquid herb extract caused significant enhancement, unlike a liquid 70% ethanolic extract of *E. purpurea* with 95% herb and 5% roots given in the same dose and duration.

In a similar trial they used a dried 50% ethanolic root extract of *E. purpurea* in doses of one 380 mg capsule three times daily for five days. In these cases the solid root extract did not show the significant improvement found with the liquid root extract, though both were made with ethanol.

Yeast Infection Adjuvant and Wound Healing Ointment

PLANT JUICE

When taken internally an alcohol-preserved *E. purpurea* juice product can improve even local therapy. In 1986 Coeugniet and Kuhnast when used the antimycotic econazole nitrate cream locally for six days to treat recurrent vaginal candidiasis, the recurrence rate after six months was 60.5%. When 30 drops of purple coneflower juice product was also given three times daily for ten weeks, the recurrence rate at six months was reduced to 16.7%. Skin tests indicated that the immune response to candida was enhanced by the *E. purpurea* juice product.

JUICE OINTMENT

In a large-scale clinical trial reported by Viehmann in 1978 involving 4598 patients, an ointment containing *E. purpurea* juice was used to treat a variety of skin conditions along with surgery or other therapies. It was determined that this ointment, free from antibiotics and corticosteroids, was a highly effective topical agent for wounds, burns, varicose ulcers of the leg, inflammatory skin conditions, eczema, and herpes simplex. The success rate was 85.5% with only 2.3% (107) of the cases having any side effects. Hobbs noted that in 1981 Gasiorowska found that topical application of juice-containing ointment produced good results with ulcerative gingivitis and other periodontal conditions.

Adverse Effects Uncommon

Mengs and others in 1991 indicated that no toxicity was demonstrated with large doses of *E. purpurea* juice stabilized with ethanol when given orally or intravenously to rats. Again in 2000 they found no toxicity in either rats or mice when given the maximum feasible single doses by these methods or when given repeated 800 mg/kg to 8,000 mg/kg doses orally for 4 consecutive weeks. No embryotoxic effects were found in rats or rabbits given up to 2,700 mg/kg, and no postnatal effects were noted in rats. Gene mutation studies were negative in test tubes for bacteria, mammal, or human cells, and no malignant transformations were caused in hamster cells.

In human oral studies no significant adverse effects have been reported, only occasional gastrointestinal upset with certain individuals. According to Parnham, four cases of adverse effects were reported in Germany from 1989 to 1995, all due to allergic skin reactions to the juice. In an unpublished study of 1231 patients reported by Parnham, *E. purpurea* lozenges taken three times daily for 4-6 weeks resulted in

Table 8   Purple Coneflower Plant and Derivatives—
Summary of Medicinal Uses and Pharmacology

PURPLE CONEFLOWER *Echinacea purpurea* Munch	Native American Uses	Folk Remedy Uses	Modern Clinical Studies	Laboratory Research Findings
Dried Root	Cough Dyspepsia	Syphilis		Increases cytokines
Root Water Extract	Gonorrhea			
Root Tincture			Flu	Increases phagocytosis
Dried Whole Plant Water Extract			Colds Flu	
Fresh Whole Plant Solid Extract			Colds	
Dried Aerial Plant				Increases cytokines, macrophage/ monocyte viability
Fresh Aerial Plant Preserved Juice in Semi-solid Base			Locally: Burns Eczema Gingivitis Herpes Varicose ulcer Wounds	Enhances wound healing Inhibits hyaluronidase Reduces exudates
Fresh Aerial Plant Preserved Juice			Internally: Candida Colds Flu	Increases phagocytosis, spleen cells, cytokines Antioxidant

Continued on next page

Table 8   *Continued*

PURPLE CONEFLOWER *Echinacea purpurea* Munch	Native American Uses	Folk Remedy Uses	Modern Clinical Studies	Laboratory Research Findings
FRACTIONS OR ISOLATED CONSTITUENTS				
Polysaccharides and/or glycoproteins				Antiviral Complement activator Inhibits hyaluronidase Increases phagocytosis, cytokines
Alkamides				Anti-inflammatory Increases phagocytosis
Phenolics				Antiviral Inhibits hyaluronidase

62 (5%) reported adverse effects. By far the most common was an unpleasant taste for 21 subjects (1.7%). Complaints of 2–6 patients each, in order of diminishing frequency, involved nausea and vomiting, recurrent infection, sore throat, abdominal pain, diarrhea, and difficulty swallowing.

In 2002 Mullins and Heddle reported anaphylaxis following oral exposure in two cases, two cases acute asthma episodes, and a severe general rash in another patient. These patients consumed one form either of echinacea tablets, tea, or tincture. Of 51 other adverse reactions reported using one of six brands of these three forms, 26 suggested allergic responses, and half of these reactions were in atopic disease patients. Of 100 other atopic patients tested, 3 had used echinacea, but 20% reacted to skin prick testing with aqueous or glycerinated extracts of echinacea.

In reviewing multiple clinical trials and considering the extensive popular use of echinacea with so few reported side effects, Barret and others concluded that the estimated risk of adverse effects from oral consumption is quite small. According to Gallo and others in 2000, those using *Echinacea* spp. products during pregnancy did not show an increased fetal risk. The German Commission E advised that oral and external use of above-ground parts of *E. purpurea* not exceed eight weeks. However, Parnham noted no adverse effects were associated with *E. purpurea* plant juice after internal use of up to twelve weeks.

Unsubstantiated Contraindications and Drug Interactions

The Commission E monograph gave no contraindications for the external use of *E. purpurea* products, but stated that the internal use is contraindicated "in principle" for progressive systemic diseases such as multiple sclerosis, collagenosis, leukosis, and tuberculosis. According to Kerry Bone, the evidence suggestive of risk when echinacea products are used in these conditions seems to be based almost entirely on test tube activity of isolated polysaccharides or water-soluble fractions of one or several species. Several of these contraindications are disputable for complex hydroalcoholic extracts used in living subjects. Based on Eclectic empirical experience, this use for tubercular conditions seems safe. Though potential allergic sensitivity suggest echinacea may be a risk to some asthmatics, it appears to many herbal prescribers to be beneficial in conditions such as asthma that can be exacerbated by infections. The current belief that echinacea extracts act primarily as a stimulus to phagocytosis in living organisms supports the argument that its use in autoimmune conditions may be safe.

Speculative reports suggesting that *E. purpurea* root extracts may lead to increased blood levels of some drugs is based on a study by Budzinski and others in 2000. They monitored the effect of commercial extracts of the roots and tops in test tubes and found these preparations ranked seventh and fourteenth, respectively, out of 19 extracts studied for inhibiting the metabolic cytochrome P450 (CYP) isozyme 3A4. However, the results of this study are preliminary and questionable, based on the simple test tube procedure used. Also, St. John's wort extract was ranked as the second greatest inhibitor, and it is known from human studies to have the opposite effect of inducing CYP 3A4, rather than inhibiting it.

References

BOOKS

Blumenthal, M (ed.). *The Complete German Commission E Monographs*, American Botanical Council., Austin, Tex., 1998.

Brinker, F. *Herb Contraindications and Drug Interactions*, 2nd ed., Eclectic Med. Pub., Sandy, OR., 1998.

Felter, HW and Lloyd, JU. *King's American Dispensatory* (1898), Eclectic Medical Pub., Sandy, OR., 1992.

Grieve, M. *A Modern Herbal*, 1931 version, Dover Pub., New York, 1971.

Lloyd, JU. *A Treatise on Echinacea*, Lloyd Brothers, Cincinnati, Ohio, 1917.

Moerman, DE. *Medicinal Plants of Native America*, vol 1, Univ. Mich. Mus. of Anthrop., Ann Arbor, 1986.

ARTICLES

Alban, S et al. Differentiation between the complement modulating effects of an arabinogalactan-protein from Echinacea purpurea and heparin. *Planta Med.*, 68:1118-24, 2002.

Al-Hassan, G et al. Low molecular substances detected in the pressed juice [1.7–2.5:1] from Echinacea purpurea herbs. *Phtyomed.*, 7(Suppl. 2):32, 2000.

Arnason, JT. North American raw materials: the case for an isobutylamide standardized product. *Echin. Past, Present Future Internat. Conf. 1999 Proc.*, Session Three, p. 5 and slide 40, Skamania, Wash., June 10–12, 1999.

Barrett, B et al. Echinacea for upper respiratory infection. *J. Fam. Pract.*, 48(8):628–35, 1999.

Barrett, B et al. Treatment of the common cold with unrefined Echinacea. *Ann. Intern. Med.*, 137: 939–46, 2002.

Bauer, R et al. Immunological in vivo and in vitro examinations of Echinacea extracts. *Arzneim.-Forsch.*, 38:276–81, 1988 [in German].

Bauer, R & Remiger P. TLC and HPLC analysis of alkamides in Echinacea drugs. *Planta Med.*, 55: 367–71, 1989.

Bauer, R et al. Alkamides from the roots of Echinacea angustifolia. *Phytochem.*, 28:505–8, 1989.

Bauer, R. Standardization of Echinacea purpurea expressed juice with reference to cichoric acid and alkamides. *J. Herbs, Spices Med Plants*, 6(3):51–62, 1999.

Berg, A et al. Influence of Echinacin (EC31) treatment on the exercise-induced immune response in athletes. *J. Clin. Res.*, 1:367–80, 1998.

Beuscher, N et al. Enhanced release of interleukin-1 from mouse macrophages by glycoproteins and polysaccharides from Baptisia tinctoria and Echinacea species. *Planta Med.*, 55:660, 1989.

Binns, SE et al. Light-mediated antifungal activity of Echinacea extracts. *Planta Med.*, 66:241–4, 2000.

Bodinet, C et al. Host-resistance increasing activity of root extracts from Echinacea species. *Planta Med.*, 59(Suppl.):A672–3, 1993.

Bone, K. Echinacea: when should it be used? *Eur. J. Herb. Med.*, 3(3):13–17, 1997/98.

Braunig, B et al.. Echinacea purpureae radix for strengthening the immune response in flu-like infections. *Z. Phytother.* 13:7–13, 1992 [in German].

Brinkeborn, RM et al. Echinaforce® and other Echinacea fresh plant preparations in the treatment of the common cold. *Phytomed.*, 6(1):1—5, 1999.

Budzinski, JW et al. An in vitro evaluation of human cytochrome P450 3A4 inhibition by selected commercial herbal extracts and tinctures. *Phytomed.*, 7(4):273–282, 2000.

Burger, RA et al. Echinacea-induced cytokine production by human macrophages. *Int. J. Immunopharmac.*, 19(7):371–9, 1997.

Busing, KH. Hyaluronidase inhibition by echinacin. *Arzneim.-Forsch.*, 2:467–70, 1952 in German].

Busing, KH. Hyaluronidase inhibition of some natural substances used in therapy. *Arzneim.-Forsch.*, 5:320–2, 1955 [in German].

Cheminat, A et al. Caffeoyl conjugates from Echinacea species: structures and biologicial activity. *Phytochem.*, 27:2787–94, 1988.

Classen, B and Blaschek, W. Gel diffusion experiments with arabinogalactan-proteins from pressed juice of Echinacea purpurea and beta-glucosyl Yariv reagent. *Phtyomed.*, 7(Suppl. 2):32, 2000.

Clifford, LJ et al. Bioactivity of alkamides isolated from Echinacea purpurea (l.) Moench. *Phytomed.*, 9:249–53, 2002.

Coeugniet, E and Kuhnast, R. Adjuvant immunotherapy with different formulations of echinacin. *Therapiewoche*, 36:3352–8, 1986.

Egert, D and Beuscher, N. Studies on antigen specifity of immunoreactive arabinogalactan proteins extracted from Baptisia tinctoria and Echinacea purpurea. *Planta Med.*, 58:163–5, 1992.

Facino, RM et al. Direct charaterization of caffeoyl esters with antihyaluronidase activity in crude extracts from Echinacea angustifolia roots by fast atom bombardment tandem mass spectrometry. *Farmaco*, 48:1447–61, 1993 (*Chem. Abs.* 120:294112w).

Gallo, M et al. Pregnancy outcome following gestational exposure to Echinacea. *Arch. Intern. Med.*, 160:3141–3, 2000.

Giger, E et al. Fructans in Echinacea and in its phytotherapeutic preparations. *Planta Med.*, 55:638–9, 1989.

Grimm, W and Muller, H-H. A randomized controlled trial of the effect of fluid extract of Echinacea purpurea on the incidence and severity of colds and respiratory infections. *Am. J. Med.*, 106: 138–43, 1999.

Heyl, FW and Staley, JF. Analyses of two Echinacea roots. *Am. J. Pharm.*, 86:450–5, 1914.

Hobbs, C. *Echinacea Monograph* from *Eclectic Dispensatory of Botanical Therapeutics* (Alstat E, comp.), vol. 1, Eclectic Medical Pub., Portland, OR., 1989.

Hoheisel, O et al. Echinagard [sic] treatment shortens the course of the common cold: a double-blind, placebo-controlled clinical trial. *Eur. J. Clin. Res.*, 9:261–8, 1997.

Johnston, BA and Malone, D. States pass legislation curtailing harvest of wild Echinacea. *HerbalGram*, 46:67, 1999.

Kaiser, E and Winkler, G. The problem of competitive inhibition in the enzymatic system of hyaluronic acid and hyaluronidase. *Arzneim.-Forsch.*, 5:322–4, 1955 [in German].

Kim, H-O et al. Retention of caffeic acid derivatives in dried Echinacea purpurea. *J. Agric. Food Chem.*, 48:4182–416, 2000a.

Kim, H-O et al. Retention of alkamides in dried Echinacea purpurea. *J. Agric. Food Chem.*, 48: 4187–4192, 2000b.

Kindscher, K. Ethnobotany of purple coneflower (Echinacea angustifolia, Asteraceae) and other Echinacea species. *Econ. Bot.*, 43(4):498–507, 1989.

Kinkel, HJ et al. Verifiable effect of echinacin ointment on wound healing *Med. Klin.* 79:580–3, 1984 [in German].

Kreuter, M. Echinacea purpurea substances, characteristics and immunological active principles. *Echin. Past, Present Future Internat. Conf. 1999 Proc.*, Session Two, p. 3 and slide 7, Skamania, Wash., June 10–12, 1999.

Letchamo, W et al. Cichoric acid and isobutylamide content in Echinacea purpurea as influenced by flower developmental stages. In: Janick J (ed.), *Perspectives on new crops and new uses*, ASHA Press, Alexandria, VA, 1999.

Li, TSC. Echinacea: cultivation and medicinal value. *HortTechnology*, 8(2):122–9, 1998.

Li, TSC and Wardle, DA. Effects of root drying temperature and moisture content on the levels of active ingredients in Echinacea roots. *J. Herbs Spices Med. Plants*, 8(1):15–22, 2001.

Lindenmuth, G and Lindenmuth, EB. The efficacy of Echinacea compound herbal tea preparation on the severity and duration of upper respiratory and flu symptoms: a randomized double-blind placebo-controlled study. *J. Alt. Compl. Med.*, 6(4):327–334, 2000.

Livesey, J et al. Effect of temperature on stability of marker constituents in Echinacea purpurea root formulations. *Phytomed.*, 6(5):347–9, 1999.

Meissner, FK. Experimental studies of the mode of action of a herba recens Echinacea purpureae on skin flap. *Arzneim.-Forsch.*, 37:17–20, 1987 [in German].

Mekkes, JR and Nahuys, M. Induction of granulation tissue formation in chronic wounds by hyaluronic acid. *Wounds*, 13(4):159–64, 2001.

Melchart, D et al. Results of five randomized studies on the immunomodulatory activity of preparations of Echinacea. *J. Alt. Compl. Med.*, 1(2):145–60, 1995.

Melchart, D et al. Echinacea root extracts for the prevention of upper respiratory tract infections.. *Arch. Fam. Med.*, 7:541–5, 1998.

Mengs, U et al. Toxicity of Echinacea purpurea. *Arzneim.-Forsch.*, 41:1076–81, 1991.

Mengs, U et al. Toxicity studies with echinacin. *Phtyomed.*, 7(Suppl. 2):32, 2000.

Moser, J Jr. Echinacea and a spurious root that appeared in the fall of 1909. *Am. J. Pharm.*, 82:224–6, 1910.

Mullins, RJ and Heddle, R. Adverse reactions associated with Echinacea: the Australian experience. *Ann. Allergy Asthma Immunol.*, 88:42–51, 2002.

Munder, PG. Immunological experiments to evaluate the activities of orally administered echinacin. *Max Planck Institut Fuer Immunbiologie*, unpublished, March, 1986 [in German].

Nusslein, B et al. Enzymatic degradation of cichoric acid in Echinacea purpurea preparations. *J. Nat. Prod.*, 63:1615–1618, 2000.

Parnham, MJ. Benefit-risk assessment of the squeezed sap of the purple coneflower (Echinacea purpurea) for long-term oral immunostimulation. *Phytomed.*, 3(1):95–102, 1996.

Perry, NB et al. Alkamide levels in Echinacea purpurea: a rapid analytical method revealing differences among roots, rhizomes, stems, leaves and flowers. *Planta Med.*, 63:58–62, 1997.

Perry, NB et al. Alkamide levels in Echinacea purpurea: effects of processing, drying and storage. *Planta Med.*, 66:54–56, 2000.

Perry, NB et al. Echinacea Standardization: analytical methods for phenolic compounds and typical levels in medicinal species. *J. Agric. Food Chem.*, 49:1702–6, 2001.

Proksch, A and Wagner, H. Structural analysis of a 4-O-methyl-glucuronoarabinoxylan with immuno-stimulating activity from Echinacea purpurea. *Phytochem.*, 26:1989–93, 1987.

Rininger, JA et al. Immunopharmacological activity of Echinacea preparations following simultated digestion on murine macrophages and human peripherall blood mononuclear cells. *J. Leukocyte Biol.*, 68:503–10, 2000.

Schoneberger, D. The influence of immune-stimulating effects of pressed juice from Echinacea purpurea on the course and severity of colds. *Forum Immunol.*, 8:2–12, 1992.

Shalaby, AS et al. Response of Echinacea to some agricultural practices. *J. Herbs, Spices Med. Plants,* 4(4):59–67, 1997.

Stimpel, M et al. Macrophage activation and induction of macrophage cytotoxicity by purified polysaccharide fractions from the plant Echinacea purpurea. *Infect. Immun.*, 46:845–9, 1984.

Stotzem, CD et al. Influence of Echinacea purpurea on the phagocytosis of human granulocytes. *Med. Sci. Res.*, 20:719–20, 1992.

Stuart, DL and Wills, RBH. Alkylamide and cichoric acid levels in Echinacea purpurea tissues during plant growth. *J. Herbs Spices Med. Plants*, 7(1):91–101, 2000.

Sun, LZ-Y et al. The American coneflower: a prophylactic role involving nonspecific immunity. *J. Alt. Compl. Med.*, 5(5):437–46, 1999.

Tunnerhoff, FK and Schwabe, HK. Studies in human beings and animals on the influence of Echinacea extracts on the formation of connective tissue following the implantation of fibrin. *Arzneim.-Forsch.*, 6:330–3, 1956 [in German].

Viehmann, P. Results of treatment with an Echinacea-based ointment. *Erfahrung.*, 27:353–8, 1978 [in German].

Vogel, G et al. The problem of the evaluation of antiexudative drugs. *Arzneim.-Forsch.*, 18:426–9, 1968 [in German].

Vomel, T. Influence of a vegetable immune stimulant on phagocytosis of erythrocytes by the reticulohistiocytary system of isolated perfused rat liver. *Arzneim.-Forsch.*, 35:1437–9, 1985 [in German].

Wacker, A and Hilbig, W. Virus inhibition by Echinacea purpurea. *Planta Med.*, 33:89–102, 1978 [in German].

Wagner, H et al. Immunostimulating polysaccharides (heteroglycans) of higher plants. *Arzneim.-Forsch.*, 35:1069–75, 1985 [in German].

Wagner, H et al. In vitro inhibition of arachidonate metablism by some alkamides and prenylated phenols. *Planta Med.*, 55:566–7, 1989.

Wagner, H. Herbal immunostimulants for the prophylaxis and therapy of colds and influenza. *Eur. J. Herb . Med.*, 3:22–30, 1997.

SAW PALMETTO—Florida Fruit for Flow and Fecundity

Serenoa repens (W.Bartram.) Small. —fruit

Summary

After use as a food by native Americans of the Southeast, saw palmetto fruit was introduced into medicine by Eclectic doctors in the late 19th century. Its primary clinical use was for benign enlargement of the prostate and for genito-urinary (GU) and other inflammatory conditions in men. Its hormonal influence was also applied to problems affecting women. Modern scientific and clinical research has established that *Serenoa repens* fruit contain effective agents for treating symptoms of benign prostatic hypertrophy (BPH) and prostatitis. In prostatic hyperplasia saw palmetto's fatty alcohol and sterol components seem to impact hormonal expression, including testosterone, dihydrotestosterone, and estrogen. Other lipid- and water-soluble components provide important beneficial effects for both prostatitis and prostatic hypertrophy. Like several popular drugs used to treat prostate problems, recently discovered relaxation effects on the smooth muscle of the bladder and prostate are due to inhibition of the alpha-1-adrenergic receptors.

Fruit as Food

Since the late 19th century Eclectic physicians have used the berries of saw palmetto (*Serenoa repens,* formerly called *Serenoa serrulata* or *Sabal serrulata*) as medicine. This plant gets its common name from its saw-toothed leaf stalk and from the Spanish term for small palms. Saw palmetto grows mostly from Florida to South Carolina and west through the coastal plain of Alabama and Mississippi. Some colonies grow in sandy soil as far west as Louisiana and Texas and in various Caribbean islands.

Dr. Edwin Hale gave the first complete description of the history of saw palmetto in 1898. He noticed that wildlife and cattle that fed on the fruit grew sleek and fat. Early descriptions of its flavor by Quakers shipwrecked in Florida in 1696 were not flattering, but saw palmetto fruit was a dietary staple of the local natives and later migrants to the region including the Creek, Seminoles and Miccosukee. The Seminoles squeeze the juice from the fruit that they sweeten to prepare a drink. However, according to Bennet and Hicklin in 1998, there is no written record of early native Americans using the fruit medicinally.

Rapid Emergence and Commercial Supply

In 1877 Dr. J.B. Read of Savannah, Georgia, introduced the use of its fruit as a nutritive tonic and a remedy for conditions with excessive mucus production, especially irritation of the nose and throat. This was followed by another report written by Dr. Isham Goss of Marietta, Georgia, that lauded it as the best remedy for sexual debility and prostatic hypertrophy. He noted its usefulness for mucous membrane inflammation of the bladder and urethra. After these articles its reputation became widespread. By the turn of the century thousands of physicians were prescribing it in one form or another. Tegarden in 1898 reported that commercial sources consisted principally of the fresh immature fruit, the mature fruit, and the sun-dried fruit.

Around 1900 it was estimated that, if it were possible to harvest the entire crop of saw palmetto fruit that about 300,000,000 pounds could be gathered semi-annually. Bennet and Hicklin in describing the current situation estimate that only one third is harvestable. Collection of the fruit on private lands and exportation of dried fruit is unregulated. Currently, it is estimated that the annual fruit harvest is over 6,800,000 kg.

While fully matured (black) or partially-ripened (orange) fruit are preferred, unripe (green) fruit are also in the mixture. Commercial fruit are dried in driers, mechanically cleaned, and then sacked for shipment. The dried fruits may be extracted with organic solvents such as ethanol, hexane, or supercritical carbon dioxide to extract the lipids and sterols. Current commercial products include bulk dried fruit, tea bags, encapsulated powders, powdered extracts with 25–30% fatty acid content, liposterolic extracts in soft gelatin capsules, and extracts standardized to a specific fatty acid or liposterol content.

Popular and Official Medicinal Forms and Doses

Common commercial preparations included tinctures made with fresh fruits in 90% alcohol, the fluid extract, and oil mixed with sugars for internal use or with cocoa butter as a suppository. Formulas combining saw palmetto with other herbs for urinary tract problems were also popular. *Serenoa* fluid extract became official in the *United States Pharmacopeia* from 1900 until 1920, then it was included in the *National Formulary* (NF) from 1926 to 1952. In addition, 3 parts of a *Serenoa* 1:5 tincture combined with 1 part sandalwood was also official in the *NF.* In 2000 the re-entry in the *NF* of the partially dried ripe fruit and powdered saw palmetto fruit occurred as a dietary supplement.

Whole Dried Fruit

In 1917 Remington noted the use of the partially dried, ripe fruit in doses of 1–2 grams as a diuretic and tonic. By 1922 Felter gave the recommended dosage range of the dried powder from 650 mg to 4 gm. The 1946 *NF* list the dose as 1 gm. In 1953 Kuts-Cheraux gave the naturopathic dosage of from 325 mg to 3.9 gms. In 2000 the USP Convention indicated the encapsulated powdered fruit dose is 1–2 grams daily.

WATER EXTRACTS

Naturopaths utilized the water extract at times. Lust infused a teaspoon of the dried berries in one cup of water and gave 1–2 cups daily. Kuts-Cheraux indicated that 4 gms of the dried berries should be decocted in 4 ounces of water and 5–9 ounces consumed daily. While from 0.35–0.7 gm decocted in a cup of water three times daily has been used according to the USP Convention, this preparation lacks the lipophilic components recognized as important for prostatic hyperplasia. However, the infusion or decoction would be rich in the polysaccharides found to be immune enhancing and anti-inflammatory.

TINCTURE

Hale stated in 1898 that the tincture should be made from the fresh ripe berries and seeds, all crushed and macerated in 90% alcohol for 14 days. The tincture should not be filtered through cotton or paper that will absorb the oil, but decanted. According to the 2000 USP Convention, using 80% alcohol to extract the berries at a 1:2 strength for fresh fruit or 1:5 for dried fruit, the dosage range is 1–2 ml taken 3–4 times daily. Modern hydroalcoholic extracts vary greatly in strength and manufacturing processes and, therefore, appropriate dosage.

SPECIFIC MEDICINE

The saw palmetto specific medicine extract used by most Eclectic physicians to treat genito-urinary tract conditions contained an abundance of oil according to WE Bloyer. It was a 1:1 extract of the fruit made with 75% alcohol, given in doses ranging from 0.7 ml to 4 ml taken in water every 3–4 hours. Though of the same weight to volume strength as the fluid extract, it underwent further undefined special processing by Lloyd Brothers Pharmacists.

In 1898 E.M. Hale quoted John Uri Lloyd from a correspondence: "In making tincture of saw palmetto berries I use the entire fruit, pulp and seed. I use official deodorized alcohol full strength, making one pint of the tincture represent sixteen ounces of the drug. I do not filter the preparation at all, but let it clarify by settling and decantation."

FLUID EXTRACT

According to the 1946 *NF* the 1:1 extract of the dried fruit powder made with 80% alcohol is normally given in doses of 1 ml. Grieve suggested 2–4 ml per dose, and Kuts-Cheraux indicated from 0.6–4.0 ml could be used. The 2000 USP Convention indicates from 0.6 ml up to 1.5 ml three times daily can be used.

LIPOSTEROLIC EXTRACTS

Hexane or supercritical fluid carbon dioxide are used to extract the lipids and sterol components from the fruit, while excluding water-soluble components. These chemical solvents are removed, leaving a solid extract form at approximately a 10:1

strength. The oral dosage of these extracts of *Serenoa* fruit standardized to 70–95% free fatty acids, esters, and sterols is typically 160 mg two times daily.

Traditional Medical Uses

WHOLE FRUIT

Hale declared in 1898 that the best means of using the berries for nutritive purposes to increase the fat of the body would be a preparation that contains all the constituents of the berries except the inert matter. In his mind neither the tincture, fluid extract, nor the oil were appropriate preparations for this. He believed that 1–2 ml of the pure oil mixed with 200–325 mg of the complete fruit and dispensed in a soft gelatin capsule seemed the ideal method for treating leanness.

In 1914 Dr. FAP Montagu in New Zealand noted that after 12 years of studying its uses closely, he found that saw palmetto given as 335 mg pills three times daily helped enlarge small undeveloped breasts in young women, sometimes as much as four inches in three months. He warned that in some cases a slight astigmatism was caused that disappeared when the herb discontinued.

Felter did not distinguish between use of the whole fruit and its Specific Medicine extract. These he used to treat enlarged prostate and prostatitis. He believed it helped reduce symptoms of the inflamed prostate by relieving the urethral irritation and increase the tone of the bladder. It was best for relieving dull, aching, throbbing pain of the prostatic urethra and controlling excessive prostatic discharges. In some cases it could relieve gonorrheal discharge. Similar to the male, Felter reported that in women it could tone an enlarged uterus that was relaxed and flabby with a leucorrheal discharge. He also noted that in some nutritive way it was asserted to enlarge the breasts.

Meanwhile, Ellingwood described how the fruit was first used to improve digestion and relieve irritation of mucous structures, especially of the breathing passages. Lust found the berries were useful for asthma, colds, and bronchitis. Kuts-Cheraux noted the naturopathic use of the powdered ripe fruit. Without indicating the specific form used for each condition, he indicated that the preparations were best known for their genito-urinary effects, especially controlling mucus discharges, reducing inflammation, and correcting prostatic hypertrophy.

WATER EXTRACTS

Kuts-Cheraux also described a decoction of the dried ripe fruit. Lust indicated that mucous congestion problems respond to the tea, and that it was used while convalescing from illness as a general tonic.

SPECIFIC MEDICINE

In 1899 Dr. Lyman Watkins treated about a dozen elderly men with this remedy.

He found it effective for frequent urination when there was difficulty starting and when frequency was worse at night. Such symptoms were eliminated in his experience with patients by giving a teaspoonful of this specific medicine at bedtime. Both Felter and Ellingwood concurred that it was useful in the treating symptoms of prostatic hypertrophy such as relieving urinary irritation and dribbling but found no evidence that prostate size was reduced. Eclectics commonly used saw palmetto Specific Medicine for prostatitis. It was indicated when there was a throbbing, aching, dull pain associated with prostatic irritation and a discharge of mucus or yellowish, watery fluid.

Ellingwood and Felter both noted that Specific Medicine saw palmetto was valued for treating impotence. Ellingwood recommends giving it in 20–30 drop doses 3–4 times daily combined with 15 drops *Avena sativa* (green oats) tincture for weeks. Testicular underdevelopment or atrophy also improved with its use, as did inflammation of the testicles and epididymus. In men and women it was claimed to increase libido and fertility, while in women it was used to help relieve inflammation and pain of the ovaries. This form was also believed to improve breast development and milk secretion in women.

FLUID EXTRACT

As recorded in the *Eclectic Medical Journal* in 1891 and confirmed by Dr. JM Showerman in 1892, the fluid extract of saw palmetto when used for months successfully treated prostatic hypertrophy in old men along with bladder symptoms associated with this condition. Impotence also responded well in a matter of weeks. For uterine atrophy dependent on ovarian dysfunction, it was found to be a useful remedy. Dr. Showerman was convinced of its efficacy in enlarging the mammary glands.

For irritation of the upper respiratory tract, laryngitis, and bronchitis the fluid extract daily was sometimes given. Felter and Lloyd likewise indicated that it acted as an expectorant and was effective for many respiratory conditions as well as genito-urinary complaints by controlling irritation of the mucous membranes. Grieve agreed with this assessment. Kuts-Cheraux reported the naturopathic use of the fluid extract that was one of its forms used for controlling urinary incontinence, mucus discharges of the genito-urinary tract, and prostatic hypertrophy.

Active Compounds of Whole Fruit

The content of beta-sitosterol (1.9%) and its glucoside (2.3%) in the dried fruit epicarp and mesocarp of *Serenoa* is an unusually high yield as shown by Schoepflin and others in 1966. Besides beta-sitosterol, other sterols of *Serenoa repens* fruit are stigmasterol and campesterol. Jommi and others in 1988 and 1989 described active components that included fatty alcohols such as docosanol, hexacosanol, octacosanol, and triacontanol. Fatty acid fractions with their methyl and ethyl esters are made up of lauric acid (21–25%), myristinic acid (11–12%), palmitic acid (9–11%), oleic acid (33–43%), linoleic acid (2–4%) and others including myristoleic acid. Additional markers identified in the *NF 19* include the methyl esters of linolenate, palmitoleate, caproate, caprylate, caprate and stearate. A 95% ethanol extract of the dried powdered berries of *S. repens* contains two active monoacylglycerides: 1-monolaurin and 1-monomyristin.

Water-soluble high molecular weight polysaccharides are also found in saw palmetto berry but not in hexane or alcohol extracts.

In 1898 Hale quoted John Uri Lloyd as follows:

"While I assert that the volatile oil is the conspicuous constituent of the fruit of the Saw Palmetto, I do not mean that it can replace the natural drug. The fact is, in many cases our chemistry is not able to determine the therapeutical value of passive bodies. The apparently inconspicuous substances seem in natural combinations to possess *decided* powers as blenders or modifiers. I call this to your attention in order that you may not fall into the error of so many men who infer that the *conspicuous* product of a drug naturally possesses the therapeutical value of the drug."

Laboratory Research—
Extracts, Lipophilic Fractions, and Components from the Fruit

Anti-inflammatory

LIPOSTEROLIC EXTRACT

Research by Tarayre and others in 1983 showed anti-edematous activity of saw palmetto hexane extract in rats, mice, and guinea-pigs.

ACID LIPOPHILIC FRACTION

Breu and others in 1992 showed that acid lipophilic compounds in a fraction separated from fatty alcohols and sterols inhibit cyclooxygenase and 5-lipoxygenase pathways in the test tube.

STEROLS

Yamada and others showed in 1987. Gupta and others found in 1980 that β-sitosterol has potent anti-inflammatory activity.

Immune Enhancement

STEROLS

Beta-sitosterol, stigmasterol, and campesterol have demonstrated potent immune-

326 Complex Herbs—Complete Medicines

potentiating activity by activating complement via both classical and alternative pathways. These components are not soluble in water but require organic chemical solvents such as ethanol.

POLYSACCHARIDES

In addition, Wagner and Flachsbarth in 1981 found saw palmetto fruit seeds have an acidic high molecular weight polysaccharide with potent anti-inflammatory activity. In 1985 Wagner and others tested high molecular weight polysaccharides from saw palmetto that also were immune enhancing agents.

Smooth Muscle Relaxant

EXTRACTS AND LIPIDS

In lab tests in 1999 Goepel and others used two powdered saw palmetto extracts and four saw palmetto oils that all inhibited binding to human prostatic alpha-1-adrenoceptors by the antagonist prazosin, while the oils also inhibited binding of the antagonist tamsulosin. These antagonist saw palmetto extracts and oils and the pharmaceutical antagonists all have the same inhibitory effects on smooth muscle contractions. The saw palmetto extracts also inhibited activity of alpha-receptors stimulated with phenylephrine. The active concentration was similar to the concentrations expected from therapeutic doses of the extracts.

LIPOPHILIC FRACTIONS

The influence on smooth muscles that control urinary outflow from the bladder through the prostatic urethra contributes to the therapeutic effect. A study by Gutierrrez and others in 1996 of total lipidic and saponifiable extracts of the fruit showed that both antagonize contractions of the urinary bladder induced by acetylcholine. In 1996 they further proved the antispasmodic activity is partially due to interference with intracellular calcium mobilization and protein synthesis.

In 1996 Odenthal found the lipophilic extract reduced smooth muscle contraction of the male rat deferens duct. Guinea-pig bladder smooth muscle contractions were also antagonized. This extract, in concentrations identical to those with anti-androgenic and anti-inflammatory effects, has both calcium-blocking and alpha-adrenergic antagonistic activities that could contribute to its spasmolytic effect and usefulness in treating BPH urinary symptoms.

Antitumor

LIPIDS

There is also evidence that the fatty acids found in the fruit have anti-tumor activity. Shimada and others showed in 1997 that the monoacylglyceride compounds 1-monolaurin and 1-monomyristin had anti-tumor effects against human tumor cells of the kidney and pancreas and borderline toxicity against human prostatic cells. Iguchi and others found in 2001 that the fatty acid myristoleic acid is another cytotoxic component of the lipid fraction active against prostatic cells by increasing apoptosis.

Hormonal

ALCOHOLIC EXTRACTS

Duker and others found the dried alcoholic extract yielded a 50% inhibition of 5-alpha-reductase conversion of testosterone using a 0.005% solution; twice this concentration was needed to penetrate cell membranes and produce the same effect. However, the alcoholic extract does not exhibit any male hormone receptor binding activity. *Serenoa* methanol extract containing beta-sitosterol and this isolated phytosterol were both shown by Elghamry and Hansel to have mild estrogenic activity in immature female mice.

LIPOSTEROLIC EXTRACT

No inhibition of binding of dihydrotestosterone (DHT) to prostatic receptors by commercial saw palmetto extracts could be detected in rat tissue lab studies by Rhodes and others. Even extremely high doses of liposterolic extract failed to show any inhibition of prostate growth in living castrated rats given DHT, further indicating a lack of anti-androgen activity. However, rat receptors may differ from human since the liposterolic extract was shown to inhibit DHT binding to androgen receptors in human foreskin fibroblasts by Sultan and others. Another study by El-Sheikh and others on the binding of DHT and testosterone on tissue samples from human patients showed that *Serenoa* liposterolic extract inhibited the binding of these hormones by 41% and 42%, respectively. In 1996 Ravenna and others found that hormone dependency of human cells make them more susceptible to the anti-androgenic action of the hexane extract, possibly by increasing the permeability of these cells to its liposterolic components.

In 1984 Sultan and others found the enzyme 5-alpha-reductase (5AR) that converts testosterone to the more potent DHT was inhibited by *Serenoa* hexane extract in human foreskin, though the extract also strongly inhibited the enzyme 3-ketosteroid reductase which converts DHT into a less potent form. Since a very high dose was used to achieve this effect, this indicated that saw palmetto produces only a weak inhibition of 5AR. Doses of saw palmetto extracts required to produce equivalent inhibition of 5AR (type not identified) in test tubes to the drug finesteride were 5600 times or more greater than the finesteride dose. Using this result as a basis for dosage in rats given testosterone, Rhodes and others showed in 1993 that *Serenoa* liposterolic extract produced no inhibition of prostate growth with even three times the hypothetical effective dose. However, Iehle and others in 1995 found saw palmetto liposterolic extract is active against both type 1 and type 2 5AR, whereas finesteride is mainly active against type 2. Delos and others in 1994 found the saw palmetto extract is three time more inhibiting to type 1 than finesteride. Type 1 is found in the prostate and prostate cancer cells and is predominant in liver and skin, while type 2 is primarily in the prostate and has a higher affinity for testosterone.

In 1992 when Otto and others used the lipophilic extract in mice given DHT and estradiol with transplanted human BPH tissue, the extract produced significant inhibition of prostate growth compared to that in mice receiving only the hormones. Paubert-Braquet and others also showed saw palmetto liposterolic extract affects prostate growth of rats given estrogen and testosterone in 1996. These findings indicate saw palmetto extract has anti-androgenic and/or anti-estrogenic effects.

LIPIDS

Steroid hormones influence the growth of tissues in the male genital tract. Jommi and others found that rats given 50 mg of the fatty alcohol fraction of *Serenoa* lipophilic extract showed a greater decrease in the weight of both the ventral prostate and seminal vesicles than rats given 400 mg of the total lipophilic extract. Debat showed that docosanol and other alcohols with more than sixteen carbon atoms were active against prostate enlargement through examination of the periphery of the prostate.

Human Pharmacology Studies

Hormonal

LIPOSTEROLIC EXTRACT

Effects in humans do not appear to occur from a strong systemic hormonal influence. Casarosa and others found in 1988 that 160 mg of liposterolic *Serenoa* extract given to 20 elderly men twice daily for 30 days did not change their plasma levels of testosterone, follicle-stimulating hormone, or luteinizing hormone. Likewise, a double blind study of healthy male volunteers by Rhodes and others in 1993 administered *Serenoa* liposterolic extract at 160 mg twice daily or placebo, each to 11 men for 7 days. There was no change in serum testosterone or dihydrotestosterone (DHT) in either group. Eleven healthy men given 160 mg of liposterolic extract twice daily for seven days had, like those given placebo but unlike those taking finesteride, no significant change in serum testosterone or DHT, as was demonstrated by Strauch and other in 1994. However, the concentration of DHT was decreased and testosterone was increased in the periurethral and intermediate tissue of the prostate by the hexane extract taken for 3 months by ten men with BPH compared with fifteen untreated, as reported in 1998 by Di Silverio and others. Epidermal growth factor was also reduced in these prostatic areas by the saw palmetto extract.

Weisser and others showed in 1997 in a 3-month randomized, double-blind trial using a lipophilic extract in 18 BPH patients that the activity of DHT-removing hydroxysteroid oxidoreductase enzymes in the prostate were moderately increased. In a 6-month double-blind study by Carraro and others in 1996 with 1,098 men over age 50 with moderate BHP, the liposterolic extract decreased symptoms equally to the drug finesteride in normal doses. Though finasteride decreased prostatic volume more than *Serenoa* extract, it also greatly reduced the cancer marker prostate-specific antigen (PSA), thereby potentially interfering with the diagnosis of prostate cancer. PSA was unaffected by saw palmetto. Furthermore, by comparison, the adverse effects on sexual function were minimal for *Serenoa*.

In a double-blind placebo-controlled study of 35 BPH patients by Di Silverio and others in 1992, liposterolic extract was given for three months before prostatectomy. The nuclear estrogen, progesterone and androgen receptors were significantly fewer in the treated group than in the placebo group. Unlike synthetic antiestrogen and antiandrogen combinations that produces severe loss of libido and reduced sexual performance, *Serenoa* liposterolic extract is well tolerated with few side effects.

LIPOSTEROLIC EXTRACT AND BETA-SITOSTEROL

In 2002 daily internal consumption of 200 mg of saw palmetto liposterolic extract together with 50 mg of beta-sitosterol was tested by Prager and others in a placebo-controlled double blind study involving 19 men with male-pattern baldness. The product also contained lecithin 50 mg, inositol 100 mg, phosphatidyl choline 25 mg, niacin 15 mg, and biotin 0.1 mg. After about 5 months 6 of 10 subjects taking the extract combination were rated as improved, compared to 1 of 9 receiving the placebo. None of those on the combination treatment perceived deterioration in their bald spot, though 3 of 9 on placebo did. Adverse effects were inconsequential. The positive results were believed to be due to the reduction in the hair follicles of dihydrotestosterone, probably by inhibition of 5-alpha reductase.

Clinical Studies—Prostate and Urinary Symptoms

LIPOSTEROLIC EXTRACT

In a study by Reece Smith and others in 1986 with 70 benign prostatic hypertrophy (BPH) patients, placebo produced subjective benefits as well as improved flow rate, so no significant difference could be detected when comparing its effects to a hexane extract of *Serenoa* (PA 109). In a double-blind, placebo-controlled multicenter study by Descotes and others in 1995 that excluded previous placebo responders, 176 men with BPH were randomized and 82 received the same extract for 30 days. Improvement in severity of painful urination (31.3%) and nocturnal urinary frequency (32.5%) for the extract group was almost twice that of the placebo group (16.1% and 17.7%, respectively). Daytime urinary frequency was significantly reduced for the extract (11.3%) but not for placebo users. Furthermore, increase in peak urinary flow rate for the extract group (28.9%) was over three times that of placebo (8.5%). Tolerability was comparable for both groups.

A systematic review in 1998 by Wilt and others of these and 16 other randomized, controlled trials (14 double-blinded) involving altogether 2,939 men and ranging in duration from 4–48 weeks was published in *JAMA* in 1998. It found that *S. repens* extract users had improved self-rating in symptoms and peak urine flow and showed a decrease in urinary tract symptom scores including nighttime urinary frequency. The clinical effects were comparable to the 5-AR inhibitor finasteride used to treat BPH, but *Serenoa* extracts produced a lower incidence of adverse effects such as erectile dysfunction. One concern expressed was the short duration of these studies. A negative comparison with the alpha-1-antagonist alfuzosin was excluded due to inadequate duration, while another negative comparison with the alpha-1-antagonist prazosin lacked randomization. A 3-year multicenter prospective study involving 89 urologists and 435 patients (315 completed the 36-month follow-up) studied the long-term efficacy and tolerability of a commercial liposterolic extract of saw palmetto fruit. A 50% reduction in urine retention and increased peak urinary flow rate were observed. Other symptoms showing improvement in a large percentage of patients on the extract included nocturia in 73%, daytime frequency in 54%, incomplete emptying in 75%, and prostate congestion in 55%. Over 80% of physicians and patients described the effects as good or very good. The extract was well tolerated by 98% of the patients.

Studies by Gerber and others in 1998 and 2001 with open label protocol in 46 men and a randomized, double-blind, placebo-controlled trial in 85 elderly men, respectively, used 320 mg liposterolic extract daily for 6 months to assess effects on urinary tract symptoms without specifically documenting BPH. The extract contained 85– 95% fatty acids and sterols. While urinary symptoms improved, changes in flow rates were not detected. No changes in sexual function or serum PSA, a marker for prostate cancer, were noted.

Clinical studies that do not employ placebo controls are commonly performed in Europe. A large (1334 patients), 12-week BPH outpatient drug monitoring study by Vahlensieck and others in 1993 showed a 50% decrease in urine retention, a 37% decrease in urinary frequency, and a 54% decrease in nocturia in patients using saw palmetto extracts, while the percentage of patients with dysuria was reduced from 75% to 37%. In a multicenter, 3-month, open study of 305 patients reported by Braeckman in 1994 that used a supercritical carbon dioxide as a solvent to selectively extract *Serenoa* fruit, 88% of both doctors and patients considered the therapy effective after three months based on subjective and objective standards. Regulatory status of the standardized extract in most of western Europe is as an over-the-counter or prescription drug.

The only study thus far using the liposterolic extract for nonbaceterial chronic prostatitis is an unpublished report by Remzi and others in 2003. They treated 32 men for 12 weeks with 160 mg twice daily, while a comparable group of 24 men served as controls but did not receive a placebo. Standard assessments of patient symptoms were done, along with measuring PSA levels and prostate volume. No change in prostate volume was detected, but PSA decreased from baseline by 22% after 6 weeks in the extract group. Of those taking the extract, 75% had some symptoms improvement, 55% had moderate or marked improvement, compared to 20% and 16% of the controls, respectively. Chronic Prostate Symptom Index scores were reduced by 30% after 6 weeks in 38% of the extract group but only 12.5% of the control group, but no difference was noted after 12 weeks.

STEROLS

An extract of phytosterols from *Hypoxis rooperi* under the trade name of Harzol was tested by Berges and others in 1995 with a follow-up published in 2000 on its effect on BPH patients. The extract contained 10 mg beta-sitosterol including 0.1 mg beta-sitosterol-beta-D-glucosidase and small amounts of campesterol, stigmasterol, other sterols and their glucosides, similar in composition to the saw palmetto phytosterol make-up. A dose of 20 mg beta-sitosterol three times daily for 6 months given to 100 men decreased the symptom scores, increased urinary flow, and decreased urine retention in comparison to 100 using placebo. No change was detected in prostate volume. These effects were maintained after another 18 months for the 65 in the open extension follow-up. Wilt and others found in their 1999 review of the research that while the three studies using beta-sitosterol showed improved urine flow measures and urinary symptom scores, the one using only beta-sitosterol-beta-D-glucoside did not.

Adverse Effects

Montagu suggested in 1914 that if the powdered fruit was used for prolonged periods, it may produce indigestion, hemorrhoids, or astigmatism that will disappear with its discontinuance.

The 18 clinical trials reviewed by Wilt and others in 1998 showed the liposterolic fraction extract produced few side effects. The most commonly reported were comparable to placebo: erectile dysfunction in 1.1% (0.7% for placebo) and gastrointestinal effects in 1.3% (0.9% for placebo). Of patients using the extracts 9.1% withdrew from the studies, compared to 7.0% of those on placebo and 11.2% for finesteride. Doses should be taken with food to reduce gastric upset.

Cheema and others in 2001 reported one case of a hemorrhage that occurred during brain surgery that the doctors associated with use of saw palmetto hexane extract. This is the only reported incident of this type.

The supercritical carbon dioxide extract reported by Braeckman had side effects in 5% of patients, half of which were gastrointestinal symptoms: stomachache, nausea, vomiting, diarrhea, and constipation. Other side effects were isolated and widely variable, but no erectile dysfunction was noted. Only 2% of patients withdrew from this study due to adverse reactions.

Drug Interactions

Saw palmetto commercial extracts and oils inhibited binding to alpha-1-adrenoceptors (A1A) by antagonists tamsulosin and prazosin in test tube studies by Goepel and others in 1999 in the same fashion as do other pharmaceutical A1A antagonists terazosin, alfuzosin, and doxazosin. Since saw palmetto shares this activity but is less potent than these drugs, it may reduce their effects somewhat if used together. In addition, the oils and extracts inhibited the action of A1A agonist phenylephrine. Odenthal and Gutierrez and others had shown in test tube studies in 1996 that saw palmetto extracts antagonized tubular smooth muscle contractions induced by the A1A agonist norepinephrine, further indicating saw palmetto's A1A antagonist activity that could block some effects of these drugs.

Table 9   Saw Palmetto Fruit and Derivatives—
Summary of Medicinal Uses and Pharmacology

SAW PALMETTO Serenoa repens (W. Bertram.) Small	Eclectic Medical Uses	Traditional Naturopathic Uses	Modern Clinical Studies	Laboratory Research Findings
Whole Fruit	BPH* Prostatitis Urethritis Mucous irritation Atonic uterus Small breasts Nutritive tonic	Asthma Colds Bronchitis GU** inflammation BPH GU discharges		
Water Extract		Mucus congestion Covalescence		

Table 9   *Continued*

SAW PALMETTO *Serenoa repens* (W. Bertram.) Small	Eclectic Medical Uses	Traditional Naturopathic Uses	Modern Clinical Studies	Laboratory Research Findings
Specific Medicine (Hydro-alcoholic)	BPH symp-toms Prostatitis Impotence Atrophic testes Inflamed testes Inflamed ovaries Sterility Small breasts			
Fluid Extract	BPH Impotence Uterine atrophy Small breasts Laryngitis Bronchitis	BPH Urinary incontinence GU discharges		5AR† inhibition
Liposterolic Extract (Hexane, Carbon dioxide)			Urinary symptoms of BPH Chronic prostatitis Baldness	5AR inhibition Spasmolytic A1A†† antag-nist Anti-androgenic Anti-estrogenic Anti-inflammatory

FRACTIONS AND ISOLATED CONSTITUENTS

Polysaccharides				Anti-inflammatory Immune enhancing
Fatty Alcohols				Anti-androgenic

Continued on next page

Table 9   *Continued*

SAW PALMETTO *Serenoa repens* (W. Bertram.) Small	Eclectic Medical Uses	Traditional Naturopathic Uses	Modern Clinical Studies	Laboratory Research Findings

FRACTIONS AND ISOLATED CONSTITUENTS

Lipids				Spasmolytic A1A antagonist Anti-inflammatory Antitumor
Sterols			Urinary symptoms of BPH	Anti-inflammatory Immune enhancing Estrogenic

*   Beneign Prostatic Hypertrophy
**   Genito-Urinary
†   5-Alpha Reductase
††   Alpha-1 Adrenergic

References

BOOKS

Anonymous. Saw palmetto monograph. The United States Pharmacopeial Convention, Inc., 2000

Ellingwood, F. *American Materia Medical, Therapeutics and Pharmacognosy,* 1919 ed., Eclectic Medical Pub., Sandy, OR., 1994.

Felter, HW. *The Eclectic Materia Medical, Pharmacology and Therapeutics,* 1922 ed., Eclectic Medical Pub., Sandy, OR., 1994.

Felter, HW & Lloyd JU. *King's American Dispensatory,* 1898 ed., Eclectic Medical Pub., Sandy, OR., 1993.

Grieve, M. *A Modern Herbal,* 1931 ed., Dover Pub., Inc., New York, 1971.

Hale, EM. *Saw Palmetto—Its History, Botany, Chemistry, Pharmacology, Provings, Clinical Experience and Therapeutic Applications,* Boericke & Tafel, Philadelphia, 1898.

Kuts-Cheraux, AW. *Naturae Medicina and Naturopathic Dispensatory,* American Naturopathic Physicians and Surgeons Assoc., Des Moines, Iowa, 1953.

Lloyd, JU. *History of the Vegetable Drugs of the Pharmacopeia of the United States,* JU & CG Lloyd, Cincinnati, Oh., 1911.

Lust, J. *The Herb Book,* Bantam Books, New York, 1974.

Remington, JP. *The Practice of Pharmacy,* 6th ed., J.B. Lippincott Co., Philadelphia, 1917.

The National Formulary, 19th ed., United States Pharmacopeial Convention, Inc., Rockville, MD, 1999.

ARTICLES

Anonymous. Saw palmetto. *Ecl. Med. J.,* 51:229–30, 1891

Bach, D, Ebeling L. Long-term drug treatment of benign prostatic hyperplasia—results of a prospective 3-year multicenter study using Sabal extract IDS 89. *Phytomed.,* 3(2):105–11, 1996.

Bennet, BC, Hicklin JR. Uses of saw palmetto (Serenoa repens, Arecaceae) in Florida. *Econ. Bot.,* 52(4):381–3, 1998.

Berges, RR et al. Randomised, placebo-controlled, double-blind clinical trial of beta-sitosterol in patients with benign prostatic hyperplasia. *Br. Med. J.,* 345:152–32, 1995.

Berges, RR et al. Treatment of symptomatic benign prostatic hyperplasia with beta-sitosterol: an 18-month follow-up. *B.J.U. Internat.,* 85:842–6, 2000.

Bloyer, WE. Saw palmetto. *Ecl. Med. J.,* 56:581–2, 1896.

Braeckman, J. The extract of Serenoa repens in the treatment of benign prostatic hyperplasia: a multicenter open study. *Curr. Ther. Res.,* 55:776–85, 1994.

Breu, T et al. Antiphlogistic activity of an extract from Sabal serrulata fruits prepared by supercritical carbon dioxide/in vitro inhibition of the cyclooxygenase and 5-lipoxygenase metabolism. *Arzneim.-Forsch.,* 42:547–51, 1992.

Carraro, JC et al. Comparison of phytotherapy (Permixon®) with finasteride in the treatment of benign prostate hyperplasia: a randomized international study of 1,098 patients. *Prostate,* 29:231–40, 1996.

Casarosa, C et al. Lack of effects of a liposterolic extract of Serenoa repens on plasma levels of testosterone, FSH, and luteinizing hormone. *Clin. Ther.,* 10:585–8, 1988.

Cheema, P et al. Intraoperative haemorrhage associated with the use of extract of saw palmetto herb: a case report and review of literature. *J. Int. Med.,* 250:167–9, 2001.

Debat, J. Higher alkanol compositions and the use thereof in treatment of prostate disorders. *Chem. Abs.,* 93:#7655w, 1980.

Delos, S et al. Inhibition of the activity of 'basic' 5-alpha-reductase (type 1) detected in DU 145 cells and expressed in insect cells. *J. Steroid Biochem. Molec. Biol.,* 48(4):347–52, 1994.

Descotes, JL et al. Placebo-controlled evaluation of the efficacy and tolerability of Permixon® in benign postatic hyperplasia after exclusion of placebo responders. *Clin. Drug Invest.,* 9(5):291–7, 1995.

Di Silverio, F et al. Evidence that Serenoa repens extract displays an antiestrogenic activity in prostatic tissue of benign prostatic hypertrophy patients. *Eur. Urol.,* 21:309–14, 1992.

Di Silverio, F et al. Effects of long-term treatment with Serenoa repens (Permixon®) on the concentrations and regional distribution of androgens and epidermal growth factor in benign prostatic hyperplasia. *Prostate*, 37:77–83, 1998.

Duker, E-M et al. Inhibition of 5-alpha-reductase activity by extracts from Sabal serrulata. *Planta Med.*, 55:587, 1989.

Elghamry, ME and Hansel, R. Activity and isolated phytoestrogen of shrub palmetto fruits (Serenoa repens Small), a new estrogenic plant. *Experientia*, 25:828–9, 1969.

Gerber, GS et al. Saw palmetto (Serenoa repens) in men with lower urinary tract symptoms: effects on urodynamic parameters and voiding symptoms. *Urol.*, 51:1003–7, 1998.

Gerber, GS et al. Randomized, double-blind, placebo-controlled trial of saw palmetto in men with lower urinary tract symptoms. *Urol.*, 58:960–5, 2001.

Goepel, M et al. Saw palmetto extracts potently and noncompetitively inhibit human alpha-1-adrenoceptors in vitro. *Prostate*, 38:208–215, 1999.

Gupta, MB et al. Anti-inflammatory and antipyretic activities of beta-sitosterol. *Planta Med.*, 39:157–63, 1980.

Gutierrez, M et al. Mechanisms involved in the spasmolytic effect of extracts from Sabal serrulata fruit on smooth muscle. *Gen. Pharmac.*,27(1):171–6, 1996.

Gutierrez, M et al. Spasmolytic activity of a lipidic extract from Sabal serrulata fruits: further study of the mechanisms underlying this activity. *Planta Med.*, 62:507–11, 1996.

Hatinguais, P et al. Composition of the hexane extract from Serenoa repens Bartram fruits. *Trav. Soc. Pharm. Montpellier*, 41:253-62, 1981. (*Chem. Abs.* 99:10736c)

Iehle, C et al. Human prostatic steroid 5-alpha-reductase isoforms—a comparative study of selective inhibitors. *J. Steroid Biochem. Molec. Biol.*, 54(5/6):273–9, 1995.

Iguchi, K et al. Myristoleic acid, a cytotoxic component in the extract from Serenoa repens, induces apoptosis and necrosis in human prostatic LNCaP cells, *Prostate*, 47:59–65, 2001.

Jommi, G et al. Alcohols isolated from lipophilic Serenoa repens extracts and their use for the treatment of prostate pathologies. *Chem. Abs.*, 111:#84073x, 1989.

Magdy, El-Sheikh M et al. The effect of Permixon on androgen receptors. *Obstet. Gynecol. Scand.*, 67:397–9, 1988.

Montagu, FAP. Serenoa serrulata—saw palmetto. *Elllingwood's Ther.*, 8:95, 1914.

Odenthal, KP. Phytotherapy of benign prostatic hyperplasia (BPH) with Curcurbita, Hypoxis, Pygeum, Urtica and Sabal serrulata (Serenoa repens). *Phytother. Res.*, 10:S141–3, 1996.

Otto, U et al. Transplantation of human benign hyperplastic prostate tissue into nude mice: first results of systemic therapy. *Urol. Int.*, 48:167–70, 1992.

Paubert-Braquet, M et al. Effect of Serenoa repens extract (Permixon®) on estradiol/testosterone-induced experimental prostate enlargement in the rat.. *Pharmacol. Res.*, 34(3/4):171–9, 1996.

Prager, N et al. A randomized, double-blind, placebo-controlled trial to determine the effectiveness of botanically drived inhibitors of 5-alpha-reductase in the treatment of androgenetic alopecia. *J. Alt. Compl. Med.*, 8(2):143–52, 2002.

Ravenna, L et al. Effects of the lipidosterolic extract of Serenoa repens (Permixon®) on human prostatic cell lines. *Prostate*, 29:219–30, 1996.

Reece Smith, H et al. The value of Permixon in benign prostatic hypertrophy. *Brit. J. Urol.*, 58:36–40, 1986.

Remzi, M et al. Abstract 103937. Am. Urolog. Assoc. 98th Annual Meeting, April 26, 2003.

Rhodes, L et al. Comparison of finasteride (Proscar®), a 5-alpha reductase inhibitor, and various commercial plant extracts in in vitro and in vivo 5-alpha reductase inhibition. *Prostate*, 22:43–51, 1993.

Schoepflin, G et al. Beta-sitosterol as a possible hormone of sabal fruits. *Planta med.*, 14:402–7, 1966. (*Chem. Abs.* 66:44265g)

Shimada, H et al. Biologically active acylglycerides from berries of saw-palmetto (Serenoa repens). *J. Nat. Prod.*, 60:417–8, 1997.

Showerman, JM. Saw palmetto (Sabula serrulata). *Ecl. Med. J.*, 52:432, 1892.

Strauch, G et al. Comparison of Finasteride) Proscar®) and Serenoa repens (Permixon ®) in the inhibition of 5-alpha reductase in healthy male volunteers. *Eur. Urol.*, 26:247–52, 1994.

Sultan, C et al. Inhibition of androgen metabolism and binding by a liposterolic extract of "Serenoa repens B" in human foreskin fibroblasts. *J. Steroid Biochem.*, 20:515–9, 1984.

Tarayre, JP et al. Anti-edematous action of an hexane extract from Serenoa repens Bartr. drupes. *Ann. Pharm. Fr.*, 41:559–70, 1983.

Tegarden, JL. Saw palmetto. *Ecl. Med. J.*, 58:653–4, 1898.

Vahlensieck, W Jr. et al. Benign prostatic hyperplasia – treatment with sabal fruit extract. A treatment study of 1,334 patients. *Fortschritte der Medizin*, 111:323–6, 1993.

Watkins, L. Saw palmetto. *Ecl. Med. J.*, 59:276–7, 1899.

Weisser, H et al. Enzyme activities in tissue of human bengin prostatic hyperplasia after three months treatment with the Sabal serrulata extract IDS 89 (Strogen®) or placebo. *Eur. Urol.*, 31:97–101, 1997.

Wilt, TJ et al. Saw palmetto extracts for treatment of benign prostatic hyperplasia. *JAMA*, 280(18): 1604–9, 1998.

Yamada, H et al. Effects of phytosterols on anti-complementary activity. *Chem. Pharm. Bull.*, 35:4851–5, 1987.

Wagner, H, Flachsbarth H. A new antiphlogistic principle from Sabal serrulata, I. *Planta Med.*, 41:244–51, 1981.

Wagner, H et al. A new antiphlogistic principle from Sabal serrulata, II. *Planta Med.*, 41:252–8, 1981.

Wagner, H et al. Immunostimulating polysaccharides (heteroglycans) of higher plants. *Arzneim.-Forsch.*, 35:1069–75, 1985.

Wilt, TJ et al. Beta-sitosterol for the treatment of benign prostatic hyperplasia: a systematic review. *B.J.U. Internat.*, 83:976–83, 1999.

6
IMMIGRANT HERBS
TRANSPLANTED TO AMERICA

When foreign herbs are adopted, their complete scope of application typically is utilized only in part. When compared to its central position in South Pacific culture and ethnic medicine, the limited applications in the West of kava illustrates this practice of reductionism. Kava has been the principle cultivated herb of the south Pacific for hundreds of years, and its multiple cultivars representing numerous phytochemical variations are appreciated for their different effects. A water maceration of a fresh pulverized root is the traditional method of preparation for kava root (*Piper methysticum*). This preparation has been used extensively with little adverse effects outside of scaly skin from chronic abuse. As a prime example of how adoption and adaptation can occur, Eclectics produced an alcoholic extract from the dried root for use in urinary tract conditions. Lately, concentrated alcohol and acetone extracts have become popular treatments for anxiety, irregardless of the variety of cultivar employed. It is unfortunate that liver problems recently associated with these concentrated extracts have sullied the reputation of all forms of preparations from this root.

Foreign herbs that have been standards in European practice through the ages also sometimes find limited use when they cross over to American shores. Even those physicians like the Physiomedicalists and Eclectics who utilized herbs exclusively or extensively did not fully incorporate knowledge of non-native plants into common practice. Herbs long popular in Europe were included in traditional American medicine, yet, understandably, these did not receive the same attention as those that are native to these shores. Naturopaths did use many Old World herbs due to the German origins of the profession. Eventually, with some herbs only certain aspects of their usefulness became magnified and widely advertised.

St. John's wort (*Hypericum perforatum*) and milk thistle or St. Mary's thistle (*Silybum marianum*, formerly *Carduus marianus*) were not considered important remedies in America until recently. However, the Eclectic physicians included these plants in their medical texts for a variety of uses, and their alcoholic extracts were manufactured by the Lloyd Brothers Pharmacists. Outside of Eclectic and naturopathic practice, their role had been relatively minor until modern science identified important pharmacological properties that enhanced the awareness of their potential in the medical realm.

St. John's wort has a long tradition in European medicine. Its topical use for wounds was among its most common applications, and this herb was considered one of the superior vulnerary remedies. Associations of this plant with the relief of morbid mental states led some to believe it possessed the power to overcome evil spirits. Such assessments were products of the worldview of medieval times. Modern appreciation of mental conditions as outcomes of disrupted neurochemistry has led to a clearer understanding of the effects of this plant. Its enhancement of detoxification reactions in the liver has led to potential problems for patients on pharmaceutical medications, but St. John's wort's own inherent safety is remarkable in comparison to similar-acting drugs.

St. Mary's thistle was long used as a food plant. However, since Rademacher designated the milk thistle fruit tincture as an organ-specific remedy for the liver in the 19th century, this has maintained its status as an important botanical medicine. However, milk thistle extract did not attain dominance in this area until fairly recently. Most liver tonics have been used for their effects on stimulating liver output of bile. As a protective and rejuvative agent for the liver, the concentrated silymarin fraction of milk thistle has been proven useful for both prevention and treatment of damage to this organ. The applications of this fraction are more limited than those of the traditional tincture and whole fruit, but its current importance is obvious in these times when exposure to a wide variety of liver toxins is becoming commonplace.

Utilization of these botanicals in European medicine has mostly gone the route of concentrated extracts. The emphasis on a single traditional application of these herbs has typically led to focusing on a particular fraction of an extract that appears most responsible for the effective treatment of that particular condition. In the process other bioactive components in the herb have been reduced, along with their therapeutic effects, to achieve a more limited composition aimed at a specific target. While retaining some of the activity of the whole complex botanical, such products have become more comparable to the isolated compounds that are the standards of medical practice than to the herbs from which they are derived.

SOUTH PACIFIC KAVA—
Challenging Facets of a Peaceful Beverage
Piper methysticum G. Forster. —roots and rhizomes

Summary

Kava juice extracted in water has long been used in the South Pacific as a tranquilizing beverage and is part of the indigenous culture on many of the islands. The people of these islands recognize the different effects of fresh versus dry root and between various kava cultivars that lead to specific preferences for different occasions and purposes. Each of the major kava lactone components has distinct properties, and the specific proportion of these lactones in each cultivar's roots largely determines the effects derived from the extract. Indiscriminate cultivar selection for product manufacturing contributes to unpredictable outcomes in spite of standardization to total kava lactones.

The growing popularity and commercialization of kava root and its extracts as an anti-anxiety agent and muscle relaxant has coincided with a lack of discrimination between the varieties and an emphasis on total kava lactone content. In addition, rather than water, chemical solvents such as acetone have been used commercially to increase extraction of kava lactones. Some manufacturers greatly concentrate the lactone content in their extracts. As a consequence, the content of non-lactone compounds in the extract are also necessarily altered, and effects are different from those produced by the traditional extract. An unfortunate example of the different effects is the liver toxicity that has been occasionally associated with use of concentrated extracts made with chemical solvents. This toxicity has not been documented with traditional preparations made by using water.

Names

The scientific name of kava, *Piper methysticum,* can be translated as "intoxicating pepper." Singh described kava, kava-kava, or kawa as the Polynesian names; it is sometimes called either ava or awa in Tahiti and Hawaii. On Polynesian islands the term kava refers to the taste that is described as sharp or pungent. Kava refers to both the plant and the drink made from the root. In Melanesia different names are used. It is called yagona in Fiji. In some islands of Vanuatu, its ancestral home, it is generally referred to as kava, while the people of other islands there call local varieties gea, gi, malohu, maluk, milik, or meruk. The spaces between the leaf stems, the leaf and stem color, and the quality of the root help determine identification by native names.

Wati is the most common term name used in Papua New Guinea, but its cultural importance on that island is not prominent.

A closely related wild species found only in the Melanesian islands of New Guinea, the Solomon Islands and Vanuatu, *Piper wichmannii*, is similar in appearance and contains active kava lactones. However, it root is harder and woody. Since *P. wichmanni* grows in the wild, it may have been the precursor for cultivated *P. methysticum*. This wild species is also called kava in some places where it grows.

Cultivars and Potency

Kava has long been cultivated, to the extent that it no longer reproduces sexually. As noted by Singh in 1992 and Lebot and others in 1997, many different cultivars are known by their outward appearance and preferred for different purposes by native users. Marked differences are noted between some cultivars regarding their psychotropic effects. In Hawaii Lebot and others in 1999 found at least 14 different names distinguish the cultivars. There are at least six cultivars in Samoa, seven in Tonga, four in Papua New Guinea, and twelve in Fiji. In Vanuatu 80 distinct cultivars known by 247 vernacular names are familiar to the traditional growers. The cultivar "borogu" is the favorite of Vanuatu native kava drinkers. All told there are about 120 distinct cultivars on 42 Pacific islands based on their structural characteristics and appearance.

Lebot and other found different cultivars grown in the same soil can vary greatly in their total kava lactone content. The Samoan varieties are considered to be much less potent. This may be due to differences in soil and climate that also affect potency. The green roots produce a much stronger drink, so for this reason the islanders in Vanuatu prefer the freshly harvested roots. Singh noted in Fiji the white varieties are considered the best but taken longer (more than 4 years) than black varieties (from 2.5–3 years) to attain maturity. As a consequence, the black varieties are more commonly cultivated for commercial sale.

Haensel and Lazar indicated that total kava lactone content of rhizomes from Fiji, Samoa, and Hawaii tested in a range from 5.5–8.8%. Lebot and others showed in 1999 that individual cultivars in Hawaii vary in total content, some rhizomes, or lateral roots, containing almost 21%. Kava lactone content diminishes steadily from the rhizomes to the rootstock, stump, and basal stem. The kava lactone content of stems and leaves is much less than the root and provide different proportions of lactones. Smaller roots have a higher concentration of lactones. Total kava lactones decrease when the plant is grown in shade but increase with soil fertility, irrigation and cultivation. Plant age is probably not a major factor after lactone content reaches it highest percentage at 18 months, though root size and total content continues to increase.

Traditional Applications

WATER EXTRACT

Kava juice in water is used in the South Pacific both ceremonially and as a relaxant for mind and body and to allay fatigue. The taste is sometimes described as bitter. After drinking kava there is a distinct numbness and astringent effect on the tongue and somewhat throughout the mouth which diminishes the sense of taste. Kava is therefore commonly used before meals, since food helps temper the effects. Kava is not consumed after eating, since the food then largely neutralizes the desired actions. Empirically, kava has a tranquilizing activity, pleasantly quieting the mind. In moderate active doses kava is not sedating, since thought processes remain clear though detached, leaving one disinclined to physical activity. Large doses produce drowsiness.

Kava's uses for medicinal purposes are many and varied. Some cultivars are used only to treat specific conditions. Many medical applications involve the leaves or stump; only the use of the root will be considered here. In Fiji kava water extract has been used for diarrhea and asthma. In Tahiti and Samoa kava drink is used for gonorrhea. In other areas of Polynesia the traditional kava root preparation has been drunk for chronic cystitis, dysmenorrhea, female puberty syndromes, weakness, headache, migraine in women's sicknesses, chills, pulmonary pains, and sleeping problems.

Eclectic Use for Genito-Urinary and Other Problems

ROOT POWDER

A paste of kava root powderon the lip produces both a burning sensation and feeling of numbness. Chewing the root for 15 minutes increases its local anesthetic effect. Kava root in doses from 325 mg up to four grams was used by Eclectic doctors for prostate troubles of old men with significant urinary discomfort. The root is used to relax menstrual cramps as well.

HYDROALCOHOLIC EXTRACTS

As indicated by Ellingwood in 1919 and Felter in 1922, besides acting as a diuretic, kava alcoholic extracts have been used for inflammation of the prostate, bladder and urethra. The efficacy is based on reducing congestion in the urinary tract and relieving inflammation. Kava lactones apparently produce a local and reflex anesthetic effect in the pelvic region by greatly diminishing the function of the pain-conducting nerves. The pain relief also helps explain the use of kava alcoholic extract for inflammation of the male genital tract and soreness or tenderness in the groin.

The basis for efficacy in these conditions is the muscular relaxation and anesthetic activity of the lactones of kava. Kava lactones and their metabolites are excreted in the urine of humans, as shown by Rasmussen and others in 1979 and Duffield and others in 1989. As the Eclectic Wilson indicated, the Specific Medicine was combined with those of saw palmetto and others to treat benign prostate enlargement. Part of its effectiveness in enlarged prostate problems is likely due to the presence of alcohol-soluble compounds identified by Gracza and Rubb in 1986 that includes five sterols and six fatty alcohols.

Eclectics also found the alcoholic extract can be helpful to enhance digestion, especially when stomach and intestinal upsets are associated with nervous irritability. The pain of different neuralgias especially involving the trigeminal nerve of the face, the eyes, ears, and other organs suffering from reflex pains can likewise be ameliorated. The alcoholic preparations are also of some value for vaginal and uterine pain, rheumatism, and chronic bronchitis.

FLUID EXTRACT

Lloyd described a standard process for manufacturing a satisfactory fluid extract using a 60% alcoholic solvent that removed the characteristic components. Shortly after kava's introduction to America around 1857, it was primarily given for treating gonorrhea in a dose from 0.3–2 ml. Ellingwood gave the dose of kava fluid extract as 10–60 minims (0.7–4 ml).

Traditional and Commercial Preparations

KAVA JUICE IN WATER

Traditionally, kava root is prepared as a cold water extract of the fresh roots. Preparation by chewing was especially common in Tonga, while pounding or grating was the first method used in Fiji. Incubation of the kava root with saliva from humans has been shown to increase kava extract potency. Pounding is now the most universally favored practice, either for an informal social setting or for a ceremonial ritual. The dried root is now sometimes used in Fiji, Samoa, and Tonga, while fresh root is demanded in Vanuatu where "nakamals" serve the fresh juice extracted in water. After kava root is scraped, it is cut into small pieces, then broken into fine particles with a mortar and pestle. After pounding, the root is placed in a bowl, and water is added. The kava maker kneads the kava as the extraction proceeds. He squeezes the soaked root through a strainer into a cup. The kava extract is then consumed.

In 1971 Csupor and Spaich demonstrated a principle with kava and several other medicinal plants known to Lloyd long before and applicable to many plant components considered to have minimal solubility in water. The solubility of the kava lactones kavain, methysticin and yangonin as isolated components was compared with their solubility as components of a complex kava extract. They showed that the solubility of these compounds in water was increased from 7–20 fold as components of the extract.

DRIED POWDERED ROOT

Drying reduces the weight of the fresh root by 80%. Commercial kava is ground. Duve and Prasad reported in 1981 that powdered roots/basal stems from Fiji were adulterated and lower in lactones than the dried unpowdered roots/basal stems. Hot water is used in Western cultures to extract the root for a quicker and stronger effect.

HYDROALCOHOLIC EXTRACTS

Kava lactones dissolve more completely in alcohol than in water. Kava root Specific Medicine used by Eclectics in the early 20th century was made by the Lloyd Brothers with 85% alcohol. Felter's dosage range was from 0.3–4 ml. Tinctures or other extracts made with water and alcohol have varied in strength and dosage but became popular kava products in Western countries.

CONCENTRATED LACTONE EXTRACTS AND FRACTIONS

Other toxic organic extracts such as acetone, chloroform, or ethyl acetate have been used to extract more of the lactone-containing resin than water which recovers only 5–10% of the amount of resin extracted by dichloromethane. In Europe a concentrated extract fraction called WS 1490, standardized to 70 mg kava lactones per 100 mg dry extract, has undergone a number of human studies.

Specific Root Lactones and Chemotypes

Kava contains over a dozen lactones, also referred to as alpha-pyrones. Of these kava lactones 96% are a mixture of kavain (K), methysticin (M), and yangonin (Y) and their major derivatives: dihydrokavain (DK), dihydromethysticin (DM), and demethoxyyangonin (DY). The four major kava lactones of any particular cultivar account for the vast majority of the total lactone content and determine the chemotype, or plants in a species with similar chemical makeup. For example, in Hawaii where kava was introduced from the South Pacific, K, M, DK, and Y (listed in decreasing order) together make up 91% of the total kava lactones in the dominant chemotype (I).

Specific kava lactones can distinguish certain island groups. Commercial samples from Vanuatu analyzed by Cheng and others contain the lactone 5-hydroxydihydrokavain that could not be found in any commercial Fijian dried (waka) or fresh roots. Fiji kava is relatively high in Y, and its cultivars have a higher percentage of M than those from Vanuatu. Most distinctions are based on profiles of kava lactones that describe different chemotypes that vary from one area to the next.

Lebot and others describe how the chemical differences between certain cultivars determine chemotypes. There are five main *P. methysticum* chemotypes (E-I) spread sporadically throughout the South Pacific and four minor ones for *P. wichmannii*

(A-D) that are only found in Melanesia. Three of the major ones (G, H, and I) are rich in K and are the more popular blends. Two (E and F) are very high in DM as well as DK, producing strong physiological effects including nausea. Chemotype E includes the cultivar referred to as "tudei" (two-day) because its potent effects can last several days, so it is not used daily. The E and F chemotypes are not widely used due to their inferior psychoactive properties.

Vanuatu has all five of the major *P. methysticum* chemotypes and one of the chemotypes of *P. wichmannii*. All four chemotypes of this wild species are very low in the lactone K and high in either varying proportions of DM and DK or in DY. Chemotype F is the only *P. methysticum* in Papua New Guinea. In Hawaii all but one of the different cultivars are of the chemotype I, though the total kava lactone content varies greatly between these cultivars.

The differences in distribution of chemotypes help map the spread of kava throughout the Pacific. The islands of Vanuatu, where chemotype G is generally preferred for daily use, are by far the most rich in chemotype diversity (A, E, F, G, H, and I). Therefore, Vanuatu was recognized by Lebot and others in 1997 as the origin of the species. These chemotypes were then introduced by migration variably through Melanesia, Micronesia, and Polynesia. While chemotype F was carried west to Papua New Guinea, the similar potent chemotype E made it east to Wallis & Futuna and Marquesas. Chemotype G was taken east with E to Tonga and along with the desirable H to Samoa. Chemotype I became established in Fiji, Samoa and Tahiti, while I and some E were transported north of Vanuatu to Micronesian Pohnpei, and via the aforementioned Polynesian islands to Hawaii.

According to Lebot and others the chemotypes used most frequently for their tranquilizing effects are G, H, and I. The "borogu" (G) and "kelai" (H) cultivars most popular with clients of Vanuatu nakamals (commercial kava vendors) are high in K and DK and low in DM. This may be due to the rapid absorption of K and DK that produces the most immediate pleasant psychoactive effects. For medicinal purposes the chemotype E cultivar "lalahk" high in DK and M is typically used.

Unless the particular chemotype is identified or relative amounts of the major lactones are documented, consistent effects from using kava cannot be expected when based on total lactone content or even a particular island of origin. To ensure consistent effects, a standard operating procedure should be followed using kava with the same chemotype and island of origin as well as established extraction and/or preservation processes.

Non-lactone Components of the Root

Besides lactones, other alcohol-soluble compounds identified by Gracza and Rubb in 1986 include five sterols, especially beta-sitosterol (16.6%), and the fatty alcohols hexadecanol (0.36%), octadecanol (0.53%), eicosanol (0.21%), docosanol (0.20%), tetracosanol (0.32%), and trans-phytol (1.05%). These compounds contribute to the prostate effects. Which other components add pharmacologically to the kava lactone effects is uncertain. The compound bornyl cinnamate has been identified in Fijian kava steam distillate and kava resin by Cheng and others. They also found two N-cinnamoyl pyrrolidine alkaloids in resin obtained from Fiji and Vanuatu. Other non-lactone compounds in kava root resin described by Hansel in 1997 include stigmasterol, flavokavin derivatives of chalcone, and an oxaporphine alkaloid they called cepharadion A. In addition a small amount of an unstable alkaloid, pipermethystine, is also in some roots, but it is found largely in the leaves.

Laboratory Animal Research—Root, Extracts, Fractions and Isolates

Hypnotic

ROOT POWDER

Animal studies by Klohs and others in 1959 provide some specific evidence about the activity of different forms of kava and its derivatives. For instance, the ground root does not protect against strychnine seizures, but it increased sleeping time induced by pentobarbital.

RESIN

Lipid-soluble extracts made with organic solvents like acetone are usually referred to as kava resin. By weight the resin extracted by dichloromethane by Jamieson and others was more active than the water extract in producing sleep in mice. Klohs and others found the resin extracted using chloroform increased sleeping time induced by pentobarbital.

LACTONES

DK and DM given orally to rodents have hypnotic effects. While Klohs and others showed all of the major lactones individually increased sleeping time induced by pentobarbital, DM was the most potent.

Tranquilizing/Depressant

WATER EXTRACT

In 1960 Hart and others injected a water extract into mice, rats and cats that reduced their activity and improved ease of handling without visible depression. Furguiele and others in 1965, injecting a water extract in mice, produced a depressant effect and reduces spontaneous motor activity.

RESIN

The dichloromethane resin extract was shown by Jamieson and others to reduce spontaneous activity in mice and the conditioned avoidance response in rats.

NON-LACTONE FRACTION

Lactone-free fractions of kava dissolved in water were shown in 1965 by O'Hara, Furgiuele and others and by Jamieson and others in 1989 to suppress spontaneous activity in mice.

Anesthetic/Analgesic

RESIN

Jamieson and others found the resin extracted by dichloromethane was more potent than the water extract in producing local anesthesia in mice. The resin reduces pain in mice and the conditioned avoidance response in rats.

NON-LACTONE FRACTION

Lactone-free fractions of kava dissolved in water were shown in 1965 by O'Hara and others and Furgiuele and others and by Jamieson and others in 1989 to produce pain relief in mice.

LACTONES

The lactone components applied by Meyer and May produced local anesthetic effects on rabbit eyes without toxicity. The lactones were shown by Jamieson and Duffield in 1990[a] to produce analgesia in mice via non-opiate pathways.

Hormonal

FATTY ALCOHOLS

Debat showed that docosanol and other alcohols with more than sixteen carbon atoms were active against prostate enlargement through examination of the periphery of the prostate.

Muscle Relaxant/Anticonvulsant

WATER EXTRACT

O'Hara and others in the same year tested the water extract and its lactones; these relaxed contractions of isolated rat uterus by blocking the transmitter serotonin. Kretzschmar and Meyer found the same for guinea-pig intestine in 1969. In 1983 Singh showed the water extract causes muscle relaxation in mice by a direct action on muscle rather than by inhibiting nerve impulse transmission to the muscle.

RESIN

The dichloromethane resin extract tested by Jamieson and others was more active than the water extract in producing muscle relaxation in mice. Klohs and others found the resin extracted using chloroform protected against strychnine seizures.

LACTONES

The most characteristic effect of the lactones is to produce muscle relaxation in all laboratory animal species tested. Skeletal muscle relaxation produced by large doses of kava lactones results in ataxia and an ascending paralysis, followed by complete recovery. M and DM were shown by Klohs and others in 1959 to protect mice from convulsive death caused by toxic doses of strychnine, while K and DK were partly effective and Y and DY almost inactive. However, synergism is shown when a combination of all six produced the same effect as DM, though it only accounted for 6% of the total content. Meyer reported that K, DK, Y, and DY are all anticonvulsants against electroshock seizures in mice. Y and DY act synergistically with the other lactones to lower body temperature, relax muscles, and prevent convulsions. While K and DK produce their maximum anticonvulsive effect rapidly (after 10 min.) and for a short period (40–60 min.), M and DM have a stronger anticonvulsive activity that is delayed (for 45–60 min.) and prolonged (2–4 hrs.) as shown by Kretzschmar and others in 1969. Y's maximum effect is much less potent and even more delayed (2 hrs.).

Cerebral Kinetics

LACTONES VERSUS RESIN

A study by Keledjian and others in 1988 exemplified the pharmacokinetic differences and demonstrated the contrast between complex extracts and isolated compounds. They measured kava pyrone concentrations in the brain after injection individually in mice. Both K and DK quickly reached high levels in the brain in 5 minutes and were rapidly eliminated, while Y and DY were slowly and poorly absorbed and eliminated in brain tissue. When kava resin was injected, K was absorbed twice as fast and Y twenty times as fast as when they were injected individually, in contrast to DK and DY for which the same percentages were absorbed.

Isozyme Inhibition

SOLID EXTRACT

Inhibition of cytochrome P450 isozymes 1A2, 2C9, 2C19, 2D6, 3A4, and 4A9/11 by powdered kava extract was demonstrated in laboratory tests by Mathews and others in 2002.

LACTONES

Mathews and others also suggested the inhibition of 2C9, 2C19, 2D6, and 3A4 as shown in laboratory tests by the kavalactones dihydromethysticin and methysticin may contribute to increased circulating levels of hepatotoxins when cultivars such as "tudei" that are high in these two kavalactones are used. Kavain did not inhibit any of these enzymes.

Human Studies—
Solid Extracts, Fractions and Kavain for Sleep/Anxiety/Menopause

STANDARDIZED EXTRACTS AND CONCENTRATED LACTONE FRACTIONS

In a study by Emser and Bartylla with twelve healthy people 100 mg three times daily of kava acetone extract fraction WS 1490 increased the amount of deep sleep and tended to decrease the time it took to fall asleep and to wake. Contrary to normal sedative effects, as shown when Munte and others compared to the benzodiazepine drug oxazepam, kava extract fraction WS 1490 improved word recognition in a test of twelve healthy volunteers.

A meta-analysis by Pittler and Ernst in 2000 of seven randomized, placebo-controlled, double-blind studies of 377 total patients with anxiety syndrome not caused by psychotic disorders showed kava extracts taken by mouth reduced anxiety symptoms. Three of these used WS 1490 at doses of 300 mg (210 mg total lactones) daily, two consume 300 mg of a different kava extract (60 mg total lactones) daily, and two used still other kava extracts of 800 mg (240 mg lactones) and 450 mg (150 mg lactones) daily. In other words four separate extracts and doses with varying kava lactone content supplying from 60–240 mg kava daily were all effective. Fourteen patients noted mild adverse side effects including restlessness, tiredness, stomach upset, and headache.

In 1997 Schultz and others described two double-blind controlled clinical studies with standardized extracts containing 15% kava lactones (30–60 mg/day total kava lactones). These doses achieved significant relief of menopausal symptoms along with improved peri-operative well-being. Four other double-blind controlled studies reviewed used the acetone-water extract fraction standardized to 70% kava lactones. These found significant relief of menopausal symptoms or anxiety syndrome when doses were 210 mg/day of kava lactones. These comparisons appears to suggest that the more the kava lactones are concentrated and purified, the higher their effective dose becomes.

Anxiety has been associated with an increased risk of heart attacks, coronary heart disease, and sudden cardiac death. In 2001 Watkins and others administered a dose of 280 mg daily for four weeks of a kava extract standardized to 30% kavalactones to observe vagal control of heart rate in 13 patients with generalized anxiety disorder. Excluding those with hypertension that interferes with baroreceptor control, they found that 4 of 5 in the kava group had increased baroreflex control of heart rate compared to 1 of 6 in the placebo group. This improved control of heart rate correlated significantly with improved anxiety scores.

KAVAIN

Schultz and others also mentioned nine double blind studies using synthetic (dl)-kavain (K), two comparing K to drugs and seven to placebos, in which therapeutic result were similar to the pharmaceutical kava extracts. However, doses of the single isolated lactone K were quite high, ranging from 200–600 mg daily.

Adverse Effects

Regular use of kava products for more than three months should be avoided unless consulting a physician to avoid developing a consumption habit. Prolonged abuse can result in a scaly eruption of the skin that occurs after several months to a year of regular use of traditional preparations as documented by Norton and Ruze. Keller and Klohs discovered that the lactone DM at doses of 300–800 mg/day caused a high percentage of patients to develop an exfoliative dermatitis similar in nature to what occurred in those who regularly consumed excessive amounts of the beverage.

Increases in a liver enzyme (GGT) indicative of potential damage were associated with very heavy, non-traditional, and essentially abusive kava beverage consumption by 35 in an Australian Aboriginal community by Mathews and others in 1988. The average use of dried kava root was from 310–440 grams/week over a long period of time (years). However, this occurred in a population where prior alcohol abuse was evident. The researchers also noted that there was no evidence of the liver enzyme being increased in four people who consumed as much as 100 grams of dried root per week as a tea, equivalent to almost a half-ounce daily. In a review by Cairney and others in 2002 they described a more recent study identifying Australian Aboriginal heavy users who were estimated to consume water extracts of at least 610 grams of kava powder per week, equivalent to about 76 grams of lactones weekly. This would exceed the recommended therapeutic dose by more than 50 times.

Cases of acute liver toxicity from the use of WS 1490, the concentrated kava lactone extract, have also been reported by Escher and others and Russmann and others in 2001. Other reports of liver damage with high-lactone extracts were reported by Strahl and others and Kraft and others in the German literature in 1998 and 2001, respectively. The exact chemical compound(s) responsible for these events has not been established. According to Neil-Jones in 2001, the "tudei" cultivar was grown in Vanuatu by the German company that produced WS 1490. Even though all reports of adverse effects were related to use of concentrated extracts made with nonpolar solvents (unlike water) from dried roots, a ban on the sale of all kava and its products by the German government in 2002 followed multi-national warnings against the use of any kava-containing products, rather than the offending extracts.

In 2003 Dragull and others describe how analysis of the stem peelings and leaves of the kava plant demonstrated that these parts contain an alkaloid identified as pipermethystine. Its concentration in freshly prepared basal stem peelings from Hawaiian kava ranged from 0.09 to 0.85%. Based on similar compounds, this alkaloid and its breakdown products are suspected of possibly contributing to liver toxicity. Reportedly, some European pharmaceutical companies traded in Fiji for basal stem peelings to extract. These inexpensive peelings are not used by the Fiji natives but contain high levels of kava lactones dihydrokavain, dihydromethysticin, and tetrahydroyangonin. No pipermethystine has been found in commercial root powders from Fiji, Tonga, or Hawaii by routine gas chromatography or high performance liquid chromatography.

Observations by Balick and Lee in 2002 confirm that any possible liver toxicity is unlikely associated with the consumption of kava lactones per se. They describe the regular use of traditionally prepared kava on the Micronesian island of Pohnpei where it is called "sakau." Sakau is prepared by pounding the fresh lateral roots for ten minutes or more, adding water, and squeezing the liquid through fibers into a coconut half-shell cup. They documented on average that women sakau drinkers consumes 7.72 cup per sitting (taking about 4.27 hours), while men drink 8.87 cups over 5.36 hours. Based on an average content of 250 mg of kava lactones per cup, the typical daily consumption is around 2,400 mg kava lactones, or eight times the recommended European dose. Based upon Dr. Lee's experience practicing medicine in Micronesia, the occurrence of hepatotoxicity is not prevalent in the region.

However, the most recent case reports by Russmann and others in 2003 indicate that two South Pacific women in their 50s from New Caledonia developed icterus after 4–5 weeks of drinking up to 4 cups daily (18 grams of kava lactones/week) of water extracts made from dried kava. Elevated serum transaminase and bilirubin levels confirmed hepatitis, and drug, alcohol, and viral causes were ruled out. Both returned to normal three months after stopping kava consumption, and neither were poor CYP 2D6 metabolizers as was associated with some German cases. The authors surveyed heavy kava drinkers (about 32 grams kava lactones/week) of New Caledonia in good general health. They found that 23 of 27 had elevated GGT liver enzyme with no liver disease, but 15 had dry skin. Four who then greatly reduced kava use had normal skin and GGT after one month. The authors concluded that the evidence suggests a rare allergenic idiosyncrasy in those who suffer liver toxicity from kava.

Contraindications

It is believed that kava products are best avoided during pregnancy and by nursing mothers. Operating a motor vehicle following excessive use of the root or its extracts should be avoided because of possible impaired driving ability. Theoretically, high doses of kava resin should be avoided in severe depression, so as not to aggravate suicidal tendencies.

Table 10   Kava Root and Derivatives—Summary of Medicinal Uses and Pharmacology

KAVA *Piper methysticum* G. Forster.	Traditional South Pacific Uses	Eclectic Medical Uses	Modern Clinical Studies	Laboratory Research Findings
Whole Root/ Rhizomes		Enlarged prostate Oral anesthetic Uterine cramps		Hypnotic
Water Extracts	Asthma Chills Cystitis Diarrhea Dysmenorrhea Fatigue Gonorrhea Headaches Insomnia Weakness			Muscle relaxant Tranquilizing
Tincture or Specific Medicine (Hydro- alcoholic)		Bronchitis Cystitis Dysmenorrhea Enlarged prostate GU* anesthetic Nervous Indigestion Neuralgias Rheumatism Urethritis		
Solid Extract (Hydro- alcoholic)			Anxiety Menopause	

Continued on next page

Table 10   *Continued*

KAVA *Piper methysticum* G. Forster.	Traditional South Pacific Uses	Eclectic Medical Uses	Modern Clinical Studies	Laboratory Research Findings
FRACTIONS AND ISOLATED CONSTITUENTS				
Lactone / Resin Concentrates (Acetone, chloroform, dichloromethane)			Anxiety Promotes sleep	Analgesic Anesthetic Anti-convulsant Tranquilizing Hypnotic Muscle relaxant
Lactone-Free Fractions				Analgesic Tranquilizing Hormonal
Kava Lactones			Anxiety	Analgesic Anti-convulsant Hypnotic Muscle relaxant

* Genito-Urinary

Heavy consumption of kava beverage can cause severe, recurrent spasmodic movements of the limbs, trunk, neck and face following kava bingeing as reported by Spillane and others in 1997. The use of WS 1490 or another concentrated kava extract led to involuntary muscle movements associated with dopamine antagonism in three patients and aggravated Parkinsonianism in a fourth. It should be avoided in Parkinson's disease and used with caution in the elderly.

Drug Interactions

Schelosky and others reported in 1995 that kava extract taken in 150 mg doses twice daily for ten days reduced the effect of the drug levodopa in Parkinson's disease in one human case, seemingly due to its dopamine antagonism. The antagonism was not evident two days after stopping the kava extract. The benzodiazepine alprazolam seemed to have been enhanced by a kava product in another isolated case report by Almeida and Grimsley in 1996.

Herberg claimed in 1993 that kava extract WS 1490 given in 100 mg doses three times daily to men and women together with alcohol showed no additional negative effects. However, in a 1997 study with forty healthy men and women Foo and Lemon compared equal numbers using kava, alcohol, both, or placebo. They found sedation, cognition, co-ordination, and intoxication produced by alcohol were increased when one gm/kg of kava was taken by mouth.

Animal studies support some human findings. Kava resin was shown by Jamieson and Duffield in 1990[b] to greatly increase the sedative effect of alcohol in mice. As previously noted, in mice kava resin (chloroform extract) and lactones both increased sleeping time from pentobarbital. In 1989 PH Duffield and others found both kava resin (dichloromethane extract) high in lactones and a lactone-free aqueous fraction reduced hypermotility in mice caused by amphetamine.

Laboratory test tube studies by Seitz and others in 1997 indicate that kava lactones inhibit monoamine oxidase in platelets and reduce monoamine uptake in brain tissue. Therefore, its use may increase certain effects of pharmaceutical monoamine oxidase inhibitors used to treat depression such as deprenyl, clorgyline and pargyline. Another test tube study by Gleitz and others in 1997 with platelets resulted in kavain reducing platelet aggregation, which may increase the potential for bleeding when taking anticoagulants like warfarin.

References

BOOKS

Anon. *Dose Book*, Lloyd Brothers, Pharmacists Inc., Cincinnati, Ohio, 1932.

Ellingwood, F. *American Materia Medica, Therapeutics and Pharmacog.*, [1919], EMP, Sandy, OR, 1994.

Felter, HW. *Eclectic Materia Medica, Pharmacology and Therapeutics* [1922], EMP, Sandy, OR, 1994.

Lebot, V, Merlin M, Lindstrom L. *Kava The Pacific Elixir*, Healing Arts Press, Rochester, VT. 1997.

Weiss, RF. *Herbal Medicine*, Beaconsfield Pub. Ltd, Beaconsfield, Eng., 1988.

Wilson, C. *Useful Prescriptions*, Lloyd Brothers, Pharmacists, Inc., Cincinnati, 1935.

ARTICLES

Almeida, JC and Grimsley, EW. Coma from the health food store: Interaction between kava and alprazolam. *Ann. Int. Med.*, 125(11):940, 1996.

Balick, MJ and Lee, R. Traditional use of sakau (kava) in Pohnpei: Lessons for intergrative medicine. *Altern. Ther.*, 8(4):96–8, 2002.

Cairney, S et al. The neurobehavioural effects of kava. *Austral. N. Zeal. J. Psychiat.*, 36:657–62, 2002.

Cawte, J. Psychoactive substances of the South Seas: betel, kava and pituri. *Austr. NZ J. Psychiatry,* 19:83–7, 1985.

Cheng, D et al. Identification by methane chemical ionization gas chromatography/mass spectrometry of the products obtained by steam distillation and aqueous acid extraction of commercial Piper methysticum. *Biomed. Environ. Mass Spectrom.,* 17(5):371–6, 1988.

Csupor, L and Spaich, W. Galenicals or pure substances. 1. Solubility tests with pure substances and dry extracts. *Pharm. Ind.,* 33(1):15–17, 1971. [in German] (*Chem. Abs.* 75:25327y).

Dayton, A. UH scientists may have solved kava mystery. *The Honolulu Advertiser,* Monday, Apr. 7, 2003.

Debat, J. Higher alkanol compositions and the use thereof in treatment of prostate disorders. *Chem. Abs.,* 93:7655w, 1980.

Dragull, K. et al. Piperidine alkaloids from Piper methysticum. *Phytochem.,* 63:193–198, 2003.

Duffield, AM et al. Identification of some human urinary metabolites of the intoxicating beverage kava. *J. Chromatogr.,* 475:273–81, 1989.

Duffield, PH et al. Effect of aqueous and lipid-soluble extracts of kava on the conditioned avoidance response in rats. *Arch. Int. Pharmacodyn.,* 301:81–90, 1989.

Duve, RN and Prasad, J. Quality evaluation of yaqona (Piper methysticum). *Fiji Agric. J.,* 43(1):1–8, 1981. (*Chem. Abs.* 98:105940h).

Emser, W and Batylla, K. Improvement in quality of sleep: Effect of kava extract WS 1490 on the sleep patterns in healthy people. *TW Neurologie Psychiatrie,* 5:636–42, 1991. [in German]

Escher, M et al. Hepatitis associated with kava, a herbal remedy for anxiety. *Br. Med. J.,* 322:139, 2001.

Foo, H and Lemon, J. Acute effects of kava, alone or in combination with alcohol, on subjective measures of impairment and intoxication and on cognitive performance. *Drug Alcohol Rev.,* 16:147–155, 1997.

Furgiuele, AR et al. Central activity of aqueous extracts of Piper methysticum (kava). *J. Pharm. Sci.,* 54:247–52, 1965.

Gleitz, AJ et al. Antithrombotic action of the kava pyrone (+)-kavain prepared from Piper methysticum on human platelets. *Planta Med.,* 63:27–30, 1997.

Gracza, L and Ruff P. Aliphatic and alicyclic alcohols of Piperis methystici rhizoma. *Arch. Pharm. (Weinheim, Ger.),* 319:475–7, 1986. [in German] (*Chem. Abs.* 104:230306z).

Haensel, R and Lazar, J. Kava pyrones. Composition of Piper methysticum rhizomes in plant derived sedatives, *Dtsch. Apoth. Ztg.,* 125:2056–8, 1985. [in German] (*Chem. Abs.* 104:74869c).

Haensel, R. Kava-kava (Piper methysticum G. Forster) in contemporary medical research. *Eur. J. Herb. Med.,* 3(3):17–23, 1997-8.

Hart, ER et al. Synaptic & behavioral actions of a water percolate of kava (Piper methysticum). *Pharmacologist,* 2:72, 1960.

Herberg, KW. Effect of Kava-Special Extract WS 1490 combined with ethyl alcohol on safety-relevant performance parameters. *Blutalkohol,* 30(2):96–105, 1993. [in German].

Jamieson, DD et al. Comparison of the central nervous system activity of the aqueous and lipid extract of kava (Piper methysticum). *Arch. Int. Pharmacodyn. Ther.,* 301:66–80, 1989.

Jamieson, DD and Duffield, PH. The antinociceptive actions of kava components in mice. *Clin. Expl. Pharmacol. Physiol.,* 17:495–507, 1990a.

Jamieson, DD and Duffield, PH. Positive interaction of ethanol and kava resin in mice. *Clin. Expl Pharmacol. Physiol.,* 17:509–14, 1990b.

Keledjian, J et al. Uptake into mouse brain of four compounds present in the psychoactive beverage kava. *J. Pharmaceut. Sci.,* 77(12):1003–6, 1988.

Keller, F and Klohs, MW. A review of the chemistry and pharmacology of the constituents of Piper methysticum, *Lloydia,* 26:1–15, 1963.

Klohs, MW et al. A chemical and pharmacological investigation of Piper methysticum Forst. *J. Med. Pharm. Chem.,* 1(1):95–103, 1959.

Kraft, M et al. Fulminant liver failure after administration of the herbal antidepressant kava-kava. *Dtsch. Med. Wschr.,* 126:970–2, 2001.

Kretzschmar, R and Meyer, HJ. Comparative studies on the anticonvulsive activity of pyrone compounds from Piper methysticum, *Arch. Int. Pharmacodyn. Ther.,* 177:261-77, 1969. [in German] (*Chem. Abs.* 72:30057c).

Kretzschmar, R et al. Spasmolytic activity of aryl substituted α-pyrones and aqueous extracts of Piper methysticum, *Arch. Int. Pharmacodyn. Ther.,* 180:475–91, 1969. [in German] (*Chem. Abs.* 72:20254a).

Kretzschmar, R et al. Strychnine antagonistic potency of pyrone compounds of the kava root (Piper methysticum Forst.). *Experientia,* 26(3):283–284, 1970.

Lebot, V et al. Morphological, phytochemical, and genetic variation in Hawaiian cultivars of 'ava (kava, Piper methysticum, Piperaceae). *Econ. Bot.,* 53(4)::407–18, 1999.

Lloyd, JU. New remedies—Piper methysticum. *Ecl. Med. J.,* 38:112–5, 1878.

Mathews, JD et al. Effects of the heavy usage of kava on physical health: summary of a pilot survey in an Aboriginal community. *Med. J. Austral.,* 148:548–55, 1988.

Mathews, JM et al. Inhibition of human cytochrome P450 activities by kava extract and kavalactones. *Drug Metabol. Dispos.,* 30(11):1153–1157, 2002.

Meyer, HJ. Pharmacology of kava. *Ethnopharmacol. Search Psychoact. Drugs, [Proc. Symp.],* pp. 133-40, 1979. (*Chem. Abs.* 92:121862r).

Meyer, HJ and Kretzschmar, R. Kawa pyrones: a new group of components in central muscle relaxing agents of the mephenesin type. *Klin. Wochschr.,* 44:902–3, 1966. [in German] (*Chem. Abs.* 65:12750g).

Meyer, HJ and May, HU. Local anesthetic properties of natural kava pyrones. *Klin. Wochschr.,* 42:407, 1964. (*Chem. Abs.* 61:9932c).

Mohr, H. Treatment of irritable bladder in women. Experiences with "Cystokapseln"—Fink. *Munch. Med. Wochens.,* 112:858–60, 1970.

Munte, TF et al. Effects of oxazepam and an extract of kava roots (Piper methysticum) on event-related potentials in a word recognition task. *Neuropsychobio.,* 27:46–53, 1993.

Neil-Jones, M. Kava industry faces liver scare. *Pacific Magazine / PINA Nius Online,* Nov. 27, 2001.

Norton, SA and Ruze, P. Kava dermopathy. *J. Am. Acad. Dermatol.,* 31:89–97, 1994.

O'Hara, MJ et al. Preliminary characterization of aqueous extracts of Piper methysticum (kava, kawa kawa). *J. Pharm. Sci.*, 54:1021–5, 1965.

Pittle, MH and Ernst, E. Efficacy of kava extract for treating anxiety: systematic review and meta-analysis. *J. Clin. Psychopharm.*, 20(1):84–9, 2000.

Rasmussen, AK et al. Metabolism of some kava pyrones in the rat. *Xenobiotica*, 9(1):1–16, 1979.

Russmann, S et al. Hepatic injury due to traditional aqueous extracts of kava root in New Caledonia. *Eur. J. Gastroenterol. Hepatol.*, 15:1033–036, 2003.

Russmann, S et al. Kava hepatotoxicity. *Ann. Int. Med.*, 135(1):68–9, 2001.

Ruze, P. Kava-induced dermopathy: a niacin deficiency? *Lancet*, 335(8703):1442–5, 1990.

Schelosky, L et al. Kava and dopamine antagonism. *J. Neurol. Neurosurg. Psychiatry*, 58(5):639–40, 1995.

Schulz, V et al. Clinical trials with Phyto-Psychopharmacological agents. *Phytomed.*, 4(4):379–387, 1997.

Seitz, U et al. [^{3}H]-Monoamine uptake inhibition properties of kava pyrones. *Planta Med.*, 63:548–9, 1997.

Sherman, SM. Piper methysticum. *Ecl. Med. J.*, 66:393-4, 1906.

Singh, YN. Effects of kava on neuromuscular transmission and muscle contractility. *J. Ethnopharmacol.*, 7:267–76, 1983.

Singh, YN. Kava: an overview. *J. Ethnopharmacol.*, 37:13–45, 1992.

Spillane, PK et al. Neurological manifestations of kava intoxication. *Med. J. Austral.*, 167:1723, 1997.

Strahl, et al. Necrotizing hepatitis after taking herbal medication (extracts of kava or of common or lesser celandine). *Dtsch. Med. Wschr.*, 123:1410–4, 1998. [in German].

Uebelhack, R et al. Inhibition of platelet MAO-B by kava pyrone-enriched extract from Piper methysticum Forster (kava-kava). *Pharmacopsychiat.*, 31:187–92, 1998.

Watkins, LL et al. Effect of kava extract on vagal cardiac control in generalized anxiety disorder: preliminary findings. *J. Psychopharmacol.*, 15:283–6, 2001.

ST. JOHN'S WORT—Driving Away the Demons of Depression
Hypericum perforatum L. —flowering tops

Summary

The use of St. John's wort in the Old World spans millennia. Throughout Western medicine the herb and its extracts have been used to enhance the function of the liver, relieve chest congestion, and relieve mental disturbances. Secondarily, it was known to ease problems with urinary and menstrual function. The oil extract has long been renowned for the topical treatment of injuries.

The rich phytochemical complexity accounts for much of its usefulness. The photosensitizing component hypericin is problematic for animals grazing the herb under the sun, but it also helps overcome the growth of multiple viruses. Another active compound, hyperforin, not only has local antimicrobial properties but affects neuotransmitters associated with depression. St. John's wort is rich in flavonoids, carotenoids, and procyanidins that enhance such activities and/or reduce the photoxicity.

Extracts and fractions vary in their effects based on the relative content of the specific phytochemicals available in St. John's wort. Those products known to contain significant amount of hyperforin appear to be most effective for depression, though other components contribute to its antidepressant efficacy. Hyperforin also appears to be largely responsible for increasing drug metabolism, while hypericin reduces drug absorption. Hypericin in very large amounts is known to increase photosensitivity. However, the powerful benefits outweigh the relative risks when other medications or photosensitizers are not being used. In other cases potential interactions must be evaluated and avoided when using this valuable herb.

Names and Distribution

The name *Hypericum* is believed to be derived from the Greek words *hyper* meaning "over" and *eikon* indicating "image." This has led to speculation as recorded by Grieve that it means "over an apparition," referring to its power over evil spirits. Lucas claimed the term described the value of the plant as beyond imagination. Others report the herb was placed above holy pictures as a talisman for keeping evil out of homes. The medicinal species name *perforatum* refers to the translucent glands on the leaves.

A common name for this plant throughout the Middle Ages was *fuga demonum*, or the "devil's scourge." Lucas recalls old German names for the herb that refer to its mysterious applications. *Jagdenteufel* refers to "chase the devil," while *teufelsflucht* means "devil's flight." The plant was hung in front of some houses in Europe to protect against evil spirits. Historically, dark thoughts that dwell in disturbed minds were ascribed to a demon. It's no wonder that the plant has been found to be effective for treating nervous and depressive states.

Its common name of St. John's wort also has a variety of explanations. Wort is the English term for plant. The flowers begin to bloom around the end of June and are associated with the June 24 feast of St. John the Baptist's birthday on the Catholic calendar. Maria Treben relates that maidens twisted the flowering plants into garlands that they wore while dancing around the fire on this St. John's night. The red drops of exudate that form when the tops are picked are also likened to the blood of the Baptist who was beheaded.

This species is native to Europe, western Asia, and North Africa. It was introduce to Australia and North America where it now flourishes as a weed and is often treated on ranches with herbicides. It is especially abundant in the Pacific Northwest, where it is known as Klamath weed. There are 370 species in the genus throughout the world. Some such as *H. maculatum* are used at times as spurious substitutes.

Ancient Greek Uses

Pitman reports that in the Hippocratic Corpus *Hypericum* was used with complementary herbs for lung conditions involving fever with blood or pus in the sputum. It was also given with other herbs for summer jaundice associated with grievances. In her review of Dioscorides herbal, *De Materia Medica*, she notes he discusses three other species besides Askuron (*H. perforatum*): Uperikon (*H. crispum*), Androsaimon (*H. perfoliatum*), and Koris (*H. coris*). The primary use indicated here was for treating wounds and burns, as well as giving it in wine for malarial fever, and the seed being used for sciatica. Uperikon was considered diuretic and an emmenagogue.

English Applications

An oil made with the flowers was listed in the first *Pharmacopoeia Londonensis* in 1618. In 1633 Gerard stated this St. John's wort balm was without equal for wounds, burns, ulcers and bites. In 1653 Culpepper noted the herb is aperative and diuretic, useful for malaria, and an excellent vulnerary. Externally it was for bruises and wounds when boiled in wine, or made into an ointment for obstructions, swellings, and closing wounds. He recommended a tincture of the flowers in wine for melancholy and madness. The decoction of herb, flowers, and seeds was drunk in wine to allay vomiting and spitting blood and the bites of venomous creatures. The seed in warm wine was taken for sciatica and palsy. English uses were in accord with Greek precedent.

Maude Grieve, a more recent British author writing in 1931, described St. John's wort as astringent, expectorant, and nervine. She recommended its external use in fomentations for hard swellings, caked breasts, and ecchymosis. She noted its use in all pulmonary complaints, dysentery, diarrhea and worms. She used it as a remedy for hemorrhages including spitting blood and for jaundice. For bladder problems and urine suppression, as well as bedwetting children, a tea can be used. She also recommends the fluid extract and oil. Its nervine properties are applicable in hysteria and nervous depression. In other words she maintained a consistent endorsement of traditional uses.

German Folk Applications

With the release of his book in 1886 Fr. Sebastian Kneipp popularized this European herbal folk remedies as part of his approach to natural healing. Regarding St. John's wort he noted that it was often referred to as "witch's herb," or *hexenkraut*, and observed: "Now-a-days both itself and its services are quite forgotten." He claimed a tea made from the herb especially influenced the liver, eliminating morbid matter observable in the urine. Head complaints associated with catarrh, stomach spasms, and lungs afflicted with phlegm were all relieved by the tea. He also recommended it for bedwetting children.

Maria Treben, a recent Austrian herbalist and follower of Kneipp's practices, expanded his application of St. John's wort tea. As a female regulator she advised 2 cups daily for a while during puberty to promote regular menstruation. She gave the tea for nerve injuries caused by trauma, as well as neuralgias, recommending 2–3 cups be sipped daily and the oil be rubbed in locally. For nervous complaints, neuritis, neurosis, and nervous debility, she gave the tincture. She used the tea for hysterics, speech disorders and depression and various night-time problems such as insomnia, fitful sleep, sleep walking, and bedwetting. For these nervous complaints, along with the tea she advocated a warm sitz bath in the dilute tea each week, followed by six consecutive days of foot baths.

In her 1980 book, Treben was an enthusiastic promoter of St. John's wort flowers infused into olive oil until it turned red. Used not only for open wounds, she also applied it to all injuries, glandular swellings, colic, sore back and lower back, sciatica, and rheumatism. For sunburns, burns, and scalds she used an infusion of the flowers in linseed oil instead.

American Adoption

Those who maintained the European herbal tradition with this plant in America in the 20th century include the Eclectics, one of the later Physiomedicalists, plus early and later naturopaths. Like others in America, the Eclectics utilized St. John's wort flowering tops and leaves but considered it a minor remedy in their armementarium. In 1898 Felter and Lloyd noted that it imparted its properties to water, alcohol or oil. For the conditions treated they noted the doses for the powdered herb, the infusion, and the tincture. The components noted were a volatile oil, resin, tannic acid and a red coloring principle. They considered it astringent, sedative, and diuretic and used it for suppressed urine, diarrhea, dysentery, worms, jaundice, spitting blood, and menorrhagia. They emphasized its power of the nervous system in is application for hysteria, throbbing of the whole body in nervous individuals, and nervous affections with depression. Ellingwood in 1919 listed doses for the powder, tincture and fluid extract and suggested 2 drops every 4 hours was valuable for treating hemorrhoids.

Felter and Lloyd noted that Scudder used it for its homeopathic indications of injuries to the spine and lacerations or puncture wounds of the limbs, and it was utilized by Webster for spinal irritation with burning pain. Ellingwood observed that homeopaths used it internally and externally for irritation, soreness, or chronic disease with tenderness of the spinal column or trauma to the spinal cord.

Externally, the Eclectics used *Hypericum* as a fomentation or ointment for hard swellings, caked breasts, bruises, ecchymosis, and ulcers. The flowers infused in oil were used as an ointment in these cases. As described by Felter and Lloyd, the fresh herb was used to produce a saturated tincture with 76% alcohol for topical application for bruises and other injuries as arnica was commonly used.

The physiomedical authority William Cook, M.D., did not include it in his *Physiomedical Dispensatory* in 1869. However, in 1905 R. Swinburne Clymer noted the use of the tea primarily for bedwetting. Picked in full bloom and used fresh or dried as a tea, he found it a favorite remedy for stomach ailments. It was also tinctured in whiskey for this use and as a liver corrector, either alone or combined with gentian. In these recommendations he appeared to be following the lead of Kneipp and foreshadowed its reputation of enhancing liver detoxification via isozyme induction.

The founder of naturopathy in America at the beginning of the 20th century, Benedict Lust, admittedly obtained his recommendations directly from his mentor, Fr. Kneipp. Along this line he noted that in the past it was known to be a herb that witches (herbally crafty women) used to banish disease. He advised its use as a liver remedy and for constipation, as well as mucus congestion in the chest and lungs. He used the tea to cure bedwetting. His nephew, John Lust, in 1974 likewise mentioned the tea of the flowers being useful for headache, insomnia, chest congestion, and jaundice, as well as uterine cramping and other menstrual difficulties. Its calming properties were considered effective for not only bedwetting but nervous conditions and some forms of melancholy. The oil extract was applied externally to burns, wounds, bruises, sores, and other skin problems, and was taken internally for stomachache, colic, and lung congestion. A consistent herbal tradition based largely on the tea and the oil was established early and maintained throughout European nations and America into modern times.

Forms and Doses

POWDER

From 65–325 mg of the powdered herb per dose was recommended by Ellingwood, while Felter and Lloyd indicated that 1–4 grams is the proper dose of the herb powder.

Water Extract

Lust describes using one teaspoon dried herb per half cup water and steeping for five minutes while covered. The half cup was consumed warm before breakfast and at bedtime. Felter and Lloyd recommend 1–2 fluid ounces of an infusion but do not describe the strength. Similarly, Grieve indicated that 1–2 tablespoons are used per dose when one ounce of herb is infused in a pint of water.

Tincture

Up to 0.7 ml per dose was recommended by Ellingwood. Felter and Lloyd confirm this for a "strong" tincture.

Fluid Extract

Up to 0.3 ml was Ellingwood's dose, though Grieve suggests 2–4 ml.

Oil Extract

Lust advised to fill a jar with fresh flowers and leaves and cover them with olive oil. The jar is then closed and this maceration left in warm or sunny spot for 6–7 weeks, shaking often. By that time the oil is red. It is strained through a cloth; if a watery layer forms on top, this is decanted off. The oil can be stored in a dark container for up to two years. Internal dose is 10–15 drops.

In 1992[b] Maisenbacher and Kovar analyzed several oil extract preparations made from buds, flowers and fruits after the standard method (using fresh flowers in olive oil for several weeks, both including or excluding sunlight) and compared these to 1:10 strength extracts of freeze-dried flowers macerated for eight days at room temperature (excluding light) using olive oil, peanut oil, sesame oil, isopropyl myristate, medium chain triglycerides or eutanol G. The 80 grams fresh flowers or 20 grams freeze-dried flowers were also macerated in 200 gm of olive oil for 3.5 hours at 95 degrees C, as well as with 17 grams of freeze-dried flowers macerated in hot olive oil and eutanol G for eight days.

Maisenbacher and Kovar found the extracts made in sunlight contained no hypericin, but the red-brown pigments in the oil were hypericin derivatives. Flavonoid content was 13 mg/100 grams of oil infused for weeks in light, but only 1-3.4 mg / 100 grams when excluding light. Apparently, the light released flavonoids from their glycoside forms. Flavonoids included quercetin, biapigenin, and up to four others; up to 4 xanthones were also discerned. A content of 63 mg hyperforin per 100 grams of olive oil was found in the freshly prepared oil, but this antimicrobial hyperforin was absent in the oil fourteen days later. Even when exposed to no light, the hyperforin and adhyperforin content was undetectable after thirty days. Using the other solvents at room temperature for eight days, 0.3% hyperforin was obtained that lasted up to ninety days. The best hyperforin retention was by hot maceration of freeze-dried flowers for several hours with oil and eutanol G in which hyperforin content lasted six months if stored in the absence of air. Following hot maceration in olive oil for several hours, the hyperforin content was 0.3%, but the hyperforin broke down after three months. So it appears the best way to assure that the oil is potent in hyperforin is to prepare the extract as needed by macerating freeze-dried flowers in hot olive oil for several hours.

STANDARDIZED EXTRACTS

These commercial products have multiplied over time as emphasis has moved from hypericin to hyperforin in studies of these extracts for depression. One of the common commercial forms studied is the methanolic extract LI 160, a 300 mg tablet standardized to 0.31% total hypericin (the sum of its hypericin and pseudohypericin content) including 0.12%–0.28% hypericin. The methanolic extract LI 160S has 0.17% hypericin and 4.67% hyperforin. A 350 mg tablet of the *Hypericum* 60% ethanolic extract STEI 300 is standardized to 0.2–0.3% total hypericins and 2–3% hyperforin. An extract designated WS 5572 consists of tablets with 300 mg of a hydroalcoholic extract of *H. perforatum* of 2.5–5.0:1 strength and containing 0.14% hypericin and a minimum 3% hyperforin. Extract Ph-50 is a 350 mg tablet standardized to 50% flavonoids with 4.5% hyperforin and 0.3% hypericin.

Components

Beginning around 1970 and increasing greatly since 1980, the content and activity of St. John's wort components have attracted much scientific attention in Eastern Europe. Analysis by Hoelzl and Ostrowski found the content of active compounds in micrograms per flower varies widely in different *H. perforatum* plants (hypericin 3–23, pseudohypericin 11–63, hyperforin 206–607, biapigenin 11–71, rutin 19–61, hyperoside 44–140, isoquercitrin 15–107, and quercitrin 21–112) with highest hypericin levels correlating with high levels of hyperforin, biapigenin, and other flavonoids. Tekel'ova and others showed in 2000 that the hypericins and flavonoids peaked during flowering, while hyperforin continued to increase during fruit formation. Costes and Thomas studied the freeze-dried petals of the flowers that contain a number of carotenoid pigments including lutein, violaxanthin, luteoxanthin, trollixanthin, and trollichrome. In 2002 Murch and others described hydroponic experiments with growing plantlet clones, but they only analyzed the content of hypericin, pseudohypericin, and hyperforin.

Hypericin and pseudohypericin are similar polycyclic naphthodianthrone components, referred to together as total hypericins or sometimes just hypericins. The hypericin content differed markedly between the herb and its extracts; 0.178% was found in the herb, 0.004% in the juice and 0.010% in intractum preparations studied by Kowalewski and others. Debska and Zmudzinska found only 10% hypericin was extracted into infusions. Hypericin loss is negligible in a dry extract or tablet stored at room temperature for one year. But after only 6 weeks at 60 degrees C, hypericin content is reduced in the juice, dry extract, and tablets by 46%, 35%, and 33%, respectively, according to Adamski and Styp-Rekowska.

Hyperforin is a phloroglucinol available in the oily extract of the flowers. In 1992 Maisenbacher and Kovar found in 1992[a] that its homologue adhyperforin is present in small quantity in the flowers, but both of these compounds are greatly increased in the unripe and ripe fruit. Hyperforin increases from 2.0% in the flowers to 4.5% in the fruit. Adhyperforin goes from 0.2% to 1.9%, and hyperforin-like polar compounds increase from 0.05% to 0.3%, as shown in freeze-dried flowers and fruit. Consequently, in seeking to maximize only the total hyperforin content, sometimes referred to as hyperforins, the fruit would be harvested in preference to the traditionally-used flower. According to Nahrstedt and Butterweck, hyperforin is unstable toward heat and light and degrades to a sedative compound found in hops, methylbutenol. Erdelmeier in 1998 pointed out that the instability results from inappropriate drying techniques and pharmaceutical preparations that expose the hyperforin to oxygen and light. Freeze-drying was used to best preserve isolated hyperforin for pharmacological studies.

Tsitsina found the highest flavonoid content of 223 species tested was in *H. perforatum* flowers (11.7%) and its leaves and stalks (7.4%). The flavonoids were highest in the leaves and lowest in the stems in the study by Razinskaite, who found they reach their highest concentration beginning and during the flowering stage. Rutin is high before flowering, while hyperin is highest afterward. Rutin (0.9–1.6%) and hyperoside (hyperin) (0.9–1.9%) are by far the most abundant, but quercetin (0.1–0.2%), quercitrin, and isoquercitrin (0.3%) are in significant amounts in the studies by Dorossiev and Grinenko. The biflavonoid biapigenin isolated by Berghofer and Holzl in 1987 is highest in concentration in the buds and flowers but very low in the fruit, while stems and leaves have no trace of this compound.

The tannins are from 5.5–6.5% in dried *Hypericum* which only yields about 1% in tinctures according to Azaryan, but the content in the fresh herb during blooming is about 15%. Derbentseva and others showed the tannins in St. John's wort contain catechins, monomeric polyphenols, and polyoxyflavone glycosides. Kitanov found these *H. perforatum* catechins (flavanols) include (+)-catechol and (-)-epicatechol. These compounds also make up the oligomeric procyanidins in St. John's wort. The phenolic acid constituents identified by Stoyanova and others along with Grujic-Vasic and Bosnic include caffeic acid, gallic acid, and chlorogenic acids.

Other compounds mentioned by Nahrstedt and Butterweck that contribute to the activity, at least in concentrations used in laboratory studies, are the amino acid gamma-aminobutyric acid (GABA) and xanthones. The xanthones are in low concentration in the dried herb (0.0004%) but are found in greater amounts in the roots. Essential oils make up from 0.1–0.25% of the dried herb. Murch and others also discovered melatonin in the leaves (1.75 mcg/gm) and flowers (4.39 mcg/gm) in 1997.

Laboratory Research—Isolates and Fractions

Kinetics

HYPERICINS

Stock and Holzl examined kinetics of radiolabeled hypericins in mice using a hydroalcoholic extract. After oral consumption in mice the levels of hypericin and pseudohypericin in the first six hours were greatest in the gastrointestinal tract, followed by the muscles. Hypericin in the blood was still on the rise after 6 hours. Hypericin and pseudohypericin also steadily accumulated in the liver in the first 6 hours after ingestion.

HYPERFORIN

Given in the context of a *Hypericum* alcoholic extract, WS5572 with a 5% hyperforin content, Biber and others studied hyperforin oral administration to rats. Hyperforin reached maximum levels after 3 hours and had a half-life of 6 hours.

Antidepressant

XANTHONES

An *in vitro* study by Suzuki and others in 1984 of an extract from *Hypericum* with 80% hypericin inhibited monoamine oxidase (MAO) type A more than type B, but 95% pure hypericin was studied by Cott in 1997 and found to be devoid of significant MAO inhibition. Xanthones had previously demonstrated potent activity of this type in a 1981 study by Suzuki and others. In 1989 test tube studies by Hoelzl and others of a hypericin-free hydroalcoholic hypericum extract for MAO inhibition indicated that active fractions against type A contained xanthones.

FLAVONOIDS

Flavonoids were shown by Sparenberg and others in 1993 to contribute to MAO-inhibiting effect in test tubes. Thiede and Walper found a MAO-inhibiting effect of an extract fraction containing flavonoids, their glycosides, and xanthones in test tube studies in 1994. This fraction also inhibited catechol-O- methyltransferase. In mice and rat studies by Butterweck and others in 1997, the flavonoid fraction of St. John's wort reduced immobility in rats undergoing a forced swimming test.

HYPERFORIN

A study by Chatterjee and others in 1998 indicated that isolated hyperforin inhibited uptake of serotonin in peritoneal cells. Further behavioral tests with rats by these researchers demonstrated that hyperforin is a major, but not the only, antidepressant component. Muller and others in 1998 likewise showed that hyperforin was the unspecific reuptake inhibitor responsible for effects on serotonin, norepinephrine and dopamine, whereas hypericin and the flavonol kaempferol were not reuptake inhibitors.

Then, in 2001 Muller and others demonstrated that hyperforin's reuptake inhibition was non-comperitive at specific binding sites of transporter molecules. Hyperforin is also non-selective, affecting GABA and L-glutamate reuptake in addition to the three bioamines. The novel mechanism responsible for its reuptake inhibition is likely due to sodium conductive pathways, since it leads to higher levels of intracellular sodium.

HYPERICIN

In 1994 Thiede and Walper studied the effect in test tubes of hypericin on MAO from pork liver. Hypericin inhibited MAO at a concentration of 0.001 moles/liter. Several extract fractions containing hypericins with some flavonols also inhibited MAO.

Butterweck and others in 2002 compared the use of hypericin and St. John's wort extract LI160 (standardized to 0.3% hypericin) to the tricyclic antidepressant imipramine. They looked at long-term (8 weeks) and short-term (2-weeks) effects on bioamine neurotransmitters in rat hypothalamus and hippocampus, since these areas are associated with motivation, emotion, learning and memory. Given orally, the hypericin dose was 0.2 mg/kg daily. All three agents studied increased serotonin concentrations and reduced homovanillic acid (a dopamine metabolite) in the hypothalamus, but not the hippocampus, only after long-term use. Hypericin also selectively reduced the norepinephrine levels in the hipposcampus after 2 and 8 weeks of treatment.

Hormonal

HYPERFORIN

In 2001 Franklin and Cowen gave 9.3 mg/kg hyperforin to rats, and acutely increased plasma corticosterones associated with increased brain cortex serotonin content, likely mediated by serotonin-2 receptors. Plasma prolactin was likewise reduced by hyperforin, an effect mediated by dopamine. However, these plasma levels did not correlate with plasma hyperforin. The hormone levels do not seem to involve noradrenaline mechanisms.

HYPERICIN

Franklin and Cowen also gave 0.4 mg/kg hypericin to rats, and it also acutely increased plasma corticosterones associated with increased brain cortex serotonin content. Hypericin caused a slight insignificant rise in prolactin. Again, these plasma levels did not correlate with plasma hypericin.

Antiviral

HYPERICINS

Along with pseudohypericin, hypericin was discovered by Meruelo and others in 1988 to have potent antiretroviral activity. Tang and others found in 1990 that these aromatic polycyclic diones in *Hypericum* are antiviral against the Friend leukemia and radiation leukemia retroviruses in test tubes and in mice in nontoxic doses. They along with Wood and others in 1990 showed hypericin is virucidal against the enveloped influenza A, parainfluenza type 3, herpes simplex types 1 and 2, vaccinia, vesicular stomatitis, and human cytomegalo-type viruses in test tube conditions. Likewise Kraus and others in 1990 found that hypericin reduced production of equine infectious anemia virus in isolated infected cells by 99.99%. Takahashi and others discovered in 1989 that these two compounds inhibit protein kinase C which may contribute to their anti-retroviral activity. Purified hypericin was shown by Cott in 1997 to have affinity for the N-methyl-D-aspartate receptor, possibly contributing to its antiviral effects.

Besides inactivating reverse transcriptase, hypericin and pseudohypericin lead to suppression of murine immunodeficiency virus as Lavie and others demonstrated in 1989. The most significant retrovirus affected by the more potent hypericin is the human immunodeficiency virus type1 (HIV-1). The reverse transcriptase inhibition for HIV-1 was shown by Schinazi and others in human lymphocytes with hypericin, suggesting a potential therapeutic value to help prevent the development of AIDS. In addition, Hudson and others in 1991 discovered that the antiviral activity of hypericin against murine cytomegalovirus, Sindbis virus, and HIV-1 is enhanced by exposure to visible light.

TANNINS

Derbentseva and others found the tannin fraction that is responsible for antiviral activity against influenza A2 virus in chicken embryos contains catechins and polyoxyflavone compounds.

PHENOLICS

Caffeic acid was shown by Herrmann and Kucera in 1967 to be antiviral against herpes simplex and vaccinia viruses, but not influenza A or B.

Antiseptic

FLAVONOIDS

In 1991 the Brantners successfully demonstrated that hyperoside is mildly antiseptic in test tubes against *E. coli*, *Klebsiella*, *Pseudomonas aeruginosa*, *Bacillus subtillus*, *Staphylococcus aureus*, *Streptococcus faecalis*, and *Candida albicans* in concentrations ranging from 250–500 mcg/ml.

RESIN

A resinous fraction isolated from the fruit, flowers, and leaves by Gaind and Ganjoo in 1959 was effective against certain bacteria. The antibacterial activity diminishes in that order, while the seeds were inactive. *Staphylococcus aureus*, *Streptococcus pneumonia*, *Strep. viridans*, *Strep. pyogenes*, *Bacillus subtilis*, and *Corynebacterium diphtheriae* were the bacteria inhibited.

HYPERFORINS

Around 1970 the constituents designated novoimanine and imanine were shown to be effective in test tubes and topically against local infections of *Staph. aureus* in mice, respectively, by Russians Negrash, Omel'chuk-Myakushko, and others. The 2–3-year-old plants in the phases of budding, flowering, and the start of fruit formation had the most imanine. The active component of novoimanine was identified by Gurevich and others as hyperforin.

Vasodilator

PROCYANIDINS

Procyanidin fractions were shown by Melzer and others to have coronary vasodilating activity in isolated guinea pig hearts in 1989 and in isolated pig arteries in 1991. These effects appear to be similar to those of *Crataegus* on coronary vessels and mimicked theophylline's phosphodiesterase inhibition.

Analgesic

FLAVONOIDS

The total flavonoids extracted from *H. perforatum* by Vasil'chenko and others in 1986 exhibited analgesic activity in mice.

Antiglioma

HYPERICIN

In 1994 Couldwell and others showed the growth of glioma in test tube studies was inhibited in a dose-related manner by hypericin, a marked effect being produced around 10 mcmol/L. This may be due to its protein kinase C inhibition. Cell death of the glioma cells occurred after 48 hours.

Photosensitizing

HYPERICIN

In 2000 Schey and others studied the effect in test tubes of hypericin on alpha-crystallin in both light and dark to determine if damage would occur to this lens protein. Changes in the protein occurred in the presence of hypericin only in light, suggesting that hypericin could lead to formation of cataracts in those who fail to protect the eye from intense sunlight while using products containing this component.

Laboratory Research—Extracts

Antidepressant

TINCTURE

A crude hydroalcoholic extract of hypericum containing 0.1% hypericin was shown by Cott to have significant receptor affinity for $GABA_A$, $GABA_B$, and benzodiazepine and to inhibit of MAO A and B in test tubes. However, the concentrations required for inhibition of the MAOs to be significant are unlikely to be attained following oral administration, unlike binding of GABA receptors. Narstedt and Butterweck note the plant contains the sedative amino acid transmitter GABA, so this could explain the laboratory effects on $GABA$ receptors.

STANDARDIZED EXTRACTS

In an animal study by Okpanyi and Weischer in 1987 the hypericum standardized extract enhanced exploratory and water wheel activity and antagonized reserpine, while decreasing aggressiveness in socially isolated male mice, all indicators of antidepressant activity. In 1994 a whole extract was shown to inhibit MAO from pork liver studied in test tubes by Thiede and Walper. This extract also inhibited catechol-O-methyltransferase. That same year Muller and Rossol found that serotonin receptor expression in a neuroblastoma cell line was reduced by the extract LI 160, an effect that was increased by interleukin-1, suggesting serotonin reuptake ability was impaired.

In 1997, Muller and others again studied the methanolic LI 160 *Hypericum* extract, standardized to 0.31% total hypericin (the sum of its hypericin and pseudohypericin content) and found it was a weak inhibitor of monoamine oxidase in isolated cells. It also inhibited serotonin, dopamine, and norepinephrine uptake by 50% at concentrations from 0.85–6.2 mcg/ml. Furthermore, while the density of beta-adrenoceptor in the frontal cortex was reduced by 16%, the 5-HT_2-receptor density was increased there by 15% (in contrast to imipramine) when LI 160 was administered orally to rats at 240 mg/kg for 14 days. The serotonin reuptake inhibition confirmed the findings of Perovic and Muller using LI 160 in 1995. In mice and rat studies by Butterweck and others in 1997, LI 160 counteracted drugs that interfered with dopamine-mediated activity. The extract also reduced immobility in rats undergoing a forced swimming test, an antidepressant indicator. Hyperforin, possibly the most important St. John's wort component for depression, was lost in the fractionation process and so was not tested.

When hyperforin was discovered to be an important contributor to the antidepressant activity of St. John's wort, an ethanolic extract with 4.5% hyperforin was compared with a carbon dioxide (CO_2) extract enriched to 38.8% hyperforin by Bhattacharya and others in 1998. The results of behavioral tests in rats and mice were similar for these two extracts based on approximately equivalent doses of hyperforin (10 times the amount of the ethanolic extract was administered). However, the ethanol extract potentiated dopaminergic responses more, while the CO_2 extract had more pronounced serotoninergic effects. This indicated that other components that varied between these extracts had additional influence on the overall effects.

A study by Chatterjee and others in 1998 indicated that a 38.8% hyperforin extract, made with supercritical carbon dioxide devoid of hypericins and numerous other *Hypericum* components, inhibited uptake of serotonin in peritoneal cells. Further behavioral tests with rats by these researchers involving comparisons with hyperforin, its concentrated extract, and an ethanolic extract demonstrated that hyperforin is a major, but not the only, antidepressant component. Muller and others in 1998 likewise showed unspecific reuptake inhibition by the methanolic extract LI 160 (0.3%, 1.5% hyperforin) on serotonin, norepinephrine and dopamine. This methanolic extract and the 38% hyperforin enriched CO_2 extract additionally caused a reduction of beta-adrenoceptor binding sites by 15%.

Another comparative study by Dimpfel and others in 1998 using the methanolic extract LI 160S with 0.17% hypericin and 4.67% hyperforin was compared with a CO_2 extract with 30.1% hyperforin on EEG effects in rats. Identical amounts of hyperforin were used in dosing the rats with these extracts, and both produced EEG changes in the first 2 hours that was similar to serotonin reuptake inhibitors. The LI 160S extract increased the delta activity later, similar to NMDA (n-methyl-d-aspartate) antagonists affecting the glutamatergic system, but the CO_2 extract did not. This provides another demonstration of different effects, associated with different components, from different extracts.

In 2001 Calapai and others used the extract Ph-50 standardized to 50% flavonoids with 4.5% hyperforin and 0.3% hypericin to discern neurotransmitter effects in rats. They found that acute oral use of Ph-50 enhanced serotonin, norepinephrine and dopamine content in the brain, while reducing immobility time during forced-swimming. The latter effect was inhibited by drugs that antagonized dopamine, serotonin and norepinephrine activity. St. John's wort's serotonin effect was the most pronounced.

Comparing the use of extract LI 160 and hypericin to the tricyclic antidepressant imipramine, Butterweck and others in 2002 looked at long-term (8 weeks) and short-term (2-weeks) effects on bioamine neurotransmitters in rat hypothalamus and hippocampus. These areas are associated with motivation, emotion, learning and memory. Given orally, the extract dose was 500 mg/kg. All three agents studied increased serotonin concentrations and reduced homovanillic acid (a dopamine metabolite) in the hypothalamus, but not the hippocampus, only after long-term use. The extract significantly reduced 5-hydroxyindoleacetic acid (a serotonin metabolite) and dopamine (a norepinephrine precursor) in the hypothalamus with long-term use.

Hormonal

STANDARDIZED EXTRACT

In 2001 Franklin and Cowen gave a single 200 mg/kg LI 160 to rats intraperitoneally by injection and found that it acutely increased plasma corticosterones associated with increased brain cortex serotonin content, likely mediated by serotonin-2 receptors. Plasma prolactin was reduced due to a dopamine-mediated mechanism.

Antiviral

WATER EXTRACT

An aqueous extract of *H. perforatum* leaves was found to be virostatic against herpes, influenza, and vaccinia virus by May and others in 1978. It was also mildly cytotoxic.

Hepatoprotective

TINCTURE

A 50% alcoholic extract of the dried aerial parts exhibited choleretic activity by increasing bile secretion in rats after intraduodenal administration by Ozturk and others in 1992. This extract also protected against carbon tetrachloride toxic liver effects in mice.

GI Sedative

HYDROALCOHOLIC EXTRACT

Jakovljevic and others showed in 2000 that when given to mice intraperitoneally, the alcohol extract high in flavonoids and hypericins reduced intestinal motility.

WATER EXTRACT

Intestinal motility reduction in mice was greater for the extract made from water that contained flavonoid glycosides and little hypericin than for the alcohol extract in the study by Jakovljevic and others.

Human Studies

Kinetics

HYPERICINS

Using a hydroalcoholic extract, Stock and Holzl studied the serum kinetics of hypericin after a single dose in one person, and hypericin in the blood was still on the rise after 8 hours. Using extract LI160, Kerb and others found in 1996 that following a single dose systemic bioavailability was about 14% for hypericin and 21% for pseudohypericin. Absorption of hypericin was faster but its distribution and elimination was much slower than for pseudohypericin.

HYPERFORIN

Given in the context of a *Hypericum* alcoholic extract, WS5572 with a 5% hyperforin content, in 1998 Biber and others found after oral administration of 300–600 mg that hyperforin reached maximum levels after 3.5 hours and had a half-life of nine hours. However, after a 900–1200 mg dose of the extract the absorption of hyperforin was not as efficient. The estimated steady state plasma concentrations after 3 doses of 300 mg daily was about 100 ng/ml.

Electroencephalograms

STANDARDIZED EXTRACTS

The effects of 4:1 strength hydroalcoholic extracts with identical hypericin but different hyperforin content (0.5% and 5.0%) were compared in a randomized, placebo-controlled study by Schellenberg and others in 1998 on their influence on EEG activity in 18 subjects. Both differed from placebo in a reproducible manner over eight days, with the 5.0% hyperforin group having a significantly higher baseline power performance than placebo at the delta (cholinergic) and beta-1 frequencies, with theta (noradrenergic) and alpha-1 (serotonergic) noticeably increased.

Antidepressant

HYDROALCOHOLIC EXTRACT

Harrer and others compared a commercial St. John's wort product in 1999 with 20 mg fluoxetine in 149 elderly patients with mild (72) or moderate (77) depression. This product was a 60% ethanolic extract in dry tablets of 5–7:1 strength; 200 mg was given twice daily in this randomized double-blind study. After 6 weeks the global scores were reduced on the Hamilton Depression (HAMD) scale from 16.60 to 7.91 for the extract and from 17.18 to 8.11 for fluoxetine. The reductions were equivalent for both medications for both mild and moderate depression. Twelve adverse drug reactions with 6 withdrawals occurred with St. John's wort extract, and 17 adverse reactions with 8 withdrawals were associated with fluoxetine.

STANDARDIZED EXTRACTS

An open-label clinical study by Muldner and Zoller in 1984 used a hypericum extract standardized to 0.15% hypericin in 15 women for 4–6 weeks for its antidepressive effects. A quantitative improvement was shown for anxiety, dysphoric mood, loss of interest, hypersomnia, anorexia, morning depression, intractable constipation, and feelings of worthlessness. No side effects or changes in EEG, ECG, or laboratory parameters were noted.

A meta-analysis of 23 randomised, placebo-controlled or active-controlled trials with 1757 outpatients by Linde and others in 1996 indicated that hypericum extracts with variable hypericin content and daily doses (from 0.4–2.7 mg total hypericin) were more effective than placebo for treatment of mild to moderate depressive disorders. A study by Lenoir and others in 1999 studied *Hypericum* preparations standardized either to 0.17 mg, 0.33 mg, or 1 mg of total hypericin. Using these with three groups three times daily for six weeks, they obtained effective responses for depression, based on at least a 50% reduction of HAMD score, by 62%, 65%, and 68% of the patients, respectively. The differences in these efficacy rates were insignificant, and tolerability of all preparations was excellent with only 7 of the 348 patients (2%) having even mild adverse reactions. The average HAMD score went from 16–17 initially to 8-9 by the end. This study and the meta-analysis suggest that the antidepressant effect is independent of hypericin content.

A series of articles published in 1997 confirmed these clinical antidepressant effects with an extract standardized to 0.3% hypericin. This extract, LI 160, is an effective therapy for patients with seasonal affective disorder, a subgroup of major depression, as studied by Kasper at a dose of 900 mg. It compared favorably with amitryptaline in a 6-week controlled clinical trial by Wheatley with 156 mild to moderately depressed outpatients. LI 160 at a dose of 1800 mg daily was equivalent to 150 mg of imipramine in a 6-week, multicenter, randomized, controlled study by

Vorbach and others with 209 severely depressed patients. The adverse effects for the hypericum extract were significantly less than for imipramine. The influence on ECG measurements actually showed improved cardiac conduction for those using hypericum compared to imipramine, according to Czekalla and others.

Then in 1999 Philipp and others compared 1050 mg daily of the *Hypericum* 60% ethanolic extract STEI 300, standardized to 0.2–0.3% total hypericins and 2–3% hyperforin, to 100 mg imipramine daily for 8 weeks in 263 patients with moderate depression. In this randomized, placebo-controlled double-blind study the resulting reduction in HAMD scores (initial average 22.6) for those using the extract (-15.4) were better than for the placebo group (-12.1) and at least as good as for those on imipramine (-14.2), while its rate of adverse effects were better than imipramine's and as good as the placebo.

LI 160 was tested by Hubner and Kirste in 2001 in children under age 12 with symptoms of mild to moderate depression. For 6 weeks the study was conducted using from 300–1800 mg per day of the extract containing 0.3% hypericin. The percentage of physicians who rated the effectiveness as good or excellent was 72% at two weeks, 97% at four weeks, and 100% at six weeks. No adverse effects were reported; 76% of the children completed the six-week course.

A randomized, double-blind, placebo-controlled multi-clinic trial by Laakmann in 1998 compared 900 mg daily of extracts containing 0.5% (WS5573) and 5% (WS 5572) hyperforin that were otherwise identical. These were used in treating 147 mild to moderately depressed patients (initial HAMD average over 20) for 6 weeks. The group receiving the 5% hyperforin extract had the largest reduction in the HAMD from the beginning of the study (-10.3), followed by WS 5573 (-8.5) and then the placebo (-7.9). Only the 5% hyperforin extract significantly improved the score in comparison with placebo. Again in 1998(b) Laackmann and others determined that those who were more severely depressed (HAMD > 22) benefited even more from the 5% hyperforin extract but not with the 0.5% hyperforin WS 5573. Kalb and others also studied WS 5572 extract with 5% hyperforin in 2001 in a clinical trial with 72 patients with mild to moderate depression using 900 mg daily for 6 weeks. Reduction of HAMD scores was over 50% for the WS 5572 group (from 19.7 to 8.9) and less than 30% for placebo (from 20.1 to 14.4). There were no adverse reactions in either group.

In 2001 Bone reported on a presentation made by Winkel and others in Munich in 2000 on their using 900 mg daily of the dry methanolic extract of St. John's wort LI 160 to treat depression in alcohol-addicted patients. The six-week randomized, placebo-controlled, double blind trial studied 119 patients with a HAMD score from 12–24 who had been treated at a detoxification unit for at least two weeks. In the final group of 85 subjects, a significant reduction in score from baseline for those using LI

160 was -10.3 compared to the placebo group with -7.4. Ernst and others in 1998 reported that another study found that there is no interaction of St. John's wort with alcohol.

In 2002 Lecrubier and others investigated an extract designated WS 5570 that consisted of tablets with 300 mg of a hydroalcoholic extract of *H. perforatum* of 4–7: 1 strength and containing 0.12%–0.28% hypericin and 3%–6% hyperforin. Three tablets daily were used in this double-blind, randomized placebo-controlled trial with 375 patients who were undergoing a mild to moderate major depressive episode of at least two weeks. Again the extract produced a significantly greater reduction in HAMD total score (–9.9 vs.–8.1) and was more effective in those with higher baseline scores. Adverse effects were comparable for the extract and placebo.

When used in major depression, Shelton and others in 2001 failed to find a significant reduction in depression from St. John's wort extract. Patients entered with a baseline HAMD score of 20 or more, the average being above 22. A positive response was considered as a final score of 12 or less. St. John's wort 300 mg standardized extract LI 160 tablets were given three times daily for the first four weeks and then increased to four times per day for the next four weeks if response was insufficient. HAMD scores were reduced to 14.2 by the extract, but placebo reduction was to 14.9. Secondary measures such as changes in the Beck Depression Inventory (BDI) score were also not significantly different for treatment. However, the extract led to 14 remissions in 98 patients, compared to 5 in 102 for placebo.

In 2002 van Gurp and others compared sertraline to a 0.3% hypericin St. John's wort extract in 87 patients diagnosed with major depression (using DSM-IV criteria) and a HAMD score of 16 or more. For the first 4 weeks patients received either 50 mg sertraline or 900 mg extract daily. The dose was doubled for the last 8 weeks for 9 patients in each group when the initial dose proved clinically insufficient. After twelve weeks the HAMD and BDI scores declined by about half and were not significantly different between the groups. Sertraline produced significantly more side effects after two and four weeks than the St. John's wort extract.

In 3-tiered study comparing an extract to placebo and sertraline, a much publicized failure in treating major depression in 2002 by the Hypericum Depression Trial Study Group occurred when using LI 160 standardized to 0.12–0.28% hypericin. However, assessing the outcome is complicated by the fact that the standard medication sertraline also failed to significantly improve the primary outcome measures (average change in HAMD score) in this trial. Entrants had a HAMD score of at least 20. After eight weeks the reduction was -9.20 for placebo, -8.68 for LI 160, and -10.53 for sertraline. Rates of full response that included HAMD plus Clinical Global Impression scores were 31.9% for placebo, 23.9% for LI 160, and 24.8% for sertraline. Though the hyperforin content of this extract was reportedly 3.1%, unfortunately this and the other studies on major depression did not use a product whose hyperforin content was standardized.

Premenstrual Syndrome

STANDARDIZED EXTRACT

In 1999 Parry reported on a woman whose premenstrual dysphoric symptoms abated considerably after taking an uncharacterized St. John's wort product. Using a single 300 mg tablet daily of St. John's wort extract standardized to 0.3% hypericin, Stevinson and Ernst in 2000 studied its effects in an open uncontrolled study with 19 women suffering from premenstrual syndrome. Symptoms were rated through validated measures (Hospital Anxiety and Depresson scale and modified Social Adjustment Scale). All outcome measures had significant reductions after treatment through two complete menstrual cycles. Overall improvement in scores at the end compared to baseline was 51%, with two thirds have at least a 50% decrease in severity of symptoms.

Hormonal

STANDARDIZED EXTRACT

In 2001 Franklin and Cowen gave healthy male subjects nine 300 mg tablets of LI 160 standardized to 0.3% hypericine (8.1 mg total hypericin per dose); this 80% methanolic dry extract of flowers and buds actually had 0.17% hypericin (4.6 mg total/dose) and 4.3% hyperforin as measured by HPLC. Significant increases occurred in salivary cortisol after 13–14 hours and in plasma growth hormone after 1-2 hours, but plasma prolactin decreased from 2–4 hours after dosing. The hormone changes did not correlate with plasma hypericin or hyperforin concentrations.

Obsessive-compulsive Disorder

STANDARDIZED EXTRACT

In a 12-week, open-label study by Talyor and Kobak in 2000, 12 patients with obsessive-compulsive disorder were treated using 450 mg or a "standard preparation of *Hypericum perforatum*" with 0.3% hypericin twice daily. Participation required a Yale-Brown Obsessive-Compulsive scale (Y-BOCS) score of 16 or more; those with HAMD scores over 13 were excluded. A significant reduction in average Y-BOCS score (-7.4 points) began after one week and continued to the end. Five subjects improved much or very much, six improved minimally, and one had no change. Side effects included diarrhea in three and restless sleep in two.

Somatoform Disorders

STANDARDIZED EXTRACT

In 2002 Volz and others administered 600 mg of LI 160 daily for six weeks in a placebo-controlled trial to treat 151 out-patients with somatoform disorders. These involve severe psychiatric illnesses that are characterized mainly by physical complaints for which no medical diagnosis can sufficiently account. To test outcomes the Hamilton Anxiety Scale subfraction for somatic anxiety (HAMA-SOM) was used. The scores were reduced from 15.39 to 6.64 for the extract and 15.55 to 11.97 for placebo. Other criteria such as clinical global impression and HAMD confirmed the positive findings. It was effective even for those without depressive symptoms.

Antiviral

STANDARDIZED EXTRACT

In 2001 Bone reported on a presentation made by Mannel and others in Munich in 2000 on their using the dry extract of St. John's wort LI160 to treat herpes. In separate randomized, placebo-controlled trials, 94 subjects with recurrent mouth/facial herpes and 110 subjects with genital herpes were treated for 90 days with three tablets daily between outbreaks and six tablets daily during herpes episodes. For the oral/facial herpes subjects the symptoms score for presence, number of blisters, intensity and size was lower for the extract group (20.3) than for placebo (32.1). Likewise, for genital herpes subjects the symptom score was lower for those using the extract (15.6) than for the placebo group (29.4). The extract significantly reduced the number of herpetic episodes in both trials.

HYPERICIN

A study by Gulick and others in 1999 with 30 patients infected with HIV and having low CD4 counts used hypericin intravenously. It was given in doses of 0.25 or 0.5 mg/kg twice weekly or 0.25 mg/kg three times each week, or it administered oral hypericin at a dose of 0.5 mg/kg daily. Consequently, sixteen discontinued treatment early due to toxic effects including severe phototoxicity in eleven of twenty-three who could be evaluated. Only two subjects who received hypericin 0.25 mg/kg intravenously 2–3 times per week completed the 24-week study. Virus markers and CD4 cell counts did not change significantly in the 14–16 patients who were assessed.

Safety Concerns

In 1993 Kako and others described the toxic effects of St. John's wort that occurred when sheep ate 250–1000 grams of the fresh plants daily for two weeks.

They developed photophobia, alopecia, skin lesions, edema of the ear, eyelids and face, mucous membrane congestion, and other symptoms. Symptoms developed sooner with higher doses. Blood biochemical changes such as decreases in hemoglobin, blood cell count, cholesterol, glucose, protein, and triglycerides along with increased elevated liver enzymes also were found in these sheep.

Numerous studies have recently been published on the effects of a hypericum extract identified as LI 160. To test its reputed photosensitizing effects, exposure to ultraviolet radiation followed consumption of the amount of hypericin present in normal therapeutic doses of this product (900 mg extract daily). This was shown to be safe by Borckmoller J and others in 1997. Twice this dose produced only a slight increased photosensitivity after fifteen days. In 2001 Schulz reviewed the reports of photosensitisation and concluded that the threshold dose of 2–4 grams per day of most commercial extracts (providing about 5–10 mg hypericin) would result in increased risk. St. John's wort extract and hypericin were both shown to have dose-dependent phototoxicity by Wilhelm and others in 2001.

However, the quercetrin flavonoid component of the extract helps reduce the phototoxicity in test tube situations, indicating the extract is probably less phototoxic than the equivalent amount of hypericin that it contains. In addition, Heinrich and others in 2003 showed that 24 mg mixed carotenoids (equal amounts of lutein, beta-carotene, and lycopein) for twelve weeks increases skin carotene content and protection from erythema from ultraviolet light as well as 24 mg of beta-carotene and better than placebo. Therefore, the carotenoid content of St. John's wort flower petals may also help to modify the photosensitizing effect of hypericin when the whole complex herb is used regularly.

According to Farnworth and others in 1975, the *Hypericum* plant has been used as an emmenagogue and abortifacient, and its leaves have shown uterine stimulant activity. Therefore, its internal use is contraindicated in pregnancy. A report by Grush and others in 1998 repeats this warning, after describing two cases in which 900 mg/day of uncharacterized St. John's wort were taken during pregnancy with no apparent adverse effects. Klier and others tested milk content in a woman after eight weeks of using 900 mg daily of a standardized extract (0.3% hypericin). Hypericin could not be detected, and hyperforin levels were low, much lower than her serum concentration. The levels in her infant were undetectable.

Contraindication in serious depression is based on the studies in 2002 by the Hypericum Depression Trial Study Group and by Shelton and others in 2001 showing 900–1500 mg daily of St. John's wort extract was not effective in the treatment of major depression. It is contraindicated in those with a history of hypomania, mania or bipolar disorder, since cases of mania have been associated by Nierenberg and others in 1999 with use of 900 mg daily of standardized St. John's wort extract. Reducing the dosage from 900 to 300 mg/day in other cases caused a reversion to depression, as reported by Moses and Mallinger in 2000.

Hypericum use is contraindicated just prior to surgery due to potential for interactions with some anesthetic agents, based on cases by Irefin and Sprung in 2000 and Crose and McKeating in 2002. It is considered wise to discontinue St. John's wort at least five days prior to surgery, based on known pharmacokinetics of hyperforin and hypericin.

Ernst and others compiled reports on adverse effects in 1998. The most common of these are dizziness or confusion, gastrointestinal symptoms, and tiredness or a sense of sedation. Though photosensitivity is considered a potential problem, reports of this problem in humans have been very rare. St. John's wort compares well with placebo in studies regarding adverse effects. In 1999 Stevinson and Ernst compared adverse effects from conventional antidepressant with those of *Hypericum* and concluded that its side effects were fewer and milder, based on clinical trials, spontaneous reporting, and drug monitoring studies. In 2001 Schulz reviewed the reports of incidences of side effects and concluded that they occur in 1%-3% of those treated, 10 times less than the rate for synthetic antidepressants.

A few additional isolated cases of adverse events have been reported since that time. Bhopal described a case of sexual dysfunction induced in a middle-aged man using an uncharacterized product in 2001. Acute psychotic delirium was reported by Laird and Webb in 2001 in a 76-year-old woman with underlying Alzheimer's dementia who used 75 mg standardized extract (0.3% hypericin) for 3 weeks. The symptoms resolved when the extract was withheld. A report by Dean in 2003 describes a 58-year-old woman who was using 1800 mg three times daily for 32 days of a St. John's wort extract standardized to 0.3% hypericin and 3% hyperforin. When she stopped suddenly due to suspected photosensitivity, she experienced nausea, dry retching, dizziness, dry mouth, thirst, anorexia, cold chills and fatigue. These suspected withdrawal symptoms peaked after 3 days and lasted for 8 days, during which time she lost about 9 pounds of weight.

Drug Interactions

A wide variety of actual and potential interactions are well documented by Brinker in 2001 and in the online Updates and Additions to his text. Henderson and others concurred most of these interactions in 2002. The major adverse interactions involve combining St. John's wort products with the antidepressant nefazodone or the selective serotonin reuptake inhibitor (SSRI) sertraline, resulting in serotonin syndrome, i.e., headache, GI upset, sweating, tremor, flushing, confusion, agitation, and myalgia. Serotonin syndrome also occurred when St. John's wort was combined with trazodone. These effects are likely due to inhibition by St. John's wort extract and its component hyperforin of synaptosomal uptake of serotonin, dopamine, and norepinephrine as shown in lab studies. Physician monitoring for additive effects with the SSRI drug fluoxetine is likewise advisable. St. John's wort taken shortly after an 8 month period of using the SSRI paroxetine caused incoherence, weakness, and lethargy. A two-week washout period between St. John's wort use and SSRI treatment is recommended.

St. John's wort extract (0.3% hypericin) 900 mg daily for fourteen days reduced plasma levels of the protease inhibitor for HIV, indinavir, by 49–99% after 8 hours. This same dose resulted in a decreased cyclosporine concentration in a heart transplant patient, resulting in transplant rejection. A renal transplant patient developed subtherapeutic blood levels of cyclosporine and also suffered transplant rejection. Dozens of other cases reportedly had a lowering of serum cyclosporine while using St. John's wort. Midazolam blood levels were reduced by 60% when the drug was given orally with St. John's wort extract, compared to levels before taking St. John's wort. Both cyclosporine and midazolam are metabolized by cytochrome P450 isozyme 3A4, a catalyst of drug metabolism enhanced by St. John's wort.

Five cancer patients receiving 900 mg daily of a St. John's wort product together with irinotecan in a randomized, unblinded crossover study had a reduction in plasma levels of the active metabolite SN-38 of 42%. Irinotecan is another CYP 3A4 substrate. The component hyperforin appears to be responsible for activating the steroid X receptor (or pregnane X receptor) and thereby increases the expression of the CYP 3A4 monooxygenase.

St. John's wort extract (0.03% hypericin, 0.09% pseudohypericin, 6.1% hyperforin) at 900 mg daily in 25 subjects did not affect stable digoxin levels after one day, but after ten days reduced the peak concentration 24% and the 24 hour post-dosing concentration by 33%, apparently due to reduced absorption and possibly through induction of P-glycoprotein. Bone in 2001 reported on a presentation by Uehleke and others in Munich in 2000 that described different impacts based on dosage and formuation of St. John's wort when used with digoxin for fourteen days. While the 900 mg daily of the extract reduced digoxin 24-hour-area-under-curve (AUC) by 24.6% compared to placebo, 4 grams of the encapsulated herb powder reduced digoxin AUC by 27.1%, and 2 grams encapsulated powder decreased AUC by 17.6%. Using 0.5–1.0 gram of powdered herb or either 2 cups of the tea (made with1.6 grams herb) or 1.2 grams of the encapsulated oil formulation caused no significant change in AUC or trough levels when compared to placebo.

When simvastatin was taken with the extract, lower plasma levels resulted.

Simvastatin is a substrate of P-glycoprotein transporter that removes agents from cells, thereby reducing absorption in the gut. Oral clearance of the HIV non-nucleoside reverse transcriptase inhibitor nevirapine, a substrate of P-glycoprotien, is increased with concurrent use of St. John's wort that should therefore be avoided. In contrast, a single dose of St. John's wort actually inhibited intestinal P-glycoprotein and increased the maximum plasma concentration of fexofenadine. However, in this case two weeks of using St. John's wort failed to produce any significant effect on fexofenadine absorption.

Since the clinically significant interactions with indinavir, cyclosporin and digoxin also may be due in part to reduced absorption from P-glycoprotein induction, a test tube study by Perloff and others in 2001 looked at this effect for both St. John's wort and hypericin. Clinically relevant, low concentrations of either St. John's wort or hypericin caused significant induction of P-glycoprotein in intestinal cells and reduced absorption of rhodamine 123.

Breakthrough bleeding reportedly occurred in three women in Switzerland using oral contraceptives together with St. John's wort. Eight other reports of intermenstrual bleeding were reported in Sweden. Most of these were women using oral contraceptives for a long period before starting on St. John's wort, in five cases beginning use one week prior to the bleeding. In addition, nine reports of unplanned preganancies from Sweden and Great Britain have occurred in association with using St. John's wort with oral contraceptives.

Seven patients reportedly had a lowering of International Normalized Ratio, indicative of increased risk of clot formation, while using St. John's wort products after being stabilized on warfarin. These cases required an increased dosage of warfarin. The oral anticoagulant phenprocoumon also had a reduced plasma concentration when taken with St. John's wort extract daily. One patient required a larger daily dose of theophylline to sustain concentration when St. John's wort standardized extract (0.3% hypericin) was used; upon discontinuing St. John's wort, the theophylline concentration in the blood increased dramatically. Chlorzoxazone metabolism by CYP 2E1 was enhanced by hypericin-standardized St. John's wort.

Jakovljevic and others showed in 2000 that when given to mice intraperitoneally, the alcohol extract high in flavonoids and hypericins prolonged the time to get to sleep after be given pentobarbital. The muscle relaxant effect of diazepam was also reduced. The effect on diazepam may be due to increasing its metabolic breakdown.

There are a number of speculative interactions in which St. John's wort products may reduce bioavailability of certain drugs based on its inducing their metabolism via cytochrome P450 isozymes, especially CYP 3A4 (and/or reducing absorption by inducing P-glycoprotein). These drugs include protease inhibitors for HIV such as amprenavir, nelfinavir, ritonavir, and saquinavir and non-nucleoside reverse

Table 11   St.John's Wort Tops and Derivatives—
Summary of Internal Uses and Pharmacology

ST. JOHN'S WORT *Hypericum perforatum* L.	Traditional And Modern European Folk Uses	American Adopted Traditional Uses	Modern Clinical Studies	Laboratory Research Findings
Flowering Tops With Leaves	Depression Hysteria Congested lungs Malaria Jaundice Worms Diarrhea Dysentery	Bloody sputum Menorrhagia Jaundice Worms Diarrhea Dysentery		Phototoxic
Water Extracts	Depression Hysteria Congested lungs Bloody sputum Insomnia Liver problems Menstrual problems Bedwetting Nasal catarrh Stomach spasms Neuralgias Vomiting Poisonous bites	Melancholy Congested lungs Constipation Insomnia Liver problems Menstrual troubles Bedwetting Headache Dyspepsia Diarrhea Dysentery Worms		Antiviral Gastro-intestinal sedative
Hydroalcoholic Extracts (wines, tinctures, fluid extracts)	Melancholy Insanity Neurosis Anxiety Malaria Neuritis	Diarrhea Dysentery Jaundice Worms Bloody sputum Menorrhagia Spinal injury Hemorrhoids	Depression	Antidepressant Liver protective Gastro-intestinal sedative
Standardized Solid Extracts (Hydroethanolic, hydro-methanolic)			Depression PMS Obsessive/ compulsive Somataform disorders Herpes	Antidepressant Phototoxic Induces P-glycoprotein

Continued on next page

Table 11 *Continued*

ST. JOHN'S WORT *Hypericum perforatum* L.	Traditional And Modern European Folk Uses	American Adopted Traditional Uses	Modern Clinical Studies	Laboratory Research Findings
FRACTIONS AND ISOLATED CONSTITUENTS				
Hypericins				Induces P-glycoprotein Antidepressant Antiviral Antigliomal Phototoxic
Hyperforins				Antidepressant Antibacterial CYP inducer
Flavonoids				Antidepressant Analgesic Antiphototoxic

transcriptase inhbitors such as delavirdine and efavirenz. Other crucial drugs possibly affected include heart disease medications such as digitoxin, diltiazem, nifedipine, and beta-blockers, antidepressants including imipramine, amoxapine, and amitriptyline, medications for seizures such as carbamazepine, phenobarbital, and phenytoin, anti-cancer drugs including cyclophosphamide, tamoxifen, taxol, and etoposide, and immune suppressants for transplants such as rapamycin and tacrolimus. In addition, the United Kingdom's Committee on Safety of Medicines also warned that St. John's wort should not be used with SSRIs citalopram and fluvoxamine or the triptans naratriptan, rizatriptan, sumatriptan, and zolmitriptan.

In 2001 after Schulz reviewed the reports of drug interactions he concluded that St. John's wort must not be used with other antidepressants, cyclosporin, and indinavir or other protease inhibitors. Use with coumarin-type anticoagulants should be closely monitored for clotting parameters if concurrent use is unavoidable. The clinical relevance of other interactions was uncertain at that time but demanded critical examination and management by doctors and pharmacist involved in the care of patients using St. John's wort preparations.

Table 12   St. John's Wort Tops and Derivatives—Summary of Local Uses and Pharmacology

ST. JOHN'S WORT *Hypericum perforatum* L.	Ancient Greek Uses	English Traditional And Modern Uses	German Traditional And Modern Uses	American Adopted Traditional Uses
Herb (poultice)	Wounds Ulcers Bruises Burns Bites			
Water Extracts (fomentation)		Hard swellings Caked breasts Ecchymosis		Caked breasts Enlarged glands Ecchymosis Bruises Hard swellings Painful ulcers
(sitz bath)			Nervous complaints	
Ointment / Oil Extract (in olive oil)		Neuralgias Wounds Injuries Gland swellings Colic Sore back Lumbago Rheumatism		Caked breasts Enlarged glands Ecchymosis Bruises Hard swellings Painful ulcers Burns Wounds Sores
(in linseed oil)			Sunburn Burns Scalds	
Hydroalcohol Extract (tincture)				Bruises Injuries

References

BOOKS

Brinker, F. *Herb Contraindications and Drug Interactions,* 3rd ed., Eclectic Medical Pub., Sandy, OR., 2001. (Online updates and additions: www.eclecticherb.com/emp).

Clymer, RS. *Nature's Healing Agents,* 1905 ed., Philosophical Pub. Co., Quakertown, Penn., 1973.

Culpeper, N. *Complete Herbal,* 1653, W. Foulsham and Co., Ltd., London.

Ellingwood, F. *American Materia Medica, Therapeutics and Pharmacognosy,* 1919 ver., Eclectic Med. Pub., Sandy, OR., 1994.

Felter, HW and Lloyd, JU. *King's American Dispensatory,* 1898 ver., Eclectic Medical Pub., Portland, OR., 1983.

Grieve, M. *A Modern Herbal,* 1931 version, Dover Publ, Inc., New York, 1971.

Kneipp, S. *My Water Cure,* Joseph Koesel, Kempten, Germ., 1897.

Lust, B. *About Herbs,* Thorsons Pub., Ltd., Wellingborough, Engl., 1961.

Lust, J. *The Herb Book*, Bantam Books, New York, 1974.

Treben, M. *Health through God's Pharmacy*, Wilhelm Ennshaler, Steyr, Austria, 1984.

ARTICLES

Adamski, R and Styp-Rekowska, E. Stability of hypericin in juice, dry extract, and tablets from Hypericum perforatum plants. *Farm. Pol.,* 27:237–41, 1971. [Pol.] (*Chem. Abs.* 75:91286k).

Azaryan, RA. Standardization of [quality indexes for the medicinal] herb Hypericum perforatum. *Farmatsiya (Moscow),* 34(5):18–21, 1985. [Russ.] (*Chem. Abs.* 104:56271x).

Ghattacharya, SK et al. Activity profiles of two hyperforin-containing Hypericum extracts in behavioral models. *Pharmacopsychiat.,* 31:22–29, 1998.

Berghofer, R and Holzl, J. Biflavonoids in Hypericum perforatum; part 1. Isolation of I3,II8-biapigenin. *Planta Med.,* 53:216–7, 1987.

Bhopal, JS. St John's wort-induced sexual dysfunction. *Can. J. Psychiat.,* 46(5):456–7, 2001.

Biber, A et al. Oral bioavailability of hyperforin from Hypericum extracts in rats and human volunteers. *Pharmacopsychiat.,* 31(Suppl.):36–43, 1998.

Bone, K. Conference report: Third International Congress on Phytomedicine. *Br. J. Phytother.,* 5(4):209–17, 2001.

Borckmoller, J et al. Hypericin and Pseudohypericin: Pharmacokinetics and Effects on Photosensitivity in Humans. *Pharmacopsychiat,* 30(Suppl):94–101, 1997.

Brantner, A and Brantner, H. Screening of flavonoid aglycones and glycosides for antimicrobial activity. *Planta Med.,* 57(Suppl.2):A43–4, 1991.

Butterweck, V et al. Effects of the Total Extract and Fractions of Hypericum perforatum in Animal Assays for Antidepressant Activity. *Pharmacopsychiat,* 117–24, 1997.

Butterweck, V et al. Long-term effects of St. John's wort and hypericin on monoamine levels in rat hypothalamus and hippocampus. *Brain Res.,* 930:21–9, 2002.

Calapai, G et al. Serotonin, norepinephrine and dopamine involvement in the antidepressant action of Hypericum perforatum. *Pharmacopsychiat.*, 34:45-9, 2001.

Chatterjee, SS et al. Antidepressant activity of Hypericum perforatum and hyperforin: the neglected possibility. *Pharmacopsychiat.*, 31(Suppl.):7-15, 1998.

Costes, C and Thomas, C. Carotenoid pigments of the petals of the inflorescence of St. John's wort (Hypericum perforatum). *Ann. Physiol. Veg.*, 9(2):157-77, 1967. [Fr.] (*Chem. Abs.* 68:66335y).

Cott, JM. In Vitro Receptor Binding and Enzyme Inhibition by Hypericum perforatum Extract. *Pharmacopsychiat*, 30(Suppl):108-12, 1997.

Couldwell, WT et al. Hypericin: a potential antiglioma therapy. *Neurosurg.*, 35(4):705-10, 1994.

Crose, S, and McKeating, K. Delayed Emergence & St. John's Wort. *Anesthesiol.*, 96:1025-1027, 2002.

Czekalla, J et al. The Effect of Hypericum Extract on Cardiac Conduction as seen in the Electrocardiogram Compared to that of Imipramine. *Pharmacopsychiat*, 30(Suppl):86-8, 1997.

Dean, AJ. Suspected withdrawal syndrome after cessation of St. John's wort. *Ann Pharmacother.*, 37:150, 2003.

Debska, W and Zmudzinska, I. Densitometric and spectrophotometric determination of hypericin in St. John's wort (Herba Hyperici) after chromatographic separation. *Herba Pol.*, 28(1-2):21-9, 1982. [Pol.] (*Chem. Abs.* 98:132414w).

Derbentseva, NA et al. Effect of tannins from Hypericum perforatum on influenza viruses. *Mikrobiol. Zh. (Kiev)*, 34(6):768-72, 1972. [Ukrain.] (*Chem. Abs.* 78:67532d).

Dimpfel, W et al. Effects of a methanolic extract and a hyperforin-enriched CO_2 extract of St. John's wort (Hypericum perforatum) on intracerebral field potentials in the freely moving rat (tele-stereo-EEG). *Pharmacopsychiat.*, 31:30-35, 1998.

Dorossiev, I. Determination of flavonoids in Hypericum perforatum. *Pharmazie*, 40:585, 1985.

Erdelmeier, CAJ. Hyperforin, possibly the major non-nitrogenous secondary metabolite of Hypericum perforatum L. *Pharmacopsychiat.*, 31(Suppl.):2-6, 1998.

Ernst, E et al. Adverse effects profile of the herbal antidepressant St. John's wort (Hypericum perforatum L.). *Eur. J. Clin. Pharmacol.*, 54:589-94, 1998.

Farnsworth, NR et al. Potential value of plants as sources of new antifertility agents I. *J. Pharm. Sci.*, 64(4):535-98, 1975.

Franklin, M and Cowen, PJ. Researching the antidepressant actions of Hypericum perforatum (St. John's wort) in animals and man. *Pharmacopsych.*, 34(Suppl. 1):S29-S37, 2001.

Gaind, KN and Ganjoo, TN. Antibacterial principle of Hypericum perforatum Linn. *Indian J. Pharm.*, 21:172-5, 1959.

Grenenko, NA. The composition of flavonoids and derivatives of anthraquinone in Hypericum perforatum L. and H. maculatum Crantz. *Rastit. Resur.*, 25:387, 1989. [Russ.] (*Chem. Abs.* 111:191524s).

Grujic-Vasic, J and Bosnic, T. Study of plant oxyaromatic acids. *Arh. Farm.*, 31(5-6):273-8, 1981. [Serbo-Croat.] (*Chem. Abs.* 96:177970z).

Grush, LR et al. St John's wort during pregnancy. *JAMA*, 280(18):1566, 1998.

Gulick, RM et al. Phase I studies of hypericin, the active compound in St. John's wort, as an antiretroviral agent in HIV-infected adults. *Ann. Intern. Med.,* 130(6):510-4, 1999.

Gurevich, AI et al. Hyperforin, an antibiotic from Hypericum perforatum. *Antibiotiki (Moscow),* 16(6):510-3, 1971. (*Chem. Abs.* 75:95625t).

Gurp, G van et al. St. John's wort of sertraline? Randomized controlled trial in primary care. *Can. Fam. Phys.,* 48:905-12, 2002.

Harrer, JG et al. Comparison of equivalence between the St. John's wort extract LoHyp-57 and fluoxetine. *Arzneim.-Forsch.,* 49(4):289-96, 1999.

Heinrich, U et al. Supplementation with beta-carotene or a similar amount of mixed carotenoids protects humans from UV-induced erythema. *J. Nutr.,* 133:98-101, 2003.

Henderson, L et al. St John's wort (Hypericum perforatum): drug interactions and clinical outcomes. *Br. J. Clin. Pharmacol.,* 54:349-56, 2002.

Herrmann, EC Jr & Kucera LS. Antiviral substances in plants of the mint family (Labiatae). II. Nontannin polyphenol of Melissa officinalis. *Proc. Soc. Exp. Biol. Med.,* 124:869-73, 1967.

Hoelzl, J and Ostrowski, E. St. John's wort (Hypericum perforatum L.). HPLC analysis of the main components and their variability in a population. *Dtsch. Apoth. Ztg.,* 129:1227-30, 1987. [Germ.] (*Chem. Abs.* 107:112686n).

Hoelzl, J et al. Investigations about Antidepressive and Mood Changing Effects of Hypericum perforatum. *Planta Med,* 55:643, 1989.

Hubner, W-D and Kirste, T. Experience with St John's wort (Hypericum perforatum) in children under 12 years with symptoms of depression and psychovegetative disturbances. *Phytother. Res.,* 15:367-70, 2001.

Hudson, JB et al. Antiviral activities of hypericin. *Antiviral Res.,* 15:101-12, 1991.

Hypericum Depression Trial Study Group. Effect of Hypericum perforatum (St. John's wort) in major depressive disorder. *JAMA,* 287(14):1807-14, 2002.

Irefin S, and Sprung, J. A Possible Cause of Cardiovascular Collapse During Anesthesia: Long-Term Use of St. John's Wort. *J. Clin. Anesth.,* 12:498-499, 2000.

Jakovljevic, V et al. Pharmacodynamic study of Hypericum perforatum L. *Phtyomed.,* 7(6):449-53, 2000.

Kako, MDN et al. Studies of sheep experimentally poisoned with Hypericum perforatum. *Vet. Hum Toxicol,* 35(4):298-300, 1993.

Kalb, R et al. Efficacy and tolerability of Hypericum extract WS5572 versus placebo in mildly to moderately depressed patients. *Pharmacopsych.,* 34:96-103, 2001.

Kasper, S. Treatment of Seasonal Affective Disorder (SAD) with Hypericum Extract. *Pharmacopsychiat,* 30(Suppl):89-93, 1997.

Kerb, R et al. Single-dose and steady-state pharmacokinetics of hypericin and pseudohypericin. *Antimicrob. Agents Chemother.,* 40(9):2087-93, 1996.

Kitanov, G. Determination of the absolute configuration of catechins isolated from Hypericum perforatum. *Farmatsiya (Sofia),* 33(2):19-22, 1983. [Bulg.] (*Chem. Abs.* 99:50290j).

Klier, CM et al. St. John's wort (Hypericum peforatum)—is it safe during breastfeeding? *Pharmacopsych.*, 35:29–30, 2002.

Kowalewski, Z et al. Quantitative determination of hypericin content in the herb Hypericum perforatum L. and its preparations. *Herba Pol.*, 27:295–302, 1981. [Pol.] (*Chem. Abs.* 98:95721w).

Kraus, GA et al. Antiretroviral activity of synthetic hypericin and related analogs. *Biochem. Biophys. Res. Commun.*,172(1):149–53, 1990.

Laakmann, G et al. St. John's wort in mild to moderate depression: the relevance of hyperforin for the clinical efficacy. *Pharmacopsychiat.*, 31:54–9, 1998.

Laakmann, G et al. Clinical significance of hyperforin for the efficacy of Hypericum extracts on depressive disorders of different severities. *Phytomed.*, 5(6):435–42, 1998.

Laird, RD and Webb, M. Psychotic episode during use of St. John's wort. *J. Herb Pharmacother.*, 1(2):81–7, 2001.

Lavie, G et al. Studies of the mechanisms of action of the antiretroviral agents hypericin and pseudohypericin. *Proc. Natl. Acad. Sci.*, 86:5963–7, 1989.

Lecrubier, Y et al. Efficacy of St. John's wort extract WS5570 in major depression: a double-blind, placebo-controlled trial. *Am. J. Psychiatry*, 159:1361–6, 2002.

Lenoir, S et al. A double-blind randomized trial to investigate three different concentrations of a standardized fresh plant extract obtained from the shoot tips of Hypericum perforatum L. *Phytomed.*, 6(3):141–6, 1999.

Linde, K et al. St John's wort for depression - an overview and meta-analysis of randomised clinical trials. *Br Med J.*, 313:253–8, 1996.

Lucas, EH. Folklore and plant drugs—Pat III. *The Naturopath*, 1(6):1,3–4, 1963.

Maisenbacher, P. and Kovar, KA. Adhyperforin: a homologue of hyperforin from Hypericum perforatum. *Planta Med.*, 58:291–3, 1992[a].

Maisenbacher, P. and Kovar, KA. Analysis and stability of hyperici oleum.*Planta Med.*,58:351–4, 1992[b].

May, G and Willuhn, G. Antiviral activity of aqueous extracts from medicinal plants in tissue cultures. *Arzneim.-Forsch.*, 28(1):1–7, 1978.

Melzer, R et al. Procyanidins from Hypericum perforatum: effects on isolated guinea pig hearts. *Planta Med.*, 55:655–6, 1989.

Melzer, R et al. Vasoactive properties of procyanidins from Hypericum perforatum L. in isolated porcine coronary arteries. *Arzneim.-Forsch.*, 41:481–3, 1991.

Meruelo, D et al. Therapeutic agents with dramatic antiretroviral activity and little toxicity at effective doses: Aromatic polycyclic diones hypericin and pseudohypericin. *Proc. Natl. Acad. Sci.*, 85:5230–4, 1988.

Moses, EL and Mallinger, AG. St. John's Wort: Three Cases of Possible Mania Induction. *J. Clin. Psychopharmacol.*, 20(1):115–117, 2000.

Muldner, H and Zoller, M. Antidepressive Effect of a Hypericum Extract Standardized to the Active Hypericin Complex / biochemistry and clinical studies. *Arzneim.-Forsch. / Drug Res.*, 34:918–920, 1984.

Muller, WEG, Rossol R. Effects of Hypericum extract on the expression of serotonin receptors. *J. Ger. Psych. Neurol.*, 7(Suppl.1):S63–4, 1994.

Muller, WE et al. Effects of Hypericum Extract (LI 160) in Biochemical Models of Antidepressant Activity. *Pharmacopsychiat*, 30(Suppl):102–7, 1997.

Muller, WE et al. Hyperforin represernts the neurotransmitter reuptake inhibiting constituent of Hypericum extract. *Pharmacopsychiat.*, 31(Suppl.):16–21, 1998.

Muller, WE et al. Hyperforin – Antidepressant activity by a novel mechanism of action. *Pharmacopsych.*, 34(Suppl 1):S98–S102, 2001.

Murch, SJ et al. Melatonin in feverfew and other medicinal plants. *Lancet*, 350:1598-9, 1997.

Murch, SJ et al. An in vitro and hydroponic growing system for hypericin, pseudohypericin, and hyperforin production of St. John's wort (Hypericum perforatum CV New Stem). *Planta Med.*, 68:1108–12, 2002.

Nahrstedt, A and Butterweck, V. Biologically Active and Other Chemical Constituents of the Herb of Hypericum perforatum L. *Pharmacopsychiat*, 30(Suppl):129–34, 1997.

Negrash, AK and Pochinok, PY. Comparative study of chemotherapeutic and pharmacological properties of antimicrobial preparations from common St. John's wort. *Firont. Mater. Sov.*,6th, pp. 198–200, 1969. [Russ.] (*Chem. Abs.* 78:66908u).

Nierenberg, AA et al. Mania Associated with St. John's Wort. *Biol. Psychiatry*, 46:1707–1708, 1999.

Okpanyi, SN and Weischer, ML. Experimental Animal Studies of the Psychotropic Activity of a Hypericum Extract. *Arzneim Forsch/Drug Res*, 37:10–3, 1987.

Omel'chuk-Myakushko, IY and Fastovskaya, AY. Dynamics of the accumulation of antimicrobic substances in Hypericum perforatum. *Rast. Resur.*, 4:346–9, 1968. [Russ.] (*Chem. Abs.* 70: 9367c).

Ozturk, Y et al. Hepatoprotective activity of Hypericum perforatum L. alcoholic extract in rodents. *Phytother. Res.*, 6:44–6, 1992.

Parry, BL. A 45-year-old woman with premenstrual dysphoric disorder. *JAMA*,281(4):368–73, 1999.

Perloff, MD et al. Saint John's wort: An in vitro analysis of P-glycoprotein induction due to extended exposure. *Br. J. Pharmacol.*, 134:1601–8, 2001.

Perovic, S and Muller, WEG. Pharmacological Profile of Hypericum Extract—Effect on serotonin uptake by postsynaptic receptors. *Arzneim Forsch/Drug Res*, 45:1145–8, 1995.

Philipp, M et al. Hypericum extract versus imipramine or placebo in patients with moderate depression: randomized multicentre study of treatment for eight weeks. *Br. Med. J.*, 319:1534–9, 1999.

Pitman, V. Dioscorides' herbal. *Eur. J. Herb. Med.*, 4(2):43–66, 1998.

Razinskaite, D. Active substances of Hypericum perforatum (St. John's wort). 2. Flavonoids and dynamics of their content. *Liet. TSR Mokslu Akad. Darb., Ser. C*, (1):89–100, 1971. [Russ.] (*Chem. Abs.* 75:72427r).

Schellenberg, R et al. Pharmacodynamic effects of two different Hypericum extracts in healthy volunteers measured by quantitative EEG. *Pharmacopsychiat.*, 31:44–53, 1998.

Schey, KL et al. Photooxidation of lens alpha-crystallin by hypericin (active ingredient in St. John's wort). *Photochem. Photobiol.,* 72(2):200–3, 2000.

Schinazi, RF et al. Anthraquinones as a new class of antiviral agents against human immunodeficiency virus. *Antiviral Res.,* 13(5):265–72, 1990.

Schulz, V. Incidence and clinical relevance of the interactions and side effects of Hypericum preparations. *Phytomed.,* 8(2):152–60, 2001.

Shelton, RC et al. Effectiveness of St John's Wort in Major Depression. *JAMA,* 285(15):1978–1986, 2001.

Sparenberg, B et al. Antidepressive constituents of St. Johns wort. *PZ Wiss,* 6:50–4, 1993.

Stevinson, C and Ernst, E. Safety of Hypericum in patients with depression. A comparison with conventional antidepressants. *CNS Drugs,* 11(2):125–32, 1999.

Stevinson, C and Ernst, E. A pilot study of Hypericum perforatum for the treatment of premenstrual syndrome. *Br. J. Obstet. Gyn.,* 107:870–6, 2000.

Stock, S and Holzl, J. Pharmacokinetic test of [^{14}C]-labelled hypericin and pseudohypericin from Hypericum perforatum and serum kinetics of hypericin in man. *Planta Med.,* 57(Suppl.2):A61, 1991.

Stoyanova, A et al. Thin-layer chromatography of extracts of Hypericum perforatum. *Farmatsiya (Sofia),* (1):8–13, 1987. [Bulg.] (*Chem. Abs.* 107:205272q).

Suzuki, O et al. Inhibition of Type A and Type B Monoamine Oxidases by Naturally Occurring Xanthones. *Planta Med,* 42:17–21, 1981.

Suzuki, O et al. Inhibition of Monoamine Oxidase by Hypericin. *Planta Med,* 1984.; 50:272–4.

Takahashi, I et al. Hypericin and pseudohypericin specifically inhibit protein kinase C: possible relation to their antiretroviral activity. *Biochem. Biophys. Res. Comm.,* 165:1207–12, 1989.

Tang, J et al. Virucidal activity of hypericin against enveloped and non-enveloped DNA and RNA viruses. *Antiviral Res.,* 13:313–25, 1990.

Taylor, LH and Kobak, KA. An open-label trial of St. John's wort (Hypericum perforatum) in obsessive-compulsive disorder. *J. Clin. Psychiatry,* 61(8):575–8, 2000.

Tekel'ova, D et al. Quantitative changes of dianthrones, hyperforin and flavonoids content in the flower ontogenesis of Hypericum perforatorum. *Planta Med.,* 66:778–89, 2000.

Thiede, H-M and Walper, A. Inhibition of MAO and COMT by Hypericum extracts and hypericin. *J. Geriatr Psychiatry Neurol.,* 7(suppl 1):S54–6, 1994.

Tsitsina, SI. Results of studying some medicinal plants containing flavone compounds. *Tr. Bot. Sadov, Akad. Nauk Kaz. SSR,* 11:111–4, 1969. [Russ.] (*Chem. Abs.* 73:32345q).

Vasil'chenka, EA et al. Analgesic action of flavonoids of Rhododendron luteum Sweet, Hypericum perforatum L. Lespedeza bicolor Turoz. and L. hedysaroides (Pall.) Kitag. *Rastit. Resur.,* 22:12–21, 1986. [Russ.] (*Chem. Abs.* 104:142140k).

Volz, H-P et al. St John's wort extract (LI 160) in somatoform disorders: results of a placebo-controlled trial. *Psychopharmacol.,* 164:294–3000, 2002.

Vorbach, EU et al. Efficacy and Tolerability of St. John's Wort Extract LI 160 Versus Imipramine in

Patients with Severe Depressive Episodes According to ICD-10. *Pharmacopsychiat*, 30(Suppl): 81–5, 1997.

Wheatley, D. LI 160, an Extract of St. John's Wort, Versus Amitriptyline in Mildly to Moderately Depressed Outpatients - A Controlled 6-Week Clinical Trial. *Pharmacopsychiat*, 30(Suppl); 77–80, 1997.

Wilhelm, K-P., Biel, S. and Siegers, C-P. Role of flavonoids in controlling the phototoxicity of Hypericum perforatum extracts. *Phytomed.*, 8(4):306–9, 2001.

Wood, S et al. Antiviral activity of naturally occurring anthraquinones and anthraquinone derivatives. *Planta Med.*, 56:651–2, 1990.

ST. MARY'S MILK THISTLE—Heavenly Mark on a Healing Herb
Silybum marianum (L.) Gaertn. —fruit/seed

Summary

Valued as a food in its native Mediteranean habitat, the milk thistle plant has also served as a medicinal agent for problems of the blood and liver since the first century. As a remedy for liver complaints, the seeds became prominent in the 19th century when Rademacher advocated their tincture as a specific for the liver and spleen. Used as a means of reducing congestion of these organs and associated hemorrhage, varicose ulcers were also found by homeopaths to respond to the decoction and tincture. Its benefits from enhancing the appetite and digestion were seen to complement its therapeutic effects.

Study by the Germans in the late 20th century identified the flavonolignan fraction as being important components for its activity in protecting the liver from damage by chemical and biological agents. Referred to as silymarin, this mixture of active components has been shown to include anti-oxidants and anti-inflammatories agents. Other flavonoid components contribute to preventing toxic hepatitis. The major flavonolignan, silybin (silibinin) also promotes regeneration through induction of nucleic acid and protein replication. The protective effects of silymarin have been shown in animals to extend to other organs such as the kidneys and stomach. Human studies have shown the value of silymarin in protecting against liver damage from toxic chemical solvents, alcohol, and medications. It may have a role in reducing undesirable cholesterol and in topical cancer prevention. Test tube studies indicate a potential for affecting the metabolism of some drugs, but no such cases have been reported. Its safety profile is remarkable, and only a few isolated adverse effects have been documented.

Names, Food Uses, and Description

In medical texts of the past Silybum marianum has been referred to primarily by the scientific name Carduus marianus, but also as Cnicus marianus. Silybum is derived from the name silybon used by the Greek physician Dioscorides for an edible thistle. Carduus and Cnicus are other genera of the Asteraceae, or composite family, comprised of similar thistles.

Its various scientific and common names such as St. Mary's thistle, Marythistle (in German Mariendistel and in French chardon-Marie), Our Lady's thistle, holy thistle, and the now common milk thistle are based on an early Christian legend. It is said that when Mary and Joseph were fleeing to Egypt with the baby Jesus from the murderous intent of King Herod, in their haste some of Mary's milk spilled on the plant while trying to nurse. The leaves of the plant are characterized by a white pattern following their veins. Interestingly, the flowers of one type of milk thistle found in Egypt are white rather than purple, and Hammouda and others discovered in 1991 that the most effective component, silybin, is highest in this less abundant white-flowered variety.

Milk thistle was formerly cultivated for the food value of its stalks and young leaves, and the large tap roots were also eaten. According to Foster, the stalks were peeled and soaked in water, as were the roots to remove the bitterness. The flower heads were boiled and eaten like the artichoke thistle. Grieve noted that the seeds are a favorite food of goldfinches.

The plant is annual or biennial and grows up to eight feet in height. Besides the long, broad leaves having a characteristic white venation, they have the prickles typical of thistles. The stem is clasp by the upper leaves at their base. The large purple flowers appear in July. They are solitary at the ends of the branches and are surrounded by bracts with spines. The fruit is the portion employed in medicine, but it is often referred to as seed. It is used when ripe and has no odor. The fruit produce a mucilaginous and oily sensation in the mouth with a somewhat bitter taste.

Distribution and Species

Milk thistle is native to the Mediterranean region but has spread northward and to America with the early colonists, growing as a weed in disturbed soil. Described in 1997 by Gliona and McAllister as "Southern California's scraggliest, nastiest weed, a foreign interloper without natural enemies." Scientists believe it was introduced to California by the Spanish centuries earlier. The best means of control of milk thistle communities there was determined to be by prescribed burns that are cheaper and more effective than chemical or mechanical attempts.

The only other species in the genus is Silybum eburneum that has completely green leaves and is distributed in the same ecological regions around the Mediterranean. According to Hertz and others in 1991, S. marianum flowers produce twice the seeds that have twice the germination rate as S. eburneum. The two species can be easily crossed-pollinated, and the plants in the second succeeding generation have variegated versus plain green leaves in a ratio of 3:1.

Traditional Medical Uses of Different Parts of the Plant

Maude Grieve quotes a number of historical authorities about different milk thistle parts' uses. The Greek Dioscorides employed a drink from the seeds as a remedy for infants "that have their sinews drawn together" and for snakebites. Foster refers to Pliny the Elder, a Roman of the first century A.D., as using the plant juice with honey for "carrying off bile." Flora and others note that the herb along with the seed was used throughout the Middle Ages and later for its liver effects, as described by Otto Brunfels (1534), Hieronimum Bock (1595), Jacobus Theodorum (1664), and Adam Lonicerus (1679).

The noted early English herbalist Gerard considered the root as the best remedy for melancholy diseases. This was his way of describing its action on the liver, from a humoral perspective of melancholy as black bile. In 1694 Westmacott called the herb and its leaves "a Friend to the Liver and the Blood" when boiled and eaten. Referred to simply as Lady's thistle by Nicholas Culpeper, a follower of the Puritan Oliver Cromwell, it was listed and described along with a dozen other thistles. Comparing it favorably to blessed thistle (Carduus, or Cnicus, benedictus) for ague and the plague, he also noted its use for the liver and spleen. The infusion of the fresh root and seeds was taken internally for jaundice and gallstones and applied externally as a fomentation over the liver. He noted that these thistles were popular among the German physicians for assisting digestion and promoting sweating, but they were not popular among the English physicians of the 17th century. Culpeper, prior to Westmacott, noted that the young tender plant, boiled after removing the prickles, could be eaten in the spring as a blood cleanser, while John Evelyn indicated that when taken in this way the plant enhanced milk production in nursing women, similar to blessed thistle. Recently, John Lust described the leaves being used as a bitter tonic to stimulate the appetite and treat indigestion.

Later Medical Popularity of the Seed Tincture

The German doctor A.A. Rademacher can be credited with promoting the value of milk thistle seeds for the liver, while influencing medical practice with his theories. He popularized the concept of organ remedies and the use of "Rademacher's Tincture" of milk thistle. In his 1841 book Erfahrungsheillehre, Rademacher designated the tincture of Carduus seed as a primary botanical remedy for congestion of the liver and spleen and in hemorrhages associated with these organs, noting its usefulness in gall stone colic as well. He also gave the tincture for hemorrhoids and for painful urination due to sores in the female urethra.

It was among the homeopaths that Carduus found the greatest initial acceptance in America, including it in the United States Homeopathic Pharmacopeia in 1878. An article from the Homeopathic Recorder, reprinted anonymously in the Ecletic Medical Journal in 1893, described a new application for varicose ulcers. The discovery was made by accident while using a decoction of the seeds to treat liver inflammation and enlargement in a housewife, in accord with Rademachers indications. The decoction was then used in other cases of varicose ulcers unassociated with liver or spleen diseases and successfully cured over 60 cases. The mother tincture of the seeds was then used on a larger scale with a dose of 5 drops three times daily. Out of 196 cases of varicose ulcers, 145 cures were achieved using only this remedy internally, along with prescribing flannel bandages and wet (water) compresses externally. About 90% of these cases were women, and most were continuing hard work daily during treatment. The 51 cases that were not recorded as cures could not be classed as failures either, since most of these patients simply failed to return for a final assessment, even though amelioration had been observed in all but a few.

The Eclectic stalwart John Scudder noted in 1892 that Rademacher and his followers had been a principle influence on his practice of medicine. However, according to Felter and Lloyd in 1898, it was the doctors and professors Drs. H.T. Webster and Finley Ellingwood who introduced milk thistle to Eclectic medical practice. These Eclectics used the tincture for venous congestion of the liver, kidneys, and spleen. Dull, aching splenic pain that refers to the left scapula, along with despondency and general debility, was the condition for which it was specifically deemed effective. Its indications included nonmalarial enlargement of the spleen, but it was useful even when splenic enlargement could not be detected.

As for the liver, the Eclectic noted that tenderness under the ribs on the right side and abdominal pain associated with gall stones, jaundice, and swollen liver were reportedly benefitted. Pelvic weight due to congestion and painful urination could be improved. It was believed to alleviate blood in the stools, urine, or sputum, as well as uterine hemorrhage. A dose of 25 drops in water twice daily was used. Ellingwood listed Carduus marianus with the special alteratives. He noted that another Eclectic, Harvey, advocated its application for venous stasis and varicose veins, often with discoloration of the skin that Harvey associated with disease of the spleen. When giving 5-drop doses 3–4 times daily, the tincture must be used persistently, since it acts slowly.

Rademacher's book was translated to English and published by the homeopathic company Boericke and Tafel in America in 1909 as Rademacher's Universal and Organ Remedies. In his 1910 book dedicated to John Uri Lloyd, Eli Jones indicated that transverse enlargement of the liver, when accompanied by uneasiness, nausea, stitching, and pains in the left lobe, along with an enlarged abdomen, would be effectively treated by a tincture of Carduus marianus using 5 drops three times daily. Likewise, he said this dose was effective for enlarged spleen with heart palpitations, nausea, uneasiness, and a distended abdomen. Jones recommended Lloyd's Specific Medicines or homeopathic tinctures from Boericke and Tafel as reliable medications.

In her 1931 herbal Maude Grieve indicated that the seeds were used for the same purpose as blessed thistle. She went on to note that it was a popular remedy in Germany for jaundice and all sorts of biliary problems. In addition it was used as a demulcent in pleurisy and catarrh. For cases of cancer a decoction could be applied externally. In 1977 the naturopath John Lust described the classic indications for the seeds, writing that they "are good for liver, gallbladder, and spleen problems, and for jaundice and gallstone colic."

Focus on Flavonolignans

Foster describes how around 1958 attempts to isolate the components that most impact liver function had begun. By 1968 Wagner and others had separated the active fraction that they designated as silymarin. Products became available for clinical use in 1969. By 1974 they had identified silymarin as a flavonolignan complex and silybin as the major active component. The silymarin fraction comprises from 4%–6% of the ripe seeds. Since the discovery of silymarin, most of the attention and research has been limited to these flavonolignans and their effects on the liver. Often, this fraction is described as milk thistle extract, though it does not represent the greater phytochemical complexity of the native extracts that accounted for its broader long-term medical usage.

The desire to optimize the liver protective effects of the milk thistle flavonolignan fraction has led to the study of the plant's genetic variation that determines silybin content. In 1995 Hertz and others looked at the flavonolignan yield of three inbred generations for eleven lines obtained from Argentina, and two distinct groups were discovered. Over three years the silymarin content of one group averaged 70% silybin, 30% silychristin, and traces of silydianin, while the other yielded 30% silybin, 57% silychristin, and 13% silydianin. The high silybin group had silymarin content ranging from 1.59–4.38% over the 3 years, while the higher silychristin/silydianin group had silymarin ranges from 0.57–2.51%. The silymarin content of each line varied yearly.

Preparations

Powdered Seed

Lust advised using 1 teaspoon of powdered seeds with water four or five times daily as a naturopathic dose.

Water Extract

One teaspoon of crushed seeds is to be steeped in a half cup of water. From one to one and a half cups are consumed each day, but only a mouthful at a time according to Lust.

Tincture

Felter and Lloyd noted that the ripe seeds were known to best yield their properties to alcohol. They described how homeopaths and others produced a strong tincture by covering one part of the whole ripe seeds with two parts of dilute (50%) alcohol. It was allowed to remain in a cool, dark place in a stoppered bottle while it was shaken twice daily. Finally, it was decanted, strained, and filtered. The dose ranged from 1–20 drops, while the traditional homeopathic dose was 5 drops three times daily. According to Grieve, homeopaths at times would make their tincture using equal parts of the root and seeds with the hull attached. Lust recommended from 15–25 drops of the tincture four or five times a day as an effective dose.

Silymarin Standardized Extract Fraction

These concentrates are typically provided in capsular form. The most common contain 140 mg of silymarin, a flavonolignan complex, per dosing unit. This can be 200 mg of an extract fraction with a 70% silymarin concentration or 175 mg of a fraction with 80% silymarin. Some of the researched silymarin standardized products whose names are registered trademarks include Thisylin in America, Legalon, Hepatron, and Carsil in Europe, and Silybor in Russia. The usual doses of silymarin in positive clinical studies range from 315 mg to 800 mg daily.

A comparative study of 7 different silymarin products by Schulz and others in 1995 found that the actual content of silymarin varied from 70% to 116% of the label claim (silybin content varied from 80% to 118% of the statement on the label). Furthermore, dissociation and liberation of the silymarin and silybin in test tubes varied greatly, with the lowest content product dissociating the least but another of the lower content products liberating the most.

Components of Fruit/Seeds

Silybum fruit/seeds contain a variety of flavonolignans that together are designated as the fraction silymarin. This separated fraction is not water soluble. Silybin (silibinin) isosilybin, silydianin, and silychristin are recognized as major components of this fraction. According to Hammouda and others in 1991 and 1993, both silybin and isosilybin are found in A and B forms, and silydianin is present in the greatest quantity in the more common purple-flowered plants. Of the flavonolignans, silybin is considered the main active compound, as described by Wagner and others in 1974. Along with the flavonolignans they identified the flavonoids taxifolin and quercitin along with dehydro-diconiferyl acholol as important components of the fruit.

In 1993 Hammouda and others compared the silymarin content of the fruit and its ethyl acetate extracts from plants cultimated under different conditions and growing wild. A 60% water regime per field capacity without fertilization led to the greatest total silymarin percentage in the extracts and the greatest silybin, isosilybin, and silychristin contents, compared to 75% and 45% capacity. Fertilization at the higher levels (100 and 150 kg nitrogen per feddan) tended to increase fruit and extract contents in a similar fashion, but this was not greatly superior to no fertilization. For the wild plants the total silymarin content was comparable, but the white-flowered variety had a much greater silybin and silychristin content, while the purple-flowered variety was very high in silydianin.

In 1984 Hikino and others identified flavonoids in minor amounts in the seeds that have significant protective effects against liver toxins such as eriodictyol, 5,7-dihydroxychromone, naringenin, and taxifolin. They also described additional flavonolignans in the white variety that contribute hepatoprotective activity such as silandrin (3-deoxyisosilybin), 3-deoxysilychristin, and silymonin (3-deoxysilydianin). Varma and others found the seeds also contain betaine hydrocloride that is used by the liver in the synthesis of choline. In 1970 Schulte and others identified polyacetylenes in the roots, flowering tops, and sprouts of the plant, but none were found in the fruit.

Laboratory Pharmacological Research

Kinetics

SILYMARIN/SILYBIN

An oral dose of 200 mg/kg of silymarin was given to rats by Morazzoni and others in 1993 and compared to an equimolar amount of the silybin-phosphatidylcholine complex silipide (IdB 1016) given orally. With silipide the silybin reached a peak in the plasma within two hours, and the biliary recovery after 24 hours was 13% of the total administered. For silymarin the total plasma level of both free and unconjugated silybin was several-fold less, and the 24-hour biliary recovery was 2% of the administered silybin. However, the plasma and bile concentrations for the isosilybin were higher than for silybin itself, and silydianin and silycristin were also present.

Liver Toxicity Prevention and Recovery

WATER EXTRACT

Milk thistle fruit infusion given orally reduces liver damage from methoxsalen when given 24 hours and 2 hours before the drug, as indicated by SGOT serum levels in mice according to Raskovic and others in 2000.

FLAVONOIDS

Besides the flavonolignans, other components were shown by Hikono and others in 1984 to have protective effects for liver cells against toxins in test tube situations. Against galactosamine induction of cytotoxicity as shown by glutamic pyruvic transaminase (GPT) levels, the flavonoids eriodityon, naringenin, taxifolin, and 5,7-dihydroxychromone were also effective, along with minor flavonolignan components including silandrin, deoxysilychristin, and silymonin. With carbon tetrachloride, the dihydroxychromone and naringenin had significant preventive effects, but eriodictyol increased the GPT levels.

SILYMARIN

Silymarin was shown by Magliulo and others in 1973 to improve the rate of regeneration of liver cells in rats that were subjected to partial liver removal. Yet, the recent interest in silymarin originated with animal studies that investigated its effects on the liver in relation to exposure to a variety of known liver toxins. In 1968 Hahn and others found that silymarin protected the liver from the mushroom poison alpha-amanitine. From 1969-1975 studies by Vogel and Temme, Schriewer, Desplaces, and others showed that silymarin protects and cures the liver from damage due to the potent hepatotoxin phalloidin from Amanita phalloides (deathcap fungus).

In 1968 Hahn and others also showed silymarin to be protective against acute carbon tetrachloride poisoning. In 1971 Rauen and Schriewer discovered that silymarin exerted both protective and curative effects on rat liver damage caused by carbon tetrachloride. Liver protection was again shown by Schriewer and others in 1973 by monitoring serum enzyme activities of sorbitol dehydrogenase, GPT, glutamic oxalacetic transaminase (GOT), and glutamic dehydrogenase (GLDH) increased by carbon tetrachloride. However, that same year Williams and Priestly failed to find diminished GPT levels in rats pretreated with silymarin prior to carbon tetrachloride exposure. Letteron and others concluded in 1990 that silymarin prevents the lipid peroxidation and hepatotoxicity caused by carbon tetrachloride in mice by decreasing its metabolic activation as well as through antioxidant effects.

Destructive changes by ethanol in the mitochondria of rat liver cells were largely prevented by silymarin in a study by Platt and Schnorr in 1971. Valenzuela and others had shown liver protective effects from ethanol toxicity by a reduction of both lipid peroxidation and malondialdehyde production in 1985[b]. In 1989 Valenzuela and others found that silymarin increases the redox state and total glutathione content in the liver of the rat preferentially due to enterohepatic circulation.

Silymarin's effects have been demonstrated with a number of other liver toxic drugs. Silymarin was shown by Hahn and others to be protective against induction of cirrhosis from chronic exposure of rats to thioacetamide. The increase in triglycerides and malic enzyme from repeated doses of halothane was prevented by silymarin in the study by Janiak and others in 1973. Liver protection was again shown by Schriewer and others in 1973 by reducing serum sorbitol dehydrogenase, GPT, GOT, and GLDH increased by deoxycholate. In 1974 Ramellini and Meldolesi showed protection from deoxycholate damage to rat the liver plasma membranes in test tubes was evident at low (0.5 mM) silymarin concentration. In 1988 Mourelle and others found silymarin helped reduce elevations of serum levels of GPT, gamma-glutamyl transpeptidase, and alkaline phosphatase from thallium exposure, along preventing liver lipid peroxidation and reduced glutathione content. Due to silymarin replenishing mitochondrial glutathione, the hepatotoxicity of methotrexate was abolished in a test tube study by Neuman and others in 1999.

In 1971 Rauen and Schriewer discovered that silymarin exerted both protective and curative effects on rat liver damage caused by D-galactosamine, a condition resembling viral hepatitis in humans. Then in 1973, Schriewer and Rauen found elevations in GOT, GPT, and GLDH caused by galactosamine hepatitis in rats were reduced by silymarin injected intraperitoneally. The injection of water-soluble silymarin in mice and rats by Gendrault and others in 1980 protected the endothelial cells of the liver from damage by the lethal frog virus 3 and prevented rupture of the sinusoidal lining.

Silybin

Silybin (silibinin) has shown a similar protective activity to the silymarin complex when using some of the same liver toxins. Water-soluble silybin (described as the dihydrogensuccinate or dihemisuccinate salt) inhibited the uptake of the Amanita poison amatoxin by rat liver cells when studied by Faulstich and others in 1980. Silybin was proven to be an effective treatment for poisoning of beagles by the deathcap fungus Amanita phalloides by markedly reducing the hemorrhagic necrosis of the liver. This was demonstrated in 1984 when Vogel and others found it reduced serum GOT and GPT, alkaline phosphatase, and bilirubin and diminished the fall in prothrombin time.

Liver damage in rats treated with carbon tetrachloride was partially or completely inhibited by silybin, when studied by Gupta and others in 1982. However, Letteron and others observed in 1990 that silybin was less effective than silymarin in reducing lipid peroxidation in carbon tetrachloride poisoning of the liver cells in test tubes, and its effects were not as long lasting as silymarin's in live mice. Halothane reduction of liver microsomal cytochrome activity and induction of fatty liver following a single exposure was diminished when silybin was given orally to mice 3 days before and 7 days after, as shown by Janiak in 1974.

Toxicity of acetaminophen (paracetamol) was reduced by silybin in rats as was shown by Campos and others in 1989 by monitoring serum enzyme activities of GOT and GPT as well as liver lipid peroxidation, malondialdehyde production, and reduced glutathione content. Garrido and others showed in 1991 that acetaminophen liver toxicity is actually due to the acetaminophen metabolite, and silybin helps reduce the oxidation of acetaminophen.

Lipid peroxidation of rat liver cells and their microsomes in test tubes was inhibited in a concentration-dependent manner (in order of potency) by silymarin > silicristin = silidianin > isosilybin = silybin in a study by Bosisio and others in 1992. However, when examining cell damage as evaluated as LDH release, they found only silybin and isosilybin had significant activity. The inhibition by silybin of 5-lipoxygenase products by the liver Kupffer cells in test tubes as shown by Dehmlow and others in 1996 contributes to its protective effects.

A primary mechanism of recovery was discovered in 1986 when Sonnenbichler and others showed that the water-soluble silybin salt enhanced liver DNA synthesis. Sonnenbichler and Zetl confirmed this in 1992 and found that regeneration is further improved by the selective activation of RNA-polymerase I by silybin that consequentially stimulates ribosomal RNA synthesis, ribosome formation, and protein synthesis.

Liver Fibrosis Protection

SILYMARIN

In 1997 Boigk and others decided to test silymarin with 60% silybin in rats whose bile ducts were occluded by a chemical injection. Treated rats received silymarin at a dose of 50 mg/kg daily for 1–6 weeks or through weeks 4–6 after the occlusion. A 30-35% reduction in total hydroxyproline, or liver collagen, was produced in this silymarin group of rats compared to those with no silymarin treatment. This action as a true antifibrotic was in addition to its decreasing alkaline phosphatase in these rats.

Non-liver Tissue Protection from Toxic Drugs

SILYMARIN

Silymarin is credited with membrane-stabilizing effects from free radical scavenging outside of the liver. This was demonstrated by Valenzuela and others in 1985[a] through protecting red blood cells against membrane lipid peroxidation by phenylhydrazine.

SILYBIN

Silybin (as a dihydrogensuccinate) helps prevent kidney damage from nephrotoxic anti-tumor agent cisplatin as shown by Gaedeke and others in 1996, when given at doses of 200 mg/kg intravenously to rats. Also in 1996 Bokemeyer and others demonstrated that this compound does not diminishing the anti-tumor activity of cisplatin or ifosfamide against human testicular cancer cell lines in test tubes. Silybin given intraperitoneally to rats at a dose of 200 mg/kg daily also protects the exocrine secretion of pancreatic amylase from being diminished by the toxicity of cyclosporin A, as observed by Schonfeld and others in 1997.

Antiulcer

SILYMARIN

In 1989 Valenzuela and others found that silymarin increases the redox state and total glutathione content in the stomach and intestines of the rat. The use of silymarin orally was shown by de la Lastra and others in 1992 to prevent stomach ulcer formation in rats caused by cold-restraint stress or by tying the pyloric valve shut, but not by pure alcohol. The stomach acid secretion was not altered by silymarin, but its histamine concentration was diminished. The effect was similar to the standard ulcer drug carbenoxolone and was believed to be due to inhibition of lipoxygenase and its production of inflammatory products. The report of their continued study in 1995 showed silymarin also protected the stomach lining from injury following ischemia and reperfusion, an indicator that it may inhibit neutrophil function that contributes to the damage.

Anti-inflammatory

SILYMARIN

As early as 1970, Zoltan and Gyori found silymarin was able to suppress inflammatory conditions outside of the liver such as reduce brain edema and functional deterioration of the CNS induced by triethyltinsulfate poisoning. In 1975 Vogel and others reported it was also shown to reduce formalin peritonitis and immune-induced polyarthritis in rats. In two articles in 1979 Fiebrich and Koch had indicated by test tube inhibition of lipoxygenase and the prostaglandin synthetase enzyme complex by silybin, silydianin, and silychristin suggests that preventing enzymatic conversion of membrane lipoids is the means by which silymarin prevents lipid peroxidation and production of inflammatory products.

In 1996 de la Puerta and others determined that giving silymarin orally significantly reduced the number of neutrophils in inflammatory exudates in mice. They also found that oral silymarin in rats reduced paw edema caused by carrageenan, and topically it was comparable in its efficacy to indomethacin in relieving inflammation caused by xylene in mice ears. In 1999 Gupta and others determined that the means by which silymarin was effective in models of induced arthritis in rats was by inhibition of 5-lipoxygenase.

Histamine Reduction

SILYMARIN

Silymarin given orally by de la Lastra and others in 1992 to rats decreased stomach histamine concentration.

SILYBIN

Miadonna and others determined that silybin significantly reduces histamine release from human basophils in a concentration-dependant manner in test tubes. They believed that further study of its potential anti-allergy activity should be done in living animals.

Cholesterol Lowering

SILYMARIN

Silymarin was compared by Krecman and others in 1998 to the anticholesterol drug probucol for lowering cholesterol in rats fed a high cholesterol diet. Oral silymarin not only had a parallel dose-dependent hypocholesterolemic effect compared to probucol, but it also increased HDL-cholesterol and decreased liver cholesterol. Both of these desirable outcomes were lacking with probucol. Silymarin also prevented the decrease in reduced glutathione in the liver associated with high cholesterol diets. By comparison, silybin was not as effective in these ways as silymarin.

Radiation Protection

SILYMARIN

Silymarin given orally to mice by Flemming in 1971 prolonged survival, sped recovery and reduced weight loss following whole-body X-ray doses described as partially lethal and minimum lethal.

Topical Tumor Prevention

SILYMARIN

The application of silymarin topically prevented tumor promotion by several chemical agents on carcinogen-initiated mouse skin, as demonstrated by Zi and others in 1997. This prevention was apparently due to inhibition of mRNA expression of tumor necrosis factor alpha, a tumor promoter found naturally in the mouse epidermis.

Human Bioavailability and Clinical Studies

Kinetics

SILYMARIN/SILYBIN

In 1984 Lorenz and others administered 560 mg of oral silymarin containing 240 mg silybin to six subjects. The resultant serum concentrations and urinary excretion of silybin over the subsequent 24 hours were low. Only 1–2% of the silybin was excreted by the kidneys during the first day. However, after giving 140 mg of silymarin containing 60 mg silybin to patients following gall bladder removal with T-tube drains, the concetration in the bile was found to be 100 times higher than in the serum.

The excretion of silybin in the bile was measured by Schandalik and others in 1992 after administration of 120 mg of silymarin to nine patients with gall bladder removal surgery. Within 48 hours only 3% of the silybin dose was recovered in the bile. Isosilybin was present in an equivalent amount, while silydianin and silychristin were found in concentrations of less than 1% of the dose or were undetectable in five and three subjects, respectively. The peak concentrations were observed within the first 6 hours. By comparison, a lipophilic silybin-phosphatidylcholine complex called silipide (IdB1016) resulted in an 11% silybin recovery in the bile and a higher plasma silybin concentration as determined in three subjects.

The low bile and plasma levels may be due to only identifying silybin in its unconjugated form. According to a study by Weyhenmeyer and others in 1992 with 6 healthy males, only 10% of total silybin (measuring both diasteromers) in the plasma is in the unconjugated form. The half-life of the unconjugated silybin was less than one hour, but for total silybin the half-life is about six hours. Excretion of 5% of the dose is through the urine. No adverse events were noted while using up to 700 mg of silymarin (254 mg silybin). The plasma levels correlated directly with the different doses consumed (102, 153, 203, and 254 mg silybin).

In 1995 10 healthy male volunteers were given 140 mg of silymarin, containing 53.2 mg silybin, in a single oral dose by Rickling and others. For the two silybin diastereomers in the plasma, 23% of diastereomer 1 and only 3% of diastereomer 2 were found in unconjugated form. The differences probably are due to stereoselective metabolism, absorption or distribution.

The pharmacokinetics of silybin in two products claiming standardization to 140 mg silymarin (actual measured silymarin content 162 mg and 122 mg) were compared by Schulz and others in 1995 together with a "higher content" 167 mg silymarin product (measured as actually 117 mg). It was shown that 2 hours after oral consumption the plasma concentration of silybin for the 122 mg silymarin-containing product was three times that of the 162 mg silymarin product and twice as high as for the 117 mg product. In other words, relative bioavailability of different products cannot be predicted even when the actual content is known.

When 80 mg silybin complexed with 160 mg phosphatidylcholine was assessed by Savio and others in 1998 for relative bioavailability, they found that the absorption of this form was 2-3 times grater when taken in a soft-gel capsule as compared with a hard shell capsule.

Liver Toxicity Protection

SILYMARIN

A clinical trial by Poser in 1971 using silymarin for toxic-metabolic liver damage, chronic-persisting hepatitis, and cholangitis hepatopathies in 67 subjects showed significant success based upon symptomatic changes, reduction in serum GOT, GPT, and glutamate dehydrogenase (GLDH), and biopsy findings. According to Blumenthal, German studies by Hammerl, Kurz-Dimitrowa, and others in 1971 also showed improvements when using up to 315 mg of silymarin daily for toxic hepatitis.

In a 1973 study following surgeries for gall bladder removal, Fintelmann studied the effects of 210 mg of silymarin daily in 20 patients and 420 mg in 31 patients daily compared to 32 controls. The use of barbiturates and the anesthetic halothane helped contribute to increased levels of these three serum enzymes associated with liver toxicity. In the group using 420 mg silymarin before and for eight days after the operation, the elevations of the serum GOT, GPT and GLDH were reduced on the first postsurgical day. The pre-operative use of silymarin by Fintelmann in1986 for a cholecystectomy resulted in a large reduction in the post-operative rise in serum enzymes, especially GLDH.

In 1981 Boari and others studied a placebo group of 20 patients whose occupational exposure to toxic substances (e.g., solvents, paints, and glues) impaired hepatic function along with 35 similar patients receiving a dose of 420 mg/day of silymarin. The silymarin group was found to have some benefits, especially with subacute toxin exposure as opposed to chronic forms. Again in 1986 Fintelmann normalized liver enzyme changes with the addition of silymarin to treatment in a patient that had hepatitis caused by dilantin.

A dose of 400 mg twice daily of the extract silymarin helped prevent liver damage from hepatotoxic butyrophenones and phenothiazines in 15 patients in a placebo-controlled double-blind study by Palasciano and others in 1994. When given with tacrine by Allain and others in 1999, 420 mg/day of oral silymarin reduced the gastrointestinal and cholinergic side effects of this drug compared with placebo. The toxicologic buffering was accomplished without interfering with tacrine's effect on cognitive performance in this 12-week randomized, placebo-controlled, double-blind study.

Alcoholic Cirrhosis and Liver Disease

SILYMARIN

Silymarin's liver protective effects in excessive ethanol consumption have been most documented. A double-blind study of alcoholic cirrhosis patients by Benda and others in 1980 showed a significantly higher survival rate in the silymarin-treated group. In 1982 its liver protective effect was confirmed by Salmi and Sarna in a placebo-controlled study with 97 patients suffering from acute and subacute liver disease due primarily to alcohol abuse. A significantly greater decrease of GOT and GPT in the silymarin-treated group was accompanied by more frequent normalization of histological changes. Salvagnini and others in 1985 performed a randomized, placebo-controlled, double-blind study with 122 patients with alcoholic liver disease using 420 mg silymarin daily. The silymarin group had significantly superior reduction in GGT levels. The use of silymarin for alcohol liver injury by Fintelmann in 1986 helped normalize lab indices such as serum GGT, GOT, and especially GPT. In a 1989 study by Trinchet and others of patients with proven alcoholic hepatitis, 57 received 420 mg silymarin orally each day for three months and 59 received placebo. Both groups had significant improvement based on liver biopsy and serum aminotransferase activity, so the authors concluded that the effect of silymarin was not clinically relevant in moderate alcoholic hepatitis. Lang and others in 1990 found that combining silymarin with amino-imidazol-carboxamide-phosphate for one month in compensated alcoholic cirrhosis was effective compared to placebo. In their double blind trial, this combination normalized elevated serum levels of aminotransferases and bilirubin, markedly reduced high GGT, decrease the CD8+ cell percentage, and suppressed lymphocytotoxicity.

Again in 1990 patients with chronic alcoholic liver disease who received 420 mg of silymarin daily for six months demonstrated a fall in serum malondialdehyde compared with those received placebo, in a study by Muzes and others. Earlier in 1989 a double-blind, randomized study was performed by Ferenci and others with 170 cirrhosis patients. In this trial the 87 patients (46 alcoholic and 41 non-alcoholic) who received 140 mg silymarin three times daily had a significantly reduced mortality rate. Their 4-year survival rate was 58%, compared to 39% in the placebo group. This effect was more pronounced for those with alcoholic cirrhosis. However, in 1998 Pares and others studied the effect of 450 mg of silymarin daily on proven alcoholic liver cirrhosis. Compared to 68 controls, 57 patients receiving silymarin for two years showed no improvement in survival rates or on the clinical course of the disease. According to the 2003 text by Blumenthal, silymarin studies using 420 mg daily for alcohol liver disease published in foreign language showed positive effects by Fintelmann and Albert (1980), as well as DiMario (1981), Feher (1989), and Deak (1990) and others. Meanwhile, Bunout and others (1992) found no advantage in morbidity or mortality with 280 mg silymarin per day in 25 patients with alcoholic liver disease compared with 34 receiving placebo.

Viral Hepatitis

SILYMARIN

Blumenthal reported a German study by Magliulo and others in 1978 that showed improved liver function tests for acute hepatitis A and B patients who used 420 mg silymarin daily. On the other hand, in 1977 Kiesewetter and others found in two double-blind studies with 24 and 12 patients that no difference in laboratory tests could be found between silymarin and placebo in treating chronic hepatitis for 3-12 months, though some histological cellular changes were noted. Again, in 1978 a double-blind clinical trial by Scheiber and Wohlzogen with 10 chronic hepatitis patients being given silymarin at a dose of 420 mg daily significantly reduced histopathological changes in the liver compared with placebo after 12 months of treatment.

SILYBIN

The silybin complex with phosphatidylcholine (IdB1016) was tested in a randomized placebo-controlled, double-blind trial by Buzzelli and others in 1993 with 20 patients suffering from chronic active hepatitis. After seven days 240 mg silybin twice daily produced a significant reduction in GGT, alanine aminotransferase, and aspartate aminotransferase levels in 10 patients, compared with 10 others on placebo. Compared to baseline value, the reductions in these enzyme levels and in total bilirubin were even more significant.

Cirrhotic Diabetes Improvement

SILYMARIN

In 1997 Velussi and others utilized 600 mg of silymarin daily in a 12-month open, controlled study with diabetic patients suffering from alcholic cirrhosis. After 4 months there were significant decreases in fasting blood glucose levels, average daily blood glucose, daily urinary sugar levels, and glycosylated hemoglobin. While the control group with standard insulin therapy had a stabilized insulin need and significant increase in fasting insulin levels, those receiving insulin and silymarin had significant decreases in average insulin requirements and fasting insulin levels. Also, the silymarin group had decreased malondialdhyde levels, indicative of improved liver status. The results suggest silymarin reduced lipoperoxidation of cell membranes and decreased insulin resistance.

Research on Drug Metabolism Influence

SILYMARIN

Contrary to a report by Kim and others in 1997, no evidence was found of an interaction of silymarin with CYP 2E1 in test tubes by Miguez and others in 1994. The reduction of hepatotoxicity appears to be due to antioxidant and free radical scavenging properties. In 2000 Venkataramanan and others provided test tube evidence that silymarin inhibits the phase I CYP 3A4 and phase II enzyme UGT. These effects contribute to inhibition of the metabolism of testosterone. However, in 2002 milk thistle extract was given by Piscitelli and others to ten human subjects at a dose of 153 mg silymarin three times daily for three weeks and did not alter CYP 3A4 metabolism of the HIV drug indinavir.

Altered metabolism of a single dose of aspirin was improved in carbon tetrachloride-induced liver cirrhosis in rats by 50 mg/kg silymarin, according to Mourell and Favari in 1988, and in portal hypertension when 150 mg/kg silymarin was given concurrently with aspirin to rats by Favari and others in 1997. Also, silymarin at doses of 210 mg daily for 4 weeks had no influence in human metabolism of phenylbutazone or aminopyrine after single doses of these drugs as shown by Leber and Knauff in 1976.

SILYBIN

As early as 1974 silybin was studied by Down and others among those involved in drug metabolism research, but the only certain influence found on the enzymes investigated was an increased demethylase activity. In 1994 Bartholomaeus and others found that silybin was a potent inhibitor of glutathione-S-transferase isoenzymes in test tubes. Contrary to earlier reports, no evidence was found of an interaction of silybin with CYP 2E1 by Miguez and others in 1994, nor on CYP 1A2, 2A6, 2C19, or 2E1 by Beckmann-Knopp and others in 2000. However, inhibition of metabolism for CYP 2C9 substrates (including S-warfarin) and CYP 3A4 substrates at therapeutic silybin concentrations could not be excluded by the latter research team.

Determinations of Relative Safety

As reported by Blumenthal in 2003, the only adverse effect reported in clinical trials with silymarin is an occasional mild laxative effect. A case report in 1999 by the Adverse Drug Reactions Advisory Committee in Australia describes an idiosyncratic response to a milk thistle product intermittently over a two-month period of time. After taking a capsule of this product a 57-year old woman would experience for up to 24 hours episodes involving sweating, nausea, vomiting abdominal pain, diarrhea, weakness and collapse. After admission to the hospital she stopped taking the product for two weeks. When it was re-introduced a violent reaction ensued. This was similar to another case in a woman who had nausea, abdominal pains, listlessness, and insomnia after using milk thistle. One other adverse effect case that involved a man with low platelet counts was associated with his use of milk thistle, but the relationship was uncertain.

Farnsworth and others reported in 1975 that the seeds and root were used as an emmenagogue in Italy. However, the silymarin fraction was safely used by six women with intrahepatic cholestasis of pregnancy for 15 days when given a dosage of 210 mg three times daily by Gonzalez and others in 1988. Hahn and others found no embryotoxic effect with silymarin in mice, rats, rabbits, and dogs in 1968.

Silymarin had a low toxicity as determined in various animals following acute, subchronic, and chronic tests by Hahn and others. Following a single intravenous injection by Desplaces and others in 1975, the median lethal dose (fatal to half the animals tested) was 970–1050 mg/kg for mice and 825–920 mg/kg for rats. The minimal lethal dose for rabbits and dogs was about 300 mg/kg. Vogel and others in the same year found that lethal intravenous doses of silymarin begin between 100–200 mg/kg depending on the species (mice, rats, rabbits, dogs, and pigs) and primarily cause a weakening effect on the heart muscle. Slow heart rate and low blood pressure occur in dogs and rats at doses of up to 30 mg/kg.

Table 13   Milk Thistle Seeds and Derivatives—
            Summary of Medicinal Uses and Pharmacology

MILK THISTLE *Silybum marianum* (L.) Gaertn. G.	Ancient Historical Uses	Traditional Medical Uses	Modern Clinical Studies	Laboratory Research Findings
Whole Fruit / Seeds		Biliary problems Jaundice Pleurisy Catarrh		
Water Extracts	Snakebites Liver tonic Jaundice Gall stones	Enlarged liver Inflamed liver Varicose ulcers External: cancer		Anti-hepatotoxic
Tincture (Hydroalcoholic)		Enlarged Liver/ spleen/kidney Painful spleen Inflamed liver Jaundice Visceral bleeding Gall stone colic Urethral sores Hemorrhoids Varicose ulcers		

FRACTIONS OR ISOLATED CONSTITUENTS

Flavonoids				Anti-hepatotoxic
Silymarin			Acute toxic hepatitis Drug induced hepatitis Acute viral hepatitis Alcoholic liver disease Cirrhosis with diabetes	Anti-hepatotoxic Anti-oxidant Antifibrotic Anti-ulcer Anti-inflamma- tory Anti-tumor promoter Membrane stabilizer Lower histamine Radiation protection

Table 13   *Continued*

MILK THISTLE *Silybum marianum* (L.) Gaertn. G.	Ancient Historical Uses	Traditional Medical Uses	Modern Clinical Studies	Laboratory Research Findings
Silybin (Silibinin)			Chronic hepatitis	Anti-hepatotoxic Antinephrotoxic Anti-oxidant Anti-inflammatory Lower histamine Enhances protein & nucleic acid synthesis

References

BOOKS

Blumenthal, M (sen. Ed.). *The ABC Clinical Guide to Herbs*, American Botanical Council, Austin, Texas, 2003.

Culpeper, N. *Complete Herbal*, 1653, W. Foulsham & Co., Ltd., London.

Ellingwood, F. *American Materia Medica, Therapeutics and Pharmacognosy*, 1919 ver., Eclectic Med. Pub., Sandy, OR, 1994.

Felter, HW and Lloyd, JU. *King's American Dispensatory*, 1898 ver., Eclectic Medical Pub., Portland, OR., 1983.

Foster, S. *Milk Thistle Silybum marianum*. Botanical Series—305, American Botanical Council, Austin, Tex., 1999.

Grieve, M. *A Modern Herbal*, 1931 version, Dover Publ, Inc., New York, 1971.

Jones, EG. *Definite Medication*, 1910, reprinted by Jain Publishing Co., New Delhi, India.

Lust, J. *The Herb Book*, Bantam Books, New York, 1974.

ARTICLES

Anonymous. Carduus marianus in varicose ulcers. *Ecl. Med. J.*, 53:362-3, 1893.

Adverse Drug Reactions Advisory Committee. An adverse reaction to the herbal medication milk thistle (Silybum marianum). *Med. J. Austral.*, 170:218–219, 1999.

Allain, H et al. Aminotransferase Levels and Silymarin in de novo Tacrine-Treated Patients with Alzheimer's Disease. *Dement Geriatr. Cogn. Disord.*, 10:181–5, 1999.

Bartholomaeus, AE et al. Inhibition of rat liver cytosolic glutathione S-transferase by silybin. *Xenobiot.*, 24(1):17–24, 1994.

Beckmann-Knopp, S et al. Inhibitory Effects of Silibinin on Cytochrome P-450 Enzymes in Human Liver Microsomes. *Pharmacol. Toxicol.*, 86:250–6, 2000.

Benda, L et al. The Influence of Therapy with silymarin on the Survival Rate of Patients with Liver Cirrhosis. [German] *Wien. Klin. Wochen.*, 92:678v9, 1980.

Boari, C et al. Occupational toxic liver diseases. Therapeutic effects of silymarin. *Min. Med.*, 72:2679–88, 1981.

Boigk, G et al. Silymarin retards collagen accumulation in early and advanced biliary fibrosis secondary to complete bile duct obliteration in rats. *Hepatol.*, 26:643–9, 1997.

Bokemeyer, C et al. Silibinin protects against cisplatin-induced nephrotoxicity without compromising cisplatin or ifosfamide anti-tumour activity. *Br. J. Cancer*, 74:2036–41, 1996.

Bosisio, E et al. Effect of the flavonolignans of Silybum marianum L. on lipid peroxidation in rat liver microsomes and freshly isolated hepatocytes. *Pharmacol. Res.*, 25(2):147–54, 1992.

Bunout, D et al. Controlled study of the effect of silymarin on alcoholic liver disease. [Spanish] *Rev. Med. Chil.*, 120(12):1370–5, 1992.

Buzzelli, G et al. A pilot study on the liver protective effect of silybinphosphatidylcholin complex (IdB1016) in chronic active hepatitis. *Int. J. Clin. Pharmacol. Ther. Toxicol.*, 31(9):456–60, 1993.

Campos, R et al. Silybin Dihemisuccinate Protects Against Glutathione Depletion and Lipid Peroxidation Induced by Acetaminophen on Rat Liver. *Planta Med.*, 55:417–9, 1989.

Dehmlow, C et al. Inhibition of Kupffer Cell Functions as an Explanation for the Hepatoprotective Properties of Silibinin. *Hepatol.*, 23:749–54, 1996.

Desplaces, A et al. The effects of silymarin on experimental phalloidine poisoning. *Arzneim.-Forsch.*, 25:89–96, 1975.

Down, WH et al. Effect of silybin on the hepatic microsomal drug-metabolising enzyme system in the rat. *Arzneim.-Forsch.*, 24(12):1986–8, 1974.

Farnsworth, NR et al. Potential Value of Plants as Sources of New Antifertility Agents I. *J. Pharm. Sci.*, 64:535–98, 1975.

Faulstich, H et al. Silybin inhibition of amatoxin uptake in the perfused rat liver. *Arzniem.-Forsch.*, 30(3):452–4, 1980.

Favari, L et al. Effect of portal vein ligation and silymarin treatment on aspirin metabolism and disposition in rats. *Biopharmaceut. Drug Dispos.*, 18:53–64, 1997.

Ferenci, P et al. Randomized controlled trial of silymarin treatment in patients with cirrhosis of the liver. *J. Hepatol.*, 9:105–13, 1989.

Fiebrich, F and Kock, H. Silymarin, an inhibitor of lipoxygenase. *Experientia*, 35:1548–50, 1979.

Fiebrich, F and Koch, H. Silymarin, an inhibitor of prostaglandin synthetase. *Experientia*, 35:1550–2, 1979.

Fintelmann, V. Postoperative behavior of serum-cholinesterase. [German] *Med. Klin.*, 68:809–15, 1973.

Fintelmann, V. Toxic-Metabolic Liver Damage and its Treatment. [German] *Zeitsch. Phytother.*, (3):65–73, 1986.

Flemming, K. Effect of silymarin on x-irradiated mice.[German] *Arzneim.-Forsch.*, 21:1373–5,1971.

Flora, K et al. Milk thistle (Silybum marianum) for the therapy of liver disease. *Am. J. Gastroenterol.*, 93:139–143, 1998.

Gaedeke, J et al. Cisplatin nephrotoxicity and protection by silibinin. *Nephrol. Dial. Transplant.*, 11:55–62, 1996.

Garrido, A et al. Acetaminophen does not induce oxidative stress in isolated rat hepatocytes: its probable antioxidant effect is potentiated by the flavonoid silybin. *Pharmacol. Toxicol.*, 69:9–12, 1991.

Gendrault, JL. Behaviour of liver sinusoidal cells obtained from silymarin-treated mice and rats after in vivo and in vitro infection with frog virus 3. *Planta Med.*, 39:247, 1980.

Glionna, J, and McALlister, S. Parks wage war against invasion of a killer weed. *Los Angeles Times*, pp. B1, B3; July 9, 1997.

Gonzalex, M et al. Effect of sylimarin [sic] on pruritus of cholestasis. *Hepatol.*, 8(5):1356, 1988.

Gupta, GK et al. Isolation of antihepatotoxic agents from seeds of Silybum marianum. *Res. Ind.*, 27(1):37–42, 1982 (*Chem. Abs.* 97:28486q).

Gupta, OP et al. Anti-inflammatory and anti-arthritic activities of silymarin acting through inhibition of 5-lipoxygenase. *Phytomed.*, 7(1):21–4, 1999.

Hahn, G et al. Pharmacology and toxicology of silymarin, the antihepatotoxic agent of Silybum marianum (L.) Gaertn. [German] *Arzneim.-Forsch.*, 18:698–705, 1968.

Hammouda, FM et al. Evaluation of the silymarin content in Silybum marianum cultivated under different agricultural conditions. *Planta Med.*, 57(Suppl. 2):A29, 1991.

Hammouda, FM et al. Evaluation of the silymarin content in Silybum marianum (L.) Gaertn. cultivated under different agricultural conditions. *Phytother. Res.*, 7:90–91, 1993.

Hertz, E et al. Genetic evidence for the existence of two varieties of Silybum marianum. *Planta Med.*, 57(Suppl. 2):A30, 1991.

Hertz, E et al. Genetic investigations on Silybum marianum and S. eburneum with respect to leaf colour, outcrossing ratio, and flavonolignan composition. *Planta Med.*, 61:54–7, 1995.

Hikino, H et al. Antihepatotoxic actions of flavonolignans from Silybum marianum fruits. *Planta Med.*, 50:248–50, 1984.

Janiak, B et al. The Effect of Silymarin on Contents and Functions of some Microsomal Liver enzymes Influenced by Carbon-tetrachloride or Halothane. [German] *Arzneim.-Forsch.*, 23(9):1322–6, 1973.

Janiak, B. Depression of microsomal activity in the liver of mice following single administration of halothane and its response to silybin. [German] *Anaesthesist*, 23(9):389–93, 1974 (*Chem.Abs.* 82:11266k).

Kiesewetter, E et al. Results of two double-blind studies on the effect of silymarine [sic] in chronic hepatitis. [German} *Leber Magen. Darm.*, 7(5):318–23, 1977.

Kim, HJ et al. Protection of Rat Liver Microsomes against Carbon Tetrachloride-Induced Lipid Peroxidation by Red Ginseng Saponin through Cytochrome P450 Inhibition. *Planta Med.*, 63:415–18, 1997.

Krecman, V et al. Silymarin inhibits the development of diet-induced hypercholesterolemia in rats. *Planta Med.*, 64:138–142, 1998.

Lang, I et al. Immunomodulatory and hepatoprotective effects of in vivo treatment with free radical scavengers. *Ital. J. Gastroenterol.*, 22(5):283v7, 1990.

Lastra, CA de la et al. Gastric anti-ulcer activity of silymarin, a lipoxygenase inhibitor, in rats. *J. Pharm. Pharmacol.*, 44:929–31, 1992.

Lastra, CA de la et al. Gastroprotection induced by silymarin, the hepatoprotective principle of Silybum marianum in ischmia-reperfusion mucosal injury: role of neutrophils. *Plant Med.*, 61:116–9, 1995.

Leber, WH and Knauff, S. Influence of Silymarin on Drug Metabolizing Enzymes in Rat and Man. *Arzneim.-Forsch.*, 26(8):1603–5, 1976.

Letteron, P et al. Mechanism for the protective effects of silymarin against carbon tetrachloride-induced lipid peroxidation and hepatotoxicity in mice. *Biochem.Pharmacol.*, 39(12):2027–34, 1990.

Lorenz, D et al. Pharmacokinetic studies with silymarin in human serum and bile. *Meth. Find. Exp. Clin. Pharmacol.*, 6(10):655–61, 1984.

Magliulo, E et al. Studies on the regenerative capacity of the liver in rats subjected to partial hepatectomy and treated with silymarin. *Arzneim.-Forsch.*, 23:161, 1973.

Miadonna, A et al. Effects of silybin on histamine release from human basophil leucocytes. *Br. J. Clin. Pharmacol.*, 24:747–52, 1987.

Miguez, MP et al. Hepatoprotective mechanism of silymarin: no evidence for involvement of cytochrome P450 2E1. *Chem. Biol. Interact.*, 91(1):51–63, 1994.

Morazzoni, P et al. Comparative pharmacokinetics of silipide and silymarin in rats. *Eur. J. Drug Metabol. Pharmacokin.*, 18(3):289–97, 1993.

Mourell, M and Favari, L. Silymarin improves metabolism and disposition of aspirin in cirrhotic rats. *Life Sci.*, 43:201–7, 1988.

Mourelle, M et al. Protection Against Thallium Hepatotoxicity by Silymarin. *J. Appl. Toxicol.*, 8:351–4, 1988.

Muzes, G et al. Effect of silimarin (Legalon) therapy on the antioxidant defense mechanism and lipid peroxidation in alcoholic liver disease (double blind protocol) [Hungarian] *Orv. Hetil.*, 131(16):863–6, 1990.

Neuman, MG et al. Inducers of Cytochrome P450 2E1 Enhance Methotrexate-Induced Hepatotoxicity. *Clin. Biochem.*, 32(7):519–36, 1999.

Palasciano, G et al. The Effect of Silymarin on Plasma Levels of Malon-Dialdehyde in Patients Receiving Long-Term Treatment with Psychotropic Drugs. *Curr. Ther. Res.*, 55:537–45, 1994.

Pares, A et al. Effects of silymarin in alcoholic patients with cirrhosis of the liver: results of a controlled, double-blind, randomized and multicenter trial. *J. Hepatol.*, 28:615–21, 1998.

Piscitelli, SC et al. Effect of milk thistle on the pharmacokinetics of indinavir in healthy volunteers. *Pharmacother.*, 22:551–6, 2002.

Platt, D and Schnorr, B. Biochemical and electronoptic studies on the possible influence of silymarin on hepatic damage induced by ethanol in rats. [German] *Arzneim.–Forsch.*, 21(8):1206–8, 1971.

Poser, G. Experience in the treatment of chronic hepatopathies with silymarin. [German] *Arzneim.–Forsch.*, 21:1209–12, 1971.

Puerta, R de la et al. Effect of silymarin on different acute inflammation models and on leukocyte migration. *J. Pharm. Pharmacol.*, 48:968–70, 1996.

Ramellini, G and Meldolesi, J. Stabilization of isolated rat liver plasma membranes by treatment in vitro with silymarin. *Arzneim.-Forsch.*, 24(5):806–8, 1974.

Raskovic, A et al. Effect of Methoxsalen and an Infusion of Silybum marianum on Enzymes Relevant to Liver Function. *Pharm. Biol.*, 49(1):70–3, 2000.

Rauen, H and Schriewer, H. The antihepatotoxic effect of silymarin on liver damage in rats induced by carbon tetrachloride, D-galactosamine, and allyl alcohol. [German] *Arzneim.–Forsch.*, 21(8):1194–1200, 1971.

Rickling, B et al. Two high-performance liquid chromatographic assays for the determination of free and total silibinin diastereomers in plasma using column switching with electrochemical detection and reversed-phase chromatography with ultraviolet detection. *J. Chromatograph. B*, 670:267–77, 1995.

Rumyantseva, ZN. The pharmacodynamics of hepatoprotectants derived from blessed milk thistle (Silybum marianum). [Russian] *Vrachebnoe Delo*, 5:15–19, 1991.

Salmi, HA and Sarna, S. Effect of silymarin on chemical, functional, and morphological alterations of the liver. A double-blind controlled study. *Scand. J. Gastroenterol.*, 17:517–21, 1982.

Salvagnini, M et al. Silymarin treatment in alcoholic liver disease: a double blind randomized clinical trial (RCT). *J. Hepatol.*, 1(Suppl):S124, 1985.

Savio, D et al. Softgel capsule technology as an enhance device for the absorption of natural principles in humans. *Arzneim.–Forsch.*, 48(11):1104–6, 1998.

Schandalik, R et al. Pharmacokinetics of silybin in bile following administration of silipide and silymarin in cholecystectomy patients. *Arzneim.-Forsch.*, 42(7):964–8, 1992.

Scheiber, V and Wohlzogen, FX. Analysis of a certain type of 2x3 tables, exemplified by biopsy findings in a controlled clinical trial. Int. *J. Clin. Pharmacol.*, 16:533–5, 1978.

Schonfeld, JV et al. Silibinin, a plant extract with antioxidant and membrane stabilizing properties, protects exocrine pancreas from cyclosporin A toxicity. *Cell. Mol. Life Sci.*, 53:917–20, 1997.

Schriewer, H et al. Pharmacokinetics of the antihepatotoxic activity of silymarine [sic] in the rat liver intoxicated by CCl4 or deoxycholate. [German] *Arzneim.–Forsch.*, 23:157–8, 1973.

Schriewer, H and Rauen, HM. Antihepatotoxic activity of parenterally applied silymarine [sic] in galactosamine hepatitis of the rat. [German] *Arzneim.–Forsch.*, 23(1a):159, 1973.

Schriewer, H et al. Antihepatotoxic effect of silymarine [sic] on phospholipid metabolism in the rat disturbed by phalloidine intoxication. *Arzneim.–Forsch.*, 23:160, 1973.

Schulte, KE et al. Polyacetylenic compounds as constituents of Silybum marianum Gaertn. [German] *Archiv Pharmazie*, 303(1):7–17, 1970.

Schulz, HU et al. Investigation of dissolution and bioequivalence of silymarin products. [German] *Arzneim.–Forsch.*, 45(1):61–4, 1995.

Scudder, J. A third study of specific medication. *Ecl. Med. J.*, 52:43–5, 1892.

Sonnenbichler, et al. Stimulatory effect of silibinin on the DNA synthesis in partially hepatectomized rat livers: non-response in hepatoma and other malign cell lines. *Biochem. Pharmacol.*, 35:538–41, 1986.

Sonnenbichler, J and Zetl, I. Biochemistry of a liver drug from the thistle Silybum marianum. *Planta Med.*, 58(Suppl. 1):A580, 1992.

Trinchet, JC et al. Treatment of alcoholic hepatitis with silymarin. A double-blind comparative study in 116 patients. [French] *Gastroenterol. Clin. Biol.*, 13(2):120–4, 1989.

Valenzuela, A et al. Inhibitory effect of the flavonoid silymarin on the erythrocyte hemolysis induced by phenylhydrazine. *Biochem. Biophys. Res. Comm.*, 126:712, 1985[a].

Valenzuela, A et al. Silymarin protection against hepatic lipid peroxidation induced by acute ethanol intoxication in the rat. *Biochem. Pharmacol.*, 34(12):2209–12, 1985.

Valenzuela, A et al. Selectivity of silymarin on the increase of the glutathione content in different tissues of the rat. *Planta Med.*, 55:420–2, 1989[b].

Varma, PN et al. Chemical investigation of Silybum marianum. *Planta Med.*, 38:377, 1980.

Velussi, M et al. Long-term (12 months) treatment with an anti-oxidant drug (silymarin) is effective on hyperinsulinemia, exogenous insulin need and malondialdehyde levels in cirrhotic diabetic patients. *J. Hepatol.*, 26:871–9, 1997.

Venkataramanan, R et al. Milk Thistle, a Herbal Supplement, Decreases the Activity of CYP3A4 and Uridine Diphosphoglucuronosyl Transferase in Human Hepatocyte Cultures. *Drug Metabol. Disposit.*, 28(11):1270–3, 2000.

Vogel, G and Temme, I. Curative antagonization of a liver damage caused by phalloidin by the aid of silymarin as a model of antiheptotoxic therapy. [German] *Arzneim.–Forsch.*, 19:613–5, 1969.

Vogel, G et al. Studies on pharmacodynamics, site and mechanism of action of silymarin, the antihepatotoxic principle from Silybum marianum (L.) Gaertn. [German] *Arzneim.–Forsch.*, 25:179–88, 1975.

Vogel, G et al. Protection by silibinin against Amanita phalloides intoxication in beagles. *Toxicol. Appl. Pharmacol.*, 73:355–62, 1984.

Wagner, H et al. Chemistry of silymarin (silybin), the active principle of the fruits of Silybum marianum (L.) Gaertn. (Carduus marianus L.). [German] *Arzneim.–Forsch.*, 18–688–96, 1968

Wagner, H et al. On chemistry and analysis of silymarin from Silybum marianum. [German] *Arzneim.–Forsch.*, 24:266–71, 1974.

Weyhenmeyer, R et al. Study on dose-linearity of the pharmacokinetics of silibinin disasteromers using a new sterospecific assay. Int. *J. Clin.Pharmacol.*, 30(4):134–8, 1992.

Williams, DE and Priestly, BG. Evaluation of prophylactic efficacy of silymarin in CCl4-induced hepatotoxicity. Res. *Comm. Chem. Pathol. Pharmacol.*, 6(1):185–94, 1973.

Zi X, et al. Novel cancer chemopreventive effects of a flavonoid antioxidant silymarin: inhibition of mRNA expression of an endogenous tumor promoter TNF-alpha. *Biochem. Biophys. Res. Comm.*, 239:334–9, 1997.

Zoltan, OT and Gyori, I. Studies on the brain edema of the rat induced by triethyltinsulfaate [sic] (TZS). *Arzneim.–Forsch.*, 20:1248–9, 1970.

Index

Addendum

Articles pertinent to the herbs covered in the last three chapters were not obtained in time to include in the text. They are summarized here because of their significance to issues discussed in the text for these herbs.

Western echinacea (Echinacea angustifolia) and purple coneflower echinacea (E. purpurea)

Test tube studies confirmed that E. angustifolia root extract and E. purpurea root extract and herb extract all enhance human monocyte cell culture gene expression of interleukin (IL)-1beta, IL-8, tumor necrosis factor-alpha, and intracellular adhesion molecule after six hours of exposure. However, when these three preparations were combined and 1.5 grams taken daily by six healthy humans for 2.3 days, the expression of all of these inflammatory compounds decreased steadily through day five, while the expression in the blood of antiviral interferon-alpha rose steadily through day twelve.

Randolph, RK. et al. Regulation of human immune gene expression as influenced by a commercial blended Echinacea product: preliminary studies. *Exp. Biol. Med.*, 228:1051-6, 2003.

Cranberry (Vaccinium macrocarpon) fruit

When compared to ten other fruit, cranberry was found to have by far the highest total antioxidant activity and antiproliferant activity against human liver cancer cells in test tube studies. The antioxidant effect was almost entirely due to phenolic components rather than vitamin C content. Cranberry has a much higher total phenolic content than (in descending order) apple, red grape, strawberry, pineapple, banana, peach, lemon, orange, pear, and grapefruit. The cranberry effects resulted in over twice the bioactivity index score for dietary cancer prevention than the next highest fruit (apple).

Sun, J. et al. Antioxidant and antiproliferative activities of common fruits. *J. Agric. Food Chem.*, 50: 7449-54, 2002 .

Black cohosh (Cimicifuga [Actaea] racemosa) rhizome

A dried 58% aqueous/ethanolic extract (CR BNO 1055) in daily doses corresponding to 40 mg of the rhizome was compared to 0.6 mg of conjugated estrogens and placebo in a study with 62 menopausal women. The extract was as potent as the estrogens and better than placebo in relieving menopausal symptoms, and it was also as beneficial as estrogens on markers in the serum for bone metabolism. While the estrogens and extract increased vaginal cell growth similarly, only the estrogens increased uterine endometrial thickness. Black cohosh hydroalcoholic extract therefore has demonstrated selective estrogen receptor modulator activity for bones and the vagina without affecting the uterus.

Wuttke, W. et al. The Cimicifuga preparation BNO 1055 vs. conjugated estrogens in a double-blind placebo-controlled study: effects on menopause symptoms and bone markers. *Maturitas*, 44 (Suppl. 1):S67-S77, 2003.

Saw palmetto (Serenoa repens) fruit

In 11 European countries 704 patients with benign prostatic hypertrophy were randomly treated in a comparative trial with either 0.4 mg of the alpha-blocker tamsulosin or 320 mg of a liposterolic extract of saw palmetto daily for one year. The scores for both irritative and obstructive symptoms diminished equally in both groups, while PSA levels remained stable. The extract group had a slight decrease in prostate volume, while ejaculation disorders were more frequent in the tamsulosin group. This was the first study to compare an alpha-blocker to saw palmetto extract.

Debruyne, F. et al. Comparison of a phytotherapeutic agent (Permixon) with an alpha-blocker (Tamsulosin) in the treatment of benign prostatic hyperplasia: a 1-year randomized international trial. *Eur. Urol.*, 41:497-507, 2002.

Kava (Piper methysticum) root

The first controlled study to test the physical and cognitive impairment of individuals intoxicated from kava beverage observed 11 individuals, each drinking kava over a 7 - 22 hour period prepared, on average, from 205 grams of powdered root. Tests were administered eight hours after consumption of kava ended. The drinkers demonstrated sedation, ataxia, tremors, and eyelid spasm, along with reduced efficiency of eye movements and accuracy in visual search tasks. The liver enzymes GGT and ALP were abnormally high among these Aboriginal chronic kava abusers who occasionally used alcohol and cannabis as well. While visual attention and movement coordination were impaired, complex mental functions remained normal.

Cairney, S. et al. Saccade and cognitive impairment associated with kava intoxication. *Hum. Psychopharm.*, 18:525-33, 2003.

St. John's wort (Hypericum perforatum) flowering tops

Reports of breakthrough bleeding in women using oral contraceptives and St. John's wort extract concurrently led to a randomized controlled trial with 17 healthy females. They were given a combination of ethinylestradiol and desogestrel for a control menstrual cycle, followed by 600 mg of a 80% methanolic standardized extract for one cycle, then 900 mg extract daily for another cycle. While taking the extract 13 and 15 women experienced intracyclic bleeding during the two cycles, respectively. This was significantly more than the six with breakthrough bleeding during the introductory control cycle when it is generally most common. Though no evidence of ovulation was noted in any women, estradiol levels were raised above control cycle levels at the higher extract dose, and significant decreases in the active metabolite 3-ketodesogestrel were detected at both doses.

Pfrunder, A. et al. Interaction of St John's wort with low-dose oral contraceptive therapy: a randomized controlled trial. *Br. J. Clin. Pharmacol.*, 56:683-90, 2003.

Milk thistle (Silybum marianum) seeds

Test tube studies suggest that the flavonolignan fraction silymarin may increase activity of cytochrome P450 isozyme 3A4, responsible for the liver and intestinal metabolism of many drugs, and increase drug removal by the cell membrane transporter P-glycoprotein. A sequential crossover trial with ten healthy adults studied the effect of milk thistle extract standardized to silymarin on the bioavailability of the CYP 3A4 and P-glycoprotein substrate indinavir, an antiretroviral agents that is part of the standard treatment for HIV/AIDS. Before and after 14 days of taking 480 mg of silymarin daily, indinavir was given. There was no apparent difference in indinavir plasma concentrations when it was taken with or without silymarin, confirming an earlier human study.

DiCenzo, R. et al. Coadministration of milk thistle and indinavir in healthy subjects. *Pharmocother.*, 23(7):866-70, 2003.

About the Author

Francis Brinker, N.D., is a 1981 graduate of the National College of Naturopathic Medicine (NCNM) in Portland, Oregon. He also completed the two-year Postgraduate Studies Program in Clinical Practice and Botanical Medicine and taught Botanical Medicine there until 1985. In addition, he has taught at the Southwest College of Naturopathic Medicine and Health Sciences in Tempe, Arizona.

Dr. Brinker's undergraduate work includes a Bachelor of Science Degree in Human Biology from Kansas Newman College and a Bachelor of Arts Degree in Biology from the University of Kansas, Phi Beta Kappa.

Currently Dr. Brinker is Clinical Assistant Professor, Department of Medicine, at the University of Arizona College of Medicine, and he serves as a botanical medicine preceptor and curriculum developer for the Program in Integrative Medicine at the University of Arizona College of Medicine. He is a reviewer for the American Herbal Pharmacopoeia monographs and maintains extensive literature research of historic, scientific and medical publications.

Dr. Brinker's work, *Herb Contraindications and Drug Interactions*, is recognized as foundational. His interest in traditional American medicines has earned him an authoritative reputation for writing and teaching on naturopathic medicine, the Eclectic Medical Era, and native American herbs of the West and Southwest. His work, *The Toxicology of Botanical Medicines*, is recognized as a classic handbook for the study of medicinal plant toxicology.

Works by Francis Brinker, N.D.

BOOKS

Complex Herbs–Complete Medicines
Herb Contraindications and Drug Interactions, Third Edition
The Toxicology of Botanical Medicines, Third Edition
Formulas For Healthful Living, Second Edition
The Eclectic Dispensatory of Botanical Therapeutics, Vol. I and II

SELECTED ARTICLES

"Enhancing Anti-inflammatory and Analgesic Drug Effects While Reducing Risks with Herbs and Their Derivatives," *Integrative Medicine,* 2004, vol. 3, no. 1, pp. 24-42.

"Potential Coagulation Effects of Preoperative Complementary and Alternative Medicines," (co-authored with Carol Norred) *Alternative Therapies in Health and Medicine,* 2001, vol. 7, no. 6, pp. 58–67. (Reprinted in *International Journal of Integrative Medicine,* Aug/Sept., 2002).

"The Role of Botanical Medicine in 100 Years of American Naturopathy," *HerbalGram,* 1998, no. 42, pp. 49-59. (Reprinted in *British Naturopathic Journal,* 1999, vol. 16, no. 4, pp. 70–73; 2000, vol.17, no. 1, pp. 8–11; 2000; vol. 17, no. 2, pp. 26–29).

"Waconda Springs: Lost Legacy?" *The Journal of Naturopathic Medicine,* 2000, vol. 9, no. 1, pp. 62–64.

"Variations in Effective Botanical Products," *HerbalGram,* 1999, no. 46, pp. 35–50. (Available as a separate Special Report from the American Botanical Council).